OXR

Royal National Institute for the Blind

Blind and partially sighted adults in Britain: the RNIB survey

Volume 1

Ian Bruce,
Aubrey McKennell
and Errol Walker

London: HMSO

This report was designed and printed by HMSO to specifications supplied by RNIB to ensure that it is legible. As the survey shows, the majority of blind and partially sighted people can read print which is clear and well designed. This report is set in 12½pt on 15pt Helvetica Regular.

The report is also available in braille and on audio tape. Enquiries about these editions should be sent direct to RNIB Customer Services, PO Box 173, Peterborough PE2 0WS, UK.

HMSO publications are available from:

HMSO Publications Centre
(Mail and telephone orders only)
PO Box 276, London, SW8 5DT
Telephone orders 071-873 9090
General enquiries 071-873 0011
(queuing system in operation for both numbers)

HMSO Bookshops
49 High Holborn, London, WC1V 6HB   071-873 0011 (counter service only)
258 Broad Street, Birmingham, B1 2HE   021-643 3740
Southey House, 33 Wine Street, Bristol, BS1 2BQ   (0272) 264306
9-21 Princess Street, Manchester, M60 8AS   061-834 7201
80 Chichester Street, Belfast, BT1 4JY   (0232) 238451
71 Lothian Road, Edinburgh, EH3 9AZ   031-228 4181

HMSO's Accredited Agents
(see Yellow Pages)

and through good booksellers

Chapter Headings

Contents

Part B Media Reading Habits   79

7 Large Print   81

8 Tapes and Tape Services   88

Foreword

This report presents the findings of the first ever nationwide survey of blind and partially sighted people in Great Britain. As the country's largest organisation working with and for visually impaired people, we considered it essential that we should obtain a more detailed profile of our 'client group' than existing statistics could provide. We wanted to know the numbers of people with visual impairments, their personal circumstances and needs, and the extent to which those needs were being met.

The survey, conducted between November 1986 and April 1987, took the form of a series of lengthy, detailed interviews with nearly six hundred blind and partially sighted adults, and three hundred children (or their parents) in their own homes by professional interviewers. The survey followed a major study by the Office of Population Censuses and Surveys on disabled people generally (also published by HMSO). It was designed to be complementary to that survey, so that comparisons could be made. This report covers our findings on adults. A separate volume will follow on children.

The findings of our survey are enlightening, but at the same time, very worrying. They show that there are roughly three times more blind and partially sighted people in Great Britain than had previously been estimated – almost a million – and this number is growing as the population ages. Of these, only a quarter are officially registered blind or partially sighted, and of the remaining three quarters, a sizeable proportion are unknown to health and social services. Many visually impaired people, in other words, receive no help at all from statutory authorities. Yet our survey shows a deep well of need, especially among older people (aged 60 and over) who make up 90% of all visually impaired people.

This report presents a major challenge to all providers of services, be they voluntary or statutory, in the fields of health, social services, housing, employment, leisure and income support. It has many implications for other spheres of activity, from building to banking, transport to television. RNIB is urgently reviewing its own policies and provision of services in the light of these findings, and we will be encouraging others – not least central and local government – to do the same.

We have collected the evidence, now we must press for action. One person in sixty depends upon it.

John A Wall MA (Oxon)
Chairman, RNIB

Acknowledgements

Social surveys of this scale and complexity are possible only with the advice, support and encouragement of many individuals and organisations. First, however, our sincere thanks must go to the hundreds of blind and partially sighted people who allowed us to intrude on their lives, and who coped with our lengthy questions with patience and good humour. Without their cooperation this survey could not have been completed. We hope that this study will result in substantial improvements to the quality and availability of services to them and to all with a visual impairment.

We are greatly indebted to our advisers, consultants and field-workers whose experience of survey work and of policy issues contributed so much to our study. Special thanks must go to the Office of Population Censuses and Surveys' team who worked on the OPCS Survey of Disability in Great Britain. The data they made available enabled us to locate and interview blind and partially sighted people not registered with the local authorities. Their advice on the survey was also invaluable. The team included: Margaret Bone, Karen Dunnell, Jean Martin, Howard Meltzer, Amanda White and Nicola Robus. We are also grateful to Mary Jobbins and Dr Annette Rawson of the (then) DHSS who allowed us to follow up the OPCS sample. The survey was piloted with the help of the London Borough of Newham Sensory Advisory Team and its clients.

The fieldwork was carried out by the British Market Research Bureau. We thank them for the immense amount of work they put into the questionnaire design and fieldwork itself. The quality of the data collected is to be commended.

Professor Gerald Hoinville of City University and Elizabeth Hoinville of the University of London worked respectively on the sampling and computational work on the sample selection. Diana Leat and Jane Ritchie of Social and Community Planning Research advised on the questionnaire content. Jane Fielding at the University of Surrey advised us on the computing and the setting up of the data. Their support has been invaluable.

An advisory committee was set up by RNIB to advise on the survey. Its members were Dr Tim Cullinan, Dr Henry Heath, Dr Adrian Hill, Colin

Low, Tom Parker, Dr Michael Tobin and Elizabeth Twining. The knowledge, experience and enthusiasm they brought to the design and development of the survey is gratefully acknowledged. Well over 20 RNIB officers also contributed their advice and experience.

Advice was sought from a number of individuals on issues to be included in the survey. Representing a wide range of disciplines and backgrounds, they brought a wealth of specialist expertise to our work for which we are most grateful. They include: Hans Cohn, Margaret Ford, Judy Baron, Elizabeth Chapman, Louise Clunies-Ross, Dr Allan Dodds, Sally Edge, Raymond Ellis (Leeds City Council), Paul Ennals (SENSE), Dr Lorimar Fison FRCS, Dr John Gill (Research Unit for the Blind, Brunel University), Lucille Hall, Roger Hinds (Dorton House School), Susan Lacroix, Graham Lomas, Tom Maley, D. Mumford (Coventry Social Services), Helen Partington (Social Services, Somerset County Council), Bill Poole, Fred Raffle (Nottinghamshire County Council), Joan Shields, Janet Silver (Moorfields Eye Hospital), Olive Stephenson (University of Nottingham) and Eric Walford.

Many organisations also commented on the scope of the survey, including charities working for visually impaired people and other statutory and private bodies with an interest in their welfare. They were: Association of Blind Asians, Association of Blind Chartered Physiotherapists, Association of Blind and Partially Sighted Teachers, Association for the Education and Welfare of the Visually Handicapped, Association of Visually Handicapped Telephonists, BBC *In Touch*, Blind Mobility Research Unit, British Retinitis Pigmentosa Society, British Telecom (Action for the Disabled), Circle of Guide Dog Owners, Disabled Living Foundation, Guide Dogs for the Blind Association, Jewish Blind Society, Leeds City Council (Social Services), National Association of Orientation and Mobility Instructors, National Association of Technical Officers for the Blind, National Blind Helpers League, National Federation of the Blind, National League of the Blind and Disabled, National Library for the Blind, North Regional Association for the Blind, Partially Sighted Society, Resource Centre for the Blind (Strathclyde Regional Council), Royal Blind Asylum and School, Royal Commonwealth Society for the Blind, Royal National College Old Students Guild, Saint Dunstan's, SENSE, Scottish National Federation for the Welfare of the Blind, South Regional Association for the Blind, Standing Conference for Ethnic Minority Senior Citizens, Wales Council for the Blind. Our thanks go to them all.

In the day-to-day tasks of managing the fieldwork and analysing the data we were ably supported by the University of Surrey, the University of London's Westfield College Computing Unit and by many RNIB staff including Elaine Dodds, David Mann, Sheena McBride and Jean White. Getting from first draft to print has been a major task and we are indebted to our editor, Christopher Pick, to Keith Riley and his colleagues of HMSO and to Hilary Todd and her team in the RNIB

Publications Unit. Their commitment, support and professionalism have enabled us to complete a work which we hope will be seen as a major landmark in the field of visual disability.

Last but by no means least we owe very special thanks to Duncan Watson who, as RNIB Chairman when the survey was commissioned, gave us every support and encouragement.

Any errors and omissions are entirely the responsibility of the authors.

Ian W Bruce

Aubrey C McKennell

Errol C Walker

Notes on the Tables and Abbreviations

1 **Percentages**
Percentages have been rounded to the nearest whole number; 0.5% is rounded up. As a result many of the tables do not total 100%. The percentages quoted in the tables and text are calculated on the basis of weighted data, not on the numbers of people interviewed (see section 2.5).

2 # = less than 0.5%.

3 **Weighted data** (section 2.4.1)
Population bases are normally given to the nearest thousand. This is the estimated population numbers for that group.

4 **Single or multiple answer questions**
Where a total % base, 'Total 100', is shown, only single answers have normally been allowed to the question. Where the population base is shown as 'Base = 100%', multiple answers have been allowed, and single responses in the body of the table cannot be added together. In a number of tables a summary figure is given which adds the respondents giving a group of answers; this represents the total number of respondents giving these answers, not the total responses themselves.

5 **Number interviewed**
This refers to the number of people actually interviewed who form the base of the column concerned. For example, (595) is the total number of people interviewed for the survey.

6 Not all questions apply to every respondent. Where respondents have not been asked a question, the total number of respondents is given as a note to the table together with a reason for their inclusion or omission. In a number of cases, respondents simply failed to answer a question, and where applicable this is also noted.

7 The question(s) that generate the answers given in a table normally forms part of the table. Where a subsequent table simply repeats the data, the question is not repeated.

Abbreviations

B	Registrable blind (see PS, also section 2.3.2.3)
BMRB	British Market Research Bureau
BPTA	Blind person's tax allowance
CAB	Citizens Advice Bureau
CCTV	Closed-circuit television magnifier
CSO	Central Statistical Office
DHSS	Department of Health and Social Security
DLS	Daily Living Skills
DOH	Department of Health
ERS	RNIB Express Reading Service
GHS	General Household Survey
HA	Housing association
HB	Housing benefit
ICIDH	International Classification of Impairments, Disabilities and Handicaps
K	000s
LA	Local Authority
LVA	Low vision aid
MSC	Manpower Services Commission
N12s	Respondents having Snellen test results 6/24 but near vision reading test results <N12 (sections 2.2.2.1, 21.1 and 21.2.1)
NHS	National Health Service
NLP	No light perception
NR	Non-registered
OPCS	Office of Population Censuses and Surveys
Popltn.	Population
PS	Registrable partially sighted (see B, also sections 2.3.2.2 and 2.4.2.3)
R	Registered
RA	Retirement age
RICA	Research Institute for Consumer Affairs
RNIB	Royal National Institute for the Blind
RP	Retinitis pigmentosa
RV	Residual vision
RVL	Residual vision level
SSD	Social Services Department
SSI	Social Services Inspectorate
STL	RNIB Student Tape Library
TB	RNIB Talking Book
VI	Registrable visually impaired, i.e. B and PS above
WA	Working age
WHO	World Health Organisation
>	Greater than
<	Less than

Summary and Policy Implications

Chapter 1, Introduction

This chapter summarises the objectives of the present survey and its relationship with other major surveys of visually impaired people.

Chapter 2, Method

This chapter reviews the procedures followed for questionnaire construction, sampling, fieldwork and analysis.

Interviews were conducted with 595 registrable visually impaired people aged 16 or over in late 1986 and early 1987. Names and addresses for the sample were obtained from two sources: the OPCS survey of general disability (Martin et al, 1988a) and local authority registers of blind and partially sighted people. Non-registered but registrable respondents were selected on the basis of sight test results obtained in the OPCS survey. The results were weighted to give estimates from the sample to population numbers.

Unless otherwise stated, the results in this report relate to registered or registrable blind or partially sighted people aged 16 and over living in private households in Great Britain. **Where the term visually impaired is used without qualification, it means all those registered or eligible for registration as blind or partially sighted.**

Chapter 3, Demographic characteristics

Size

This is the first study to produce reliable estimates of the numbers of visually impaired people living in private households in Great Britain. According to Department of Health (DOH) registration figures (section 21.3.2), there are 94,000 blind and 54,000 partially sighted people in Great Britain aged 16 or over. Our results (Table 3.1) suggest 300,000 blind people (319% over official registration figures) and 457,000 partially sighted people (846% over official registration figures) aged 16 or over in private households. Including residential institutions (section 21.3.3) increases the estimates for the numbers of blind people aged 16 or over to 380,000 compared with the DOH figure of 119,000; and for partially sighted people to 579,000, compared with the official figure of 69,000. Our estimated total for all those registered or eligible for registration as blind or partially sighted people in Great Britain in 1987 is 959,000.

Age, sex and marital status

Compared with the general population the age distribution of the registrably visually impaired population is heavily skewed towards the older age groups. Sixty-six per cent are aged 75 or over compared with 8% of the general population.

While women form 52% of the general population, they comprise 72% of the visually impaired population. The total increases across the three age groups 16 – 59, 60 – 74 and 75 + , from 57 to 68 and 75 per cent.

Fewer visually impaired people are married than among the general population – 56 and 74 per cent. The discrepancy widens in the older age group, largely because of widowhood. Fifty-five per cent of visually impaired people aged 60 or over are widowed compared with 30% of the general population of the same age.

Single person households

A surprisingly large number (346,000, 45%) of visually impaired people live on their own (Table 3.5). About a third of the 60 – 74 age group and half the 75 + age group who live alone have done so for 16 years or more.

The higher percentages of older people living alone have important implications. The chapters in which we enquire about who provides help, for example with reading (9), shopping (14) and with daily living tasks (15), show clearly that as a visually impaired person grows older the sources of help change from someone within the home to a relative or friend outside the home, and on to someone from a statutory or voluntary welfare organisation. This change is also influenced by the decrease in the proportion of older people who have close relatives (Chapter 13).

The implication for the new community care initiative is most striking. The informal care network (relatives and friends) provides help with the support of the statutory agencies. However, for a significant proportion of older visually impaired people, particularly those aged 75 + who require most support, this network simply does not exist.

It is reasonable to assume that the ability of older blind and partially sighted people to live alone is finely balanced. Any reduction in statutory domiciliary support services for this group could well result in a significant increase in demand for residential care.

Income and savings

Fifty-seven per cent of visually impaired people live at the extremes of poverty with a household income of less than £70 per week (1987 prices). The proportion increases across the three age groups 16 – 59, 60 – 74 and 75 + from 31 to 49 and 65 per cent (Table 3.5). Over half have savings of less than £500.

Few visually impaired people have any savings with which to cushion their low income and have to meet any extra costs their disability creates out of their already low income. The OPCS survey revealed the low income of disabled people. Our survey shows that it may have underestimated the true cost of disability. The high level of unemployment (Chapter 17) and the dependency on social security allowances and benefits (Chapter 18) illustrates the need for adequate levels of allowances and benefits to compensate visually impaired people for the extra costs they incur because of their disability.

Registration status

Only 23% of the 757,000 visually impaired people living in private households eligible to be registered as blind or partially sighted are in fact registered. Younger people are more likely to be registered, as are blind people. For example, 60% of blind people aged 16 – 59 are registered compared with only 13% of partially sighted people aged 75 + (Table 3.14).

While a larger percentage of younger people is registered, in terms of total population numbers the number of older registered people is far greater than the number of younger registered people.

Although the survey covers people who are registered or who would qualify for registration, people with lower residual vision are more likely to be registered than those at the higher end of the registrable residual vision range (section 3.9.4).

The most significant consequence of registration is its role as a trigger or catalyst in the awareness and receipt of services. This theme recurs whenever respondents are asked about their awareness and use of services. Registered people and younger people are always proportionately more aware of services and use them more. This important finding requires providers of services to visually impaired people to reassess their perspective on registration.

Chapter 4, Accommodation

As might be expected, older respondents have resided longer in their present dwelling. Twenty-five per cent of younger compared with 40% of older visually impaired people have lived in their present dwelling for 21 or more years.

Blind and partially sighted people, especially those aged under 60, are more likely to live in local authority rented accommodation than the general population. Twenty-three per cent of people under 60 in the general population but 40% of visually impaired people are local authority tenants. Among 60 – 74 year olds the figures are 37 and 54 per cent respectively, among those aged 75 +, 37 and 42 per cent.

Since higher-income groups tend to be owner-occupiers this pattern is explained by the lower income level of visually impaired people. If they are unable to buy into the property market, this suggests a need for affordable rented accommodation for visually impaired people.

Chapter 5, The onset of visual impairment

Reported causes

Respondents were often vague about the causes of their visual impairment. One in five of those aged 75 and over mentioned nothing more specific than 'old age'. Most of those answering in this way regard the slow deterioration of their vision as part of the natural process of growing old. Cataracts was the specific cause mentioned most often (35%) by those aged 60 or over (Table 5.1).

In so far as the causes of impairment mentioned represent disorders with a known natural history, their distribution across the age groupings reflects facts about the onset of visual impairment. We would expect to find cataracts, a disease of slow onset, most prevalent in the oldest age group. However, it is worth noting that cataracts are by no means insignificant even among the youngest age group, being mentioned by about 1 in 7 of respondents under 60. The numbers saying that their sight problem started at birth declined sharply with increased age.

Time of onset

The length of time over which the eyesight of visually impaired people deteriorates and the age at which they experience deterioration are both important factors in determining the ability to adjust and the kind of help outside agencies are likely to provide. We distinguish between sudden onset, onset at birth, and loss of sight over a more extended period.

Sudden, traumatic loss of vision (the 'military model') is the experience of a small minority of visually impaired people. Fewer than 1 in 10 said that their condition was the result of an accident (including 'falling over'), and only 1 in 20 mentioned another sudden occurrence ('happened suddenly/for no reason at all'). Overall the combined mentions in these two categories amounted to 13% (Table 5.1).

Only 8% reported that their sight loss was 'from birth'. The total was 30% among those aged 16 – 59, and because of the massive increase in age-related visual impairment decreased to 3% of those aged 75 + .

Progressive deterioration rather than sudden traumatic loss of vision is the onset experience of a large majority (86%). Those whose sight loss had become worse from birth, or was not the result of an accident, were asked at what age they first realised that their vision was causing them problems in everyday life. The age skew among visually impaired people might lead us to assume that all those aged 75 + would be recently visually impaired. This is not so; 22% experienced onset under the age of 60; 36% in the previous 15 years; and 37% in the recent past (the rest could not say).

Medical treatment received for sight

A large majority (81%) had seen a specialist about their eye problem. A substantial but smaller majority (58%) had been hospital outpatients, 33% hospital inpatients, and 49% had received some other form of medication (Table 5.4).

Visually impaired people aged 16 – 59 and 60 – 74 are more likely either to have undergone an eye-operation or to have been hospital in-patients than those aged 75 + . In the same age groups blind people are more likely to have had one of these 'treatments' than partially sighted people.

Ninety-six per cent of registered people compared with 77% of the non-registered (but registrable) had seen an eye specialist. The fact that so many registrable but non-registered people had visited an eye specialist is significant. It confirms anecdotal evidence that eye specialists do not always initiate the process of registration for many of their eligible patients, i.e. the non-registered (but registrable) are known, but not acknowledged by, the statutory authorities. This suggests that eye specialists could do more to ensure and encourage registration, particularly given its trigger effect. This is especially important for blind people receiving social security benefits, where registration is a passport to higher levels of payments.

Chapter 6, Residual vision

Distance vision

Respondents were asked eight carefully graded questions about how much they could see in everyday situations involving distance vision.

Once lay people and even some professionals realise that all registered blind people are not totally blind, they ask 'how many blind people are totally blind?' Our survey answers this question for the first time, but not before one defines 'totally blind'. If sighted readers shut their eyes they will quite reasonably think of themselves as, temporarily, totally blind. However, with their eyes shut they can still sense 'from the light where the windows are'. Thus our definition of 'totally blind' includes people who have perception of light but nothing more. On this definition, we can say that 18% of blind people are totally blind; this figure consists of 25% of those under 60 and 14% of those 60 or over.

While only a minority of visually impaired people (19% – 12 and 23 per cent of blind and partially sighted people respectively) can recognise a friend across a road, a majority (66% – 49 and 80 per cent of blind and partially sighted people) can at least recognise a friend at arms length (section 6.1.1). However, the importance of distance recognition should not be over-emphasized by sighted readers who may not realise the extent to which visually impaired people use shape and movement for recognition purposes.

Near vision

Two assessments of respondents' near vision capabilities were made. First, we asked about their visual ability to read newspapers, and, second, we administered a simple large-print reading test.

A surprisingly large proportion of blind and partially sighted people (46% – 27 and 57 per cent of blind and partially sighted people respectively) reported that they could read ordinary newspaper print (Table 6.2).

Seventy-two per cent of respondents asked to take our simple test were able to read the card, and 58% (36 and 75 per cent of blind and partially sighted people) could read it comfortably. Only 22% of blind people age 16 – 59 could read it comfortably.

One of the key questions faced by service-giving organisations is how far it is necessary to produce large-print documents for visually impaired people, especially blind people. The traditional argument runs that, 'as very few blind people can read, it is not necessary'. Our survey suggest otherwise and quantifies the gains of using large print. This is not a panacea, since reading large print is far more tiring than a sighted person would find. Nevertheless the large-print argument seems proved for substantial numbers of blind people.

These results also point to the importance of low vision aids (LVAs), such as hand-held and stand magnifiers, as well as closed-circuit television magnifiers (CCTVs).

Distance and near vision should be considered in tandem. Because of the wide range of causes of sight loss, some visually impaired people enjoy better distance vision than near vision and vice versa. Many blind and partially sighted people experience a significant reduction in their field of vision. Assessing the field of vision loss was beyond the scope of this survey.

Use of spectacles

Eighty-five per cent of blind and partially sighted people with light perception wear glasses (Tables 6.4 and 6.5), including 78% of blind people aged 16 – 59. Because glasses are so common among the general population, it is important to understand that for visually impaired people spectacles are a prosthesis. Their effect is of a quite different order than for sighted people. They are more like a one-legged person's crutch, allowing some amelioration of the condition, not total correction.

People use their glasses for more than one purpose. About 50% use them for each of the following reasons: reading, other close-up work, and distance vision (Table 6.5).

Use of low vision aids

The hand magnifier is the most-used LVA after spectacles (Table 6.6), by 59% overall. However, the total using a hand magnifier is lower among the younger age group (28 and 44 per cent of blind and partially sighted people respectively). Use of all other LVAs runs at under 5%.

During the reading test the interviewer was asked to code any LVAs actually used. The results in Table 6.10 confirm that the LVA predominantly used for reading is spectacles (59%), followed by hand magnifier (13%); other types of LVA were used by no more than 1 or 2 per cent. Young partially sighted people and older blind and partially sighted people used LVAs most.

The results give some quantitative indication of the substantial under-use of LVAs. While 59% had a hand magnifier, only 13% used it in the test (Table 6.7). Although the test card was printed in 16 point bold, there is no doubt that more respondents would have been able to read it using their magnifier had they been trained and supported in its use.

7

When we asked respondents if they had the simplest LVA, adequate lighting in the home, only 20% said 'yes'. The reasons given for not having adequate lighting – never having thought about it and not thinking it would help – confirm that many visually impaired people are not aware of the positive benefit of improving lighting levels. The large total (80%) who have done nothing about lighting levels is a public education opportunity for service-providers. The simple use of adequate lighting alone would bring a marked improvement in the use of residual vision for many visually impaired people.

Chapter 7, Large print

This chapter provides further evidence of the importance of large print. For partially sighted people large print is absolutely crucial. Eighty-nine per cent could read the large-print test card, and 82% normally read print (Table 7.1).

While only 12% of blind people under 60 can read ordinary newspaper print (Table 7.2), 42% read the large-print test card (Table 7.1).

These figures provide a strong argument for organisations serving visually impaired people to produce information material, not merely leisure reading, in print as well as in other media. Most important of all is large print, which doubles the access rate to almost half the blind population.

Chapter 8, Tapes and tape services

Nearly half (46%) of all visually impaired people possess a tape player. Ownership is highest among younger people and decreases across the three age groups, 16 – 59, 60 – 74 and 75 + , from 83 to 53 and 38 per cent. Twelve per cent have an RNIB Talking Book machine; the figures range from 32% of blind people under 60 to an average 6% of partially sighted people of all ages (Tables 8.1 and 8.2).

RNIB Talking Book Service

These data point to the need for further expansion of the RNIB Talking Book Service. A large number of visually impaired people do not know about Talking Books. Fifty-four per cent (over 400,000 people) have not heard of the service, of whom 23% (90,000 people) would like to try it (section 8.3.3.1).

Social services workers will play a crucial role in increasing membership of the RNIB Talking Book Service. Some 43% of existing members were introduced by social services workers.

The reading-rate among Talking Book members, especially those aged 60 and over, is impressively high. Almost half the older group read four or more books per month. Given that each book takes about 12 hours to listen to, book-listening is clearly a major activity of elderly RNIB Talking Book members and indicates the importance of this service.

Some 46% of visually impaired people have a tape player of some kind, 4% only have an RNIB Talking Book player, 34% only have an ordinary tape player and 8% have both. These averages mask some interesting and extreme variations. For example, as many as 60% of registered blind people have or have had a Talking Book machine, compared with as few as 3% of non-registered partially sighted people (Table 8.9.b.). This contrast emphasises once again the importance of registration as a trigger of service delivery.

Use of ordinary tape-players also varies widely. For example, 78% of blind people under 60 use one compared with 29% of partially sighted people aged 60 or over.

The use of tape-players varies considerably. While those who have a Talking Book player (12%) of course use it to listen to books, only 3% of blind and partially sighted people use ordinary tape-players to listen to books. The main uses of ordinary tape-players are music (32% of blind and partially sighted people) and information material such as local talking newspapers, national magazines, letters on tape, telephone numbers (14%).

Chapter 9, Readers

Forty per cent of visually impaired people have printed material read to them by a sighted person. The total varies with age, residual vision and registration status. For instance, 74% of blind people aged under 60 but only 28% of partially sighted people aged 60 or over are read to. Seventeen per cent of all blind people under 60 would like to have reading support for the first time or to have more of it. The data suggest that reading support services should be increased significantly for blind non-readers under 60, and to a lesser extent for older blind non-readers as well.

The most frequent reader is someone else in the house (53%), followed by another relative (27%) and a friend/colleague (17%). Readers vary considerably according to the age of the person read to. Eighty-four per cent of young visually impaired people are read to by 'someone in the household', to the virtual exclusion of all other categories. Among older people, 48% are read to by someone in the household, while another relative (30%) and friend or colleague (19%) now feature significantly.

The extent of informal reading is remarkable. Visually impaired people identify printed material as one of the biggest challenges to daily life. Given the frequent need for access to printed material such a crucial service should be available as of right either as a direct service or indirectly through a financial cost allowance.

Chapter 10, Braille

Our study answers another long-standing question, 'How many people read braille?' We estimate that 19,000 blind and partially sighted people have learnt braille well enough to be able read a braille magazine or book. Thirteen thousand remain active braille readers; 10,000 write in braille (section 10.3).

Braille users are proportionately most numerous among the registered blind aged 16 – 59 (81%), and lowest among the non-registered partially sighted aged 60 and over, none of whom have learnt braille (Tables 10.2.a, and 10.2.b.).

There is a comparable success rate of braille learning among adults who experience onset of their sight loss under the age of 17 years and between 17 and 59 years. Given that a significant number of successful learners are at the upper end of the latter age range, these figures suggest two conclusions. First, increased teaching among adults aged under 60 would be likely to produce a fair degree of successful braille readers. Second, since only 1% of visually impaired people aged 60 + are offered braille teaching increased provision for this age group would be likely to produce a reasonable number of successful braille readers.

Seventy-five per cent of braille users read magazines in braille, 72% letters and 70% books; 42% read the braille *Radio Times* (Table 10.8). Nearly half of working blind people use braille. Approximately 80% of readers also write in braille; a third use a writing-frame, half a writing-machine such as a Perkins, and 1 in 5 use both.

Only 11% of blind and partially sighted people who had not learnt braille said that they would like to. About one-third of these had not learnt because they had not been given the opportunity or did not know how to go about it.

Awareness of braille and Moon

More than 9 in 10 visually impaired people had heard of braille, while Moon was known by fewer than 1 in 10 (Table 10.7). Awareness of Moon was concentrated among younger respondents, and was highest (48%) among blind people aged 16 – 59. Since Moon is considered to be much easier to learn than braille, particularly for older visually impaired people, this low level of awareness gives cause for concern.

Our data suggest that for Moon to become a viable embossed tactile medium, awareness of it must be developed among elderly registrably blind people, the penetration and quality of its teaching must be increased and the supply of relevant magazines and books to learners and readers improved.

Chapter 11, Overview of reading habits and communication media

Reading habits

While Chapters 7 to 10 discussed individual methods of reading, this chapter provides data on their use in combination, thus allowing some judgement on the preferred reading media of visually impaired people.

Blind and partially sighted people differ in the reading media they use most and prefer. Among blind people the most used forms were 'personal reader' (33%), 'ordinary print' (29%) and 'tapes' (24%) (Table 11.1). Statutory and voluntary organisations should note the high mentions of a 'personal reader'; this receives little or no outside support and encouragement and is almost always left to the individual initiative of the blind person. While such initiative should not be discouraged it is important for the statutory and voluntary sectors to expand services in this area, especially given the evidence of unmet need among younger blind people (see Chapter 9).

For 2% of registrably blind people, increasing to 12% of those aged 16 – 59, braille was the most frequent reading form. There are two reasons why braille is not the most popular reading form, even among young people. First, as Chapter 10 shows, only a minority of blind people use braille; second, insufficient braille material is produced.

Among partially sighted people ordinary print is the dominant reading form (60%), followed by large print (30%). Preference for large print was higher among partially sighted people aged 75 + (34%). Personal readers and tapes trailed at 12 and 6 per cent respectively.

It is worth noting that so many partially sighted people benefit from large print. Although the commercial sector recognises the demand for large-print books, they still represent only a small percentage of the total numbers of books printed. Indeed it may justifiably be claimed that the print size on much printed material is not large enough even to qualify being called 'ordinary print'; forms are a prime example.

The fact that 12% of partially sighted people use personal readers strengthens the argument in favour of statutory and voluntary sector involvement in promoting this service.

How much do blind and partially sighted people read?

Respondents were asked whether they read more, less or about the same as before their sight problem began. Overall, 9% said that they read more, 21% the same and 69% less. There was relatively little variation in the responses across age groups, except that 77% of blind people aged 75 + said that they read less.

These data are quite startling. Almost one third (30%) of blind and partially sighted people read the same or more than before. Indeed just over one third (35%) of blind people under 60 said they read more than before. While we should not be complacent about the 69% who read less, that so many read the same or more is a remarkable tribute to the people concerned and to the organisations that supply their needs.

Communication media

Writing media

An estimated 10,000 registered blind people write in braille, 70% of whom are aged 16 – 59.

Although fewer than 5% overall use a typewriter, this figure hides an uneven distribution. For example, 25 and 21 per cent of blind and partially sighted people aged 16 – 59 use a typewriter. Almost all the registered blind who write in braille also use a typewriter.

Although we did not ask specific questions about hand-writing, the 58% of blind people aged 16 – 59 unable to read our large-print card (Table 6.3) suggests the approximate number who either might not be able to write at all or who might find it extremely difficult to write legibly. Furthermore, only 25% of blind people under 60 use a typewriter. These statistics indicate a major unmet need, in our literate world, for typewriter or keyboard training for younger blind people.

Telephones

Telephone ownership among the registered and non-registered is 86 and 67 per cent respectively, compared with 81% among the general population (section 11.2.3.2).

A not-insignificant minority said that the telephone was the 'most' and 'second most' important way of finding things out, 16 and 20 per cent respectively. This suggests that the 28% of visually impaired people without a telephone are at a major disadvantage.

The low income of visually impaired people and the relatively large proportion they spend on a telephone demonstrate its importance.

Relative importance of different sources of information

Personal communication – asking people (85%) and telephoning people (54%) – were the most important sources of information mentioned (Table 11.4). Personal communication divides into informal and formal contacts. The informal category, mentioned about four times as often as the formal, includes 'someone in the household' (32%), 'other relative' (32%) and 'friend or colleague' (21%) (Table 11.6). For younger visually impaired people the dominant source of personal communication is within the household, but moves to someone outside the house for older people.

Social services were the main source of formal information contacts, particularly among the registered. The registered also mentioned voluntary welfare organisations notably more often than the non-registered.

Radio and television were mentioned more often by the younger registered than by other sub-groups. The telephone was mentioned by 12% with little variation across sub-groups.

Chapter 12, Visual impairment and other disabilities

The OPCS study of disability shows that 1,384,000 people in private households have a 'seeing disability'. Our data give a figure of 757,000 registrably visually impaired people. The difference arises because OPCS included about 600,000 people with a seeing disability who could see well enough not to reach the registrable level for partial sight.

The OPCS survey compares the incidence of visual impairment with that of other disabilities. It ranks fifth after locomotion, hearing, personal care and dexterity. Eight other disabilities are less prevalent, including mental handicap and mental illness.

Prevalence rates for registrable visual impairment (i.e. blind and partially sighted) are 3 per 1,000 among those aged 16 – 59; 23 per 1,000, 60 to 74 years; and 152 per 1,000, 75 and over. In other words, 0.3% of the population aged 16 – 59 is registrably blind and partially sighted; 2.3% of 60 to 74 year-olds; and 15% of those aged 75 and over. The prevalence rate among the 75 + group is startlingly high, and can be assumed to be even higher among people in their 80s.

Vision and hearing are the two senses crucial to communication, one of the most critical functions of humankind. When both vision and hearing are impaired, the individual suffers a truly massive handicap, whose total impact is far greater than the sum of the two individual impairments.

Thirty-five per cent of visually impaired people suffer the additional disadvantage of experiencing difficulties in hearing normal speech in a quiet room, even when wearing a hearing aid. The total increases across the three age groups, 16 – 59, 60 – 74 and 75 +, from 22 to 34 and 37 per cent. Our interviewers noted that 45% of those aged 75 + had difficulty hearing the interview.

These figures suggest that people and organisations in contact with very old registrably visually impaired people are justified in assuming that half of the individuals they deal with will be hard of hearing. The communication process adopted by staff will need to be assessed and modified in the light of this finding.

Excluding hearing problems, 67% of visually impaired people have another permanent illness or disability, and 45% say that this illness or disability limits their daily activities (section 12.3.2.2). The illnesses or disabilities most frequently mentioned were arthritis (25%), heart condition (18%), legs/mobility (14%) and diabetes (9%).

These figures represent a major underestimate (section 12.3.2.4). For example, among people aged 75 + hearing impairment averaged 36% by self-report, but rose to 45% as reported by the interviewers.

Chapter 13, Mobility

Orientation and mobility are vital areas of limitation and challenge to visually impaired people, particularly so to blind people. We found that 87% of blind people under 60 had gone out in the week before our interview, although only 51% had gone out alone and on foot. Further analysis of our data and the OPCS survey reveals that the independent mobility of visually impaired people is more restricted than that of the broader disabled population. Only 43% compared with 78% were able to go out on their own (section 13.1.2.2).

Visually impaired people also suffer the added disadvantage of orientation and mobility in unfamiliar surroundings. Seventy-nine and forty-eight per cent expressed confidence in their mobility inside and outside their immediate neighbourhood respectively.

Younger people, partially sighted people, those without other disabilities and the registered are the groups most likely to have gone out alone in the previous week.

Among younger visually impaired people, we found a startling correlation between registration and independent mobility. Among blind people aged 16 – 59, 70 and 45 per cent of the registered and non-registered respectively had been out alone on foot during the previous week. This is all the more remarkable because the non-registered enjoy slightly better residual vision levels.

There is an expected correlation between mobility training and independent mobility. Among the registered blind aged 16 – 59, 64% of those who had been trained were independently mobile compared with 45% who had not been trained (section 13.4.1.2).

A comparison with the Gray and Todd survey of 1965 (Gray and Todd, 1968) shows that among young registered blind people the level of independent mobility has not increased over time. This is puzzling given the relative success of mobility training, which was not as widely available in 1965. One hypothesis is that without increased training provision mobility might have declined, perhaps because of actual and perceived increased environmental dangers, e.g. traffic.

Age influences the frequency with which people go out. Across the three age groups, 16 – 59, 60 – 74 and 75 + , 90, 88 and 75 per cent had been out in the previous week. Among the two younger age groups, 58 and 59 per cent had gone out alone, compared with 33% of people aged 75 + .

The mobility of older visually impaired people was more restricted than that of elderly people in general. According to Hunt's (1978) study of elderly people, 87% of the general population aged 65 + had been out, while we found that only 42% of blind and partially sighted people aged 60 and over had been out alone in the previous week (section 13.1.2.1). The reasons are both the visual impairment itself and the increased prevalence of other disabilities among visually impaired people.

Visually impaired people are less mobile than disabled people in general (section 13.1.2.2). Even more significant is that 52% of visually impaired people but only 14% of disabled people need help to go out. This finding gives important support to the argument for making visually impaired people eligible for financial help in the form of the mobility allowance.

One vulnerable group identified was blind and partially sighted people living alone. We were shocked to find that 26% (90,000 people) of people living alone say that they are never visited by friends or neighbours and 11% (38,000 people) say that they are never visited by a relative. In addition, blind and partially sighted people living alone were visited no more frequently than people living with a sighted friend or relative. These data say much for the independence of blind and partially sighted people who live alone. They also reveal the apparent absence of an informal support network of a vulnerable sector of society.

In addition, these findings identify elderly blind and partially sighted people living alone as a crucial target group for increased formal and informal support. Lack of such support will hasten an individual's entry into costly residential care.

Mobility training and mobility aids

Use of a white cane or white stick was concentrated heavily among registered (74%) compared with non-registered (8%) people (section 13.4).

Only 5% of visually impaired people overall have received significant mobility training. For registered people aged 16 – 59 the figure rises to 40%, and to 55% for those registered blind.

These findings indicate a drastic lack of mobility training, which is a fundamental requirement for blind and partially sighted people. Given this shortage it is perhaps understandable – but not excusable – that training is offered on an age-related basis. Of blind people in the three age groups, 16 – 59, 60 – 74 and 75 +, 33, 18 and 5 per cent had received training.

Thirteen per cent of blind people under 60, and 4% of all blind people, used a guide dog as a specific mobility aid.

The most positive picture to emerge from our study is that an over-whelming majority of blind people under 60 get out and about, and that half are able to do so alone and on foot. This is a reflection not only of youth and determination but also of the greater degree of service offered to this age group.

The most negative picture is of the large number of blind people aged 60 or over and partially sighted people of all ages who receive no significant support in their attempts to be more mobile. These lost opportunities become all the more tragic when set against the relative success of younger blind people. They represent both an indictment of the lack of statutory resourcing and also an underestimate of the capabilities of the people concerned, particularly of the 'young elderly' blind. This chapter contains many pointers for service planners and providers.

Chapter 14, Shopping and transport

We explored some basic aspects of shopping and the use of transport. While three-quarters of visually impaired people live within a 15-minute walk of the nearest food shop, 59% rely on others to do their food shopping.

Over half those who do their own shopping reported some difficulty. Old age rather than residual vision was the major variable determining the level of difficulty reported with shopping. The main source of help with shopping was a household member, but as age increased the helper was more likely to come from outside the home.

Blind and partially sighted people use a variety of forms of transport. The main modes are buses and taxis. Among occasional users of transport (i.e. those who did not go out in the last week), the car was most used. In the week before the interview, 59% of respondents had been out by car, 33% by bus, 15% by taxi, 3% by train, 3% by coach and 1% by tube.

Chapter 15, Daily living skills

We asked respondents about three areas of daily living skills: personal care (e.g. getting in and out of bed, washing and bathing, dressing); domestic tasks (e.g. cutting up food, making hot meals, tidying up around the house); and dealing with mail and other tasks (e.g. paperwork including bills and letters, and post and leaflets through the door).

Ninety-one per cent of all blind and partially sighted people experienced difficulty with at least one of these areas. In the three areas, 75, 54 and 59 per cent respectively needed help. For blind people the corresponding totals were 78, 60 and 75 per cent.

We asked who helped in these three areas. As far as personal care tasks were concerned, help came mainly from someone in the house or from the health service. For those aged 16 – 59, someone in the house (78%) was the main source, the health service (25%) the other frequently mentioned source. With increasing age the source shifted to someone outside the home, quite often to someone from one of the statutory welfare services; for respondents aged 75 + , the totals were 26 and 77 per cent respectively (Table 15.3).

Help with domestic tasks showed a similar pattern but with home-helps from social services departments substituting for the health service. However, while 68% of those who needed assistance with personal care were helped by the health service, only 39% of those who needed assistance with domestic tasks were helped by home-helps.

Help with dealing with the mail and other tasks showed a dramatically different pattern. Help from the statutory welfare services was practically non-existent. Someone in the household was the major source of help while other relatives, friends and neighbours filled the subsidiary role occupied by the statutory services in the other two areas.

While the degree of informal support provided by relatives and friends is recognised, the lack of any statutory service alternative is a major gap in provision. The fact that such assistance is required solely by visually impaired people reveals significant, if unwitting, discrimination which should be urgently addressed through a combination of service provision and financial help. (See also Chapter nine.)

Aids and gadgets

Technical aids and gadgets make an important contribution to helping visually impaired people to cope with everyday living. The range and sophistication of these aids varies widely. We examined awareness, ownership and usage of a few of the more popular aids and gadgets available, largely those of interest to blind people and partially sighted people with lower residual vision levels. While awareness of these typical aids was reasonably high among young blind people, it was particularly low among blind people aged 75 +. For example, awareness of special clocks and watches was 75 and 37 per cent among the two groups. Usage of aids runs at a much lower level than awareness. This is to be expected since aids are a personal matter; while some people have no need of them, others are unable to use them.

The impact of registration on awareness and possession of technical aids is remarkable. Taking special clocks and watches as an example, 84% of the registered but only 48% of the non-registered aged 16 – 59 were aware of them; 31% of the registered but only 2% of the non-registered owned at least one device. These findings provide evidence of the importance of registration as a triggering mechanism.

The overwhelming majority of visually impaired people have difficulty doing everyday tasks. As they age, the combination of the sight problem and other illnesses or disabilities compounds the difficulties they experience. Although aids and gadgets offer only limited help, lack of awareness of them is a failing which needs to be corrected.

Chapter 16, Leisure

Our most notable findings demonstrate that visually impaired people enjoy the same media as the general population. They are, first, that 94% of visually impaired people have a television, and that 90% listen to or watch it, with little variation between blind and partially sighted people. Second, 81% listen to the radio.

The extent of television usage emphasises its significance as a communications medium. It also indicates the importance of encouraging broadcasters not to expand 'vision only' information on programmes (e.g. the use of sub-titles to translate interviews in foreign languages). This also applies to the significant minority of other people who find it difficult or impossible to absorb written or graphic information.

Radio

The radio stations most listened to are local radio (34%), Radio 2 (23%), and Radio 4 (21%). A larger proportion of the two younger age groups listens to local radio (48 and 44 per cent). Proportionately Radio 1's largest audience was the 16 – 59 age group (11%).

Television and radio are both vital media through which service-giving organisations reach the visually impaired population. However, BBC Radio 4's *In Touch* programme, which is designed specifically for visually impaired people, is a highly effective targeted means of communication. Approximately one fifth of all blind and partially sighted people listen to *In Touch* either occasionally or regularly, and this rises to 75% among those who have heard of the programme. This suggests the need for both the BBC and statutory and voluntary organisations to do much more to promote knowledge of the programme's existence.

Hobbies and leisure activities

Gardening is by far the most popular hobby of visually impaired people. Although it was mentioned by 32%, this rating is in fact lower than among the general population, which suggests that more could be done to promote gardening, especially since it is equally popular among all age groups.

Although knitting would seem an unlikely hobby for blind and partially sighted people, 26%, almost all women, enjoy it. Given the popularity of this hobby it is vital that organisations give this hobby the support that its popularity deserves.

Outdoor sports are widely played by younger visually impaired people. About one-fifth of blind people and one-tenth of partially sighted people under 60 take part in sports such as walking, sailing, skiing and water-skiing, riding, fishing, archery and many others. One reason for the relatively high participation rate is the encouragement provided by schools for blind people and by a wide variety of active specialist sports organisations for blind people. The extent of the success of these organisations, and the fact that a still higher percentage of sighted people participate, suggests that these activities would benefit from further support and encouragement.

Social clubs and centres

Almost half (45%) of blind and partially sighted people go out to clubs, societies, social centres or churches (sections 16.3 and 16.4). Most visited are church or church groups (22%), followed by clubs for the elderly (15%); ordinary social centres/clubs (10%); working men's clubs (7%, men and women); clubs or day centres for visually impaired people (3%); and sports clubs/centres (2% overall, but 17% among young blind people). Frequency of attendance is quite high, over half going at least once a week to all the clubs listed except working men's clubs and blind clubs/centres.

Nevertheless, the 55% who do not visit any club or centre is an unacceptably high figure. A quarter of non-attenders said that they had 'difficulty getting there'. Just over half (56%) said that they were 'not interested'. While this is undoubtedly true in many cases, in a significant number this explanation may have been given for reasons of self-defence and self-esteem as the individuals concerned lacked ready access to such activities. The challenge facing the organisations involved is to ensure that visually impaired people are able to make a real choice between participating and not participating.

Only 3% of all blind and partially sighted people attend clubs and centres specifically for visually impaired people, although this figure rises to 27% among the registered blind. Once again, registration acts as a passport, although in this case not with a wholly benign effect. This is because we found that, among elderly people, while only 17% of the registered blind went to integrated clubs this rose to 37% among non-registered blind people. We conclude that clubs and centres for visually impaired people should be seen as providing extra opportunities, not as a substitute for attending general clubs.

Social and leisure activities predominate at these separate clubs and centres; 45% of attenders mentioned music and singing; 44%, meeting friends for a chat; 38%, talks; 28%, lunch and lunch clubs; and 23% each, indoor games and handicrafts. However, rehabilitation and training activities were rarely mentioned, even though these might be considered one of the strongest (even the only) argument in favour of separate clubs and centres. We therefore conclude that there is a major opportunity for separate clubs and centres to provide more rehabilitation and low-key training activities, especially for elderly people who have recently experienced visual impairment.

Holidays

As many as 38% of visually impaired people have not had a holiday during the last five years. This figure rises to 55% of blind people aged 75+ (Table 16.8), the equivalent of some 113,000 people, mainly women, many of whom live alone. The lack of holidays is not solely age-related, since only 36% of partially sighted people aged 75+ have not had a holiday in the past five years.

Blind people aged 75+ (mostly non-registered) form a key target group for specialised holiday providers.

Overall, 62% of visually impaired people (compared with 40% of the general population) have not taken a holiday in the previous 12 months. This figure includes 68% of those aged 75+ and less than half the

16 – 59 age group. Only 4% (all registered) said that their most recent holiday was one specially organised for visually impaired people; this figure rises to 16% of registered blind people aged 60 or over. It is older visually impaired people who show the largest preference for hotels catering specially for their needs. This strengthens the case for special-ised hotels, which are largely run by voluntary organisations, to attempt to reach the large number of older visually impaired people who have not taken a holiday in the last five years.

Access to leisure services

Visually impaired people follow an exciting variety of leisure and hobby pursuits. However, with the exception of television and radio, there is plenty of room for expansion. Our research also identifies a substantial number of mainly very elderly visually impaired people living alone who never go out for leisure or hobby pursuits and who never go on holiday. Organisations of blind people, and particularly statutory and voluntary service-giving agencies (including those not primarily aimed at visually impaired people) must give these people higher priority.

This group contains a significant number of non-registered blind people. The very act of registration dramatically increases their chances of access to leisure services and activities. All those concerned – ophthalmologists, social service departments and voluntary organisations – must reassess their attitudes towards the registration of older people in the light of the role that registration is shown to play.

Chapter 17, Employment

The OPCS disability survey shows that 31% of disabled people under retirement age are in employment. Our findings reveal that, while the same proportion of partially sighted people are working, far fewer blind people have a paid job (17%). A sighted person is about four times more likely to be employed than a blind person.

Two points should be stressed. First, that 17% of blind people hold a job demonstrates that paid work is feasible for blind people. Second, nearly three-quarters of blind people (72%) who are currently not work-ing have worked in the past, in the vast majority of cases after the onset of visual handicap (Table 17.1).

We discovered one alarming fact about the duration of unemployment. For the general population, short periods of unemployment are inter-spersed with periods of work. Once out of work, however, visually impaired people find it hard to get another job. Eighty-eight per cent have been out of work for over a year and 55% for more than five years (section 17.3). In addition the last job of 58% of those not working was the one in which their sight failed (section 17.8).

Just over a quarter of visually impaired people lost their last job within two years of onset, and a similar number left their job five years or more after onset.

The data suggest that retention of employment should be a high priority, given the high proportion of visually impaired people in work at the time of onset (section 17.3.1, Table 17.4). At present statutory provision concentrates on finding jobs for unemployed visually impaired people and creating the initial conditions (for example, provision of equipment and training) under which they can take them up.

Our findings suggest that job retention is a neglected area, with support needed to both employers and employees in the crucial period around the onset of the sight problem when the majority of visually impaired people will lose the last job they may ever hold (section 17.3.1).

Statutory and voluntary organisations should devote increased attention and resources to a public education campaign designed to explain to employers, employees and unions the positive steps that can be taken to enable newly visually impaired employees to stay in work. In particular, retraining should be provided free of charge, as already happens with technical aids and the personal reader service (see below).

Occupational structure of visually impaired people

Not only do proportionally fewer visually impaired people work, they also hold fewer professional and managerial jobs and more semi-skilled and unskilled jobs. They are not merely disadvantaged in relation to the general population, but also in relation to disabled people in general. For example, 14% of visually impaired workers hold professional jobs, compared with 25 and 34 per cent of the disabled and general populations respectively.

These findings suggest that additional firm positive action is needed to help visually impaired people to obtain and retain work.

Technical aids and other employment services

The survey provides very clear evidence of the importance of special equipment, aids and additional clerical services in helping visually impaired people to find and retain jobs. Working blind and partially sighted people are between three and six times more likely to be using aids and services in their job compared with their out-of-work counterparts in the job they lost.

This reflects the welcome increased attention and resources provided by the Department of Employment and RNIB. However, their very success suggests that additional efforts to publicise and resource this area are urgently needed. For example, only 23% of working blind people use the additional clerical services including the personal reader service. While the use of special equipment and aids is already high (45%), provision may need to be increased to help blind workers to meet technological change.

Future prospects are not unreasonable for those who manage to stay in employment after onset (Table 17.16). One quarter of people changing jobs gained promotion, one third (32%) moved to a job with similar status and under half (43%) moved to a lower-status job. This is encouraging evidence that, so long as visually impaired people are able to stay in the job market, they can enjoy reasonable expectations and also that employers find their contribution useful.

Chapter 18, Allowances and benefits

Seventy-eight per cent of visually impaired people of working age received some form of state benefit (Table 18.1). Fifty-five per cent of those of retirement age received some form of income maintenance benefit (excluding retirement pension) reflecting their low income level (Table 18.6). Fifty-five percent of those of working age received one or more of the disability-based benefits or allowances. Most strikingly, two-thirds of those not currently in work receive a benefit, which suggests that they are no longer able to work.

In general, visually impaired people depend heavily on state benefits, and a little more so than the disabled population in general.

In view of this heavy dependency, the very low proportion (21%) who have received expert advice on entitlements to benefits is disturbing (Table 18.4). This finding reveals an urgent need to expand benefits advice and support to a group that, besides being vulnerable in them-selves, also has particular difficulty in gaining access to information on benefits and completing claim forms.

Chapter 19, Local authority social services

Awareness of relevant social services

While awareness of 'social services or welfare services' in general was high at 84%, awareness of specific services for visually impaired people was extremely low. One-third of the registered but two-thirds of the non-registered were unaware of the availability of such basic services as white sticks and canes, talking books and local social and day centres.

Once again, registration acts as a trigger, with twice as many registered people knowing about these services. Almost three-quarters of non-registered people (71%) said that they were unaware of the benefits of being registered. Service planners and providers face a substantial and urgent task of increasing awareness of the social services available. If statutory agencies are unable to do this, the voluntary sector should consider taking up this role. In practice, service delivery to the registrable but non-registered must be improved, and registration must be promoted heavily.

Visits by and satisfaction with social services

Overall, only 17% of visually impaired people were visited by their social services department at or shortly after the time of their sight loss. Forty-five per cent of those newly registered said that they had not been visited by social services. Some social services departments may find it difficult to believe these figures. At the very least, we can say that some of those who claim not to have been visited were in fact visited, but the visit made such insignificant impact that they could not remember it.

Another very significant finding is that over 98% of the non-registered (but registrable) were not visited. This is important because a small proportion of social services departments claim that they offer their services equally to the registered and non-registered. While some departments may claim this policy in theory, in practice they are not delivering it.

Forty-five per cent of those registered received a first visit from social services within three months of their examination by an eye specialist. However, 42% were not, or could not remember being, visited (section 19.4.2).

Satisfaction with the first visit was poor. Thirty-four per cent were 'very' or 'a bit' dissatisfied. This represents a very high dissatisfaction rating (see note 5 to Chapter 19) and ties in with low awareness of services.

Rehabilitation

Four per cent of visually impaired people (35 and 11 per cent of those registered aged 16 – 59 and 60 + respectively) have been offered formal rehabilitation training (section 19.5), although not all offers were necessarily taken up. Only 4% have had a home visit when they were given practical advice and instruction on coping with their sight problem; this increases to 24% among the registered blind aged 16 – 59. All these are depressingly low numbers.

Since vision loss of registrable severity can take some time to develop, the long interval between initial onset of vision loss and the delivery of practical instruction and advice in the home is worrying. Only 12% received practical instruction within a year, 27% in one to five years, and 42% after 10 years (Table 19.6).

Unsatisfied demand

One-fifth (19%) of the 96% who have not received any practical advice or instruction in the home would like such help. One reason for this relatively low percentage, which reflects a slightly defensive response, is that many respondents, having had to make do on their own, might well have been disinclined to acknowledge their need for help. In absolute terms, however, the 19% represents a massive number of people wanting help.

Fewer than 1% of visually impaired people have received counselling, while a further 23% would have liked it. Demand was greatest among blind people aged under 75 (36%). One in three of this group would have welcomed counselling, but less than one in a hundred received it.

Overall this chapter presents a bleak picture of provision by social services departments. The vast majority of non-registered blind and partially sighted people receive no services, nor do a substantial minority of those registered. Furthermore, client satisfaction with services is low. This evidence combines with other studies of social services departments (Shore 1985, DHSS 1988) to reveal a worrying and unacceptable situation. While good practice certainly exists, it is the exception rather than the norm. The resources available for unmet need appear to be totally inadequate by a factor of three to five. Thus reorganisation or restructuring of services will not provide a solution unless significant additional resources are made available.

Chapter 20, Voluntary organisations involved with visually impaired people

Half our respondents (49%) could not spontaneously name any organisations that help blind people and people with sight problems. Those organisations named by the others included RNIB (22%), St Dunstans (9%), Guide Dogs for the Blind Association (7%) and various local societies for the blind (2%). The figure for RNIB is likely to be inflated because RNIB was mentioned at the start of the interview. A more accurate awareness level would fall between 10 and 22 per cent. (See also note 1 to Chapter 20.)

More registered and younger people named various organisations than non-registered and older people.

Our findings do not confirm the long-standing worry within RNIB that the organisation's title gives the impression that it only helps blind people. The following responses were received to a question about whom RNIB might help: blind people, 93%; partially sighted people, 77%; people who can't see well enough to read, 62%; and anyone who is worried about their sight, 60%.

While understanding of the broad thrust of RNIB's work and the groups it helps is accurate, detailed knowledge is poor. Half were unable to name even one service; this figure varies from 21% of the registered aged 16 – 59 to 60% of the non-registered aged 60 + (Table 20.2).

The best-known RNIB services among the registered aged 16 – 59 were: aids and gadgets, 39%; RNIB Talking Books and braille, 24% each; schools 22%; and holidays and hotels, 20%. Nevertheless, RNIB should be concerned that half of all blind and partially sighted people cannot name a single RNIB service. This suggests a need for a major promotional campaign to increase knowledge of RNIB services.

Users of RNIB services

Eighty per cent of those who know about RNIB make use of one or more of its services. This represents 13% of the visually impaired population living in private households, an estimated 100,000 people. Use of services varies. For instance, 72 and 47 per cent among the registered aged 16 – 59 and 60 + use RNIB services compared with 14 and 5 per cent of the non-registered in the same age groups.

Sources of information about RNIB services

Social services workers represent the most important source of information. A quarter (26%) of visually impaired people learned about RNIB from this source. Social workers are thus an important target group if RNIB is to make its services better known. But since they tend to concentrate on registered rather than non-registered people alternative ways of reaching the latter group must be found.

Eleven per cent found out about RNIB via Radio 4's *In Touch* and other media. These sources offer some scope for development. Opticians may be another key intermediary group. Currently they contribute 4% of introductions. The same applies to doctors (2%).

Although not mentioned above, hospital based 'eye specialists' are in contact with a considerable number of visually impaired people, notably the non-registered (section 5.3). Clubs and centres for elderly people are another possible information source.

Chapter 21, Methodological appendix

This chapter provides detailed technical information about the survey, including a definition of residual vision; the residual vision scale; the questionnaire questions; estimating population numbers from the data; and testing for statistically significant differences between percentages.

Part A

Background

1 Introduction

1.1 Objectives of the survey

The purpose of the survey was to assess the needs and views of a nationally representative sample of visually impaired people on a wide range of topics. A number of specific objectives were identified:

- To provide a national picture of the characteristics of the visually impaired population

- To examine how the needs of the visually impaired population are being met from whatever source

- To provide information which will enable RNIB to evaluate, develop and promote its services

- To give evidence of significant areas of unmet or inadequately met need so that RNIB or other agencies can take steps to ensure that those needs are met

- To identify problems in obtaining information about services or access to them

- To identify areas for further investigation

- To extend and complement the information on severely visually impaired people available from existing data sources, and in particular the OPCS disability survey.

The survey was intended to encompass visually impaired people of all age groups; however, it was felt that the under-16s would require a different questionnaire, so this report concentrates on adults. A survey of children's needs was carried out separately and is the subject of a further report, published as Volume 2.

1.2 Previous major surveys of visually impaired people

There have of course been several previous surveys, the best of which we were able to draw on with considerable advantage in designing our own. The RNIB survey, however, aimed both to collect wide-ranging information on needs and to do so on a nationally representative sample. Previous surveys have achieved one or other of these two aims but never the two together.

Tobin and Hill's (1984) 'pilot' survey of blind people in Birmingham, for example, ranged richly over need topic areas and knowledge of available services. Surveys carried out by local authorities and voluntary societies have been based on much larger samples, and some, like the Hampshire survey (Edge, 1987) have covered a wide range of topic areas, but still on a regional basis.

The surveys that have yielded national statistics, on the other hand, have only done so for a restricted range of topic areas. Hall's (1982) survey covered a large sample at modest cost by drawing from members of the British Talking Book Library. Cullinan's (1977) survey provides useful national data, but it included relatively few visually impaired people who were registered or registrable. The main government sponsored survey of the blind, that by Gray and Todd (1968), in contrast, was limited entirely to registered blind people. The latter survey is still the most thorough study of the mobility and reading habits of blind people, but the coverage was confined to just these two topic areas. Moreover, in what now seems a curious reflection on the welfare priorities of the time, the sample selected for the inquiry had an upper cut off point at 80 years old.

The RNIB survey was timely in that it coincided with the survey of disability undertaken by the Office of Population Censuses and Surveys (OPCS) for the (then) Department of Health and Social Security (Martin et al, 1988a, 1988b, 1989). In the foreseeable future, following its publication, the OPCS survey can be expected to provide the frame of reference for legislation and action on disability. The previous national survey of disabled people took place in 1969 (Harris, 1971). In order to identify a random but representative national sample of people with disabilities both these government surveys involved massive and costly screening operations. Such screening is well beyond the resources of most organisations outside central government. Because of the wide range of disabilities covered, the amount of information collected on the special needs of visually impaired people is necessarily very limited. If the latest OPCS survey is to be used as a starting point for future action on disability, then more information is desirable on the situation of visually impaired people. We hope our survey, growing as it does out of the OPCS survey, will provide this. Our use of the OPCS survey to provide part of the sampling frame for our own study is described in Chapters 2 and 21, and was possible because of the helpful cooperation and agreement of the DHSS and OPCS.

2 Method

Methodological decisions have a vital impact on the form of results, and for this reason we report fully on these both here and in Chapter 21, the methodological appendix. Those interested primarily in service delivery may wish to omit this chapter, although reading sections 2.4.1, 2.4.3.3 and 2.5 will aid interpretation. However, this chapter is crucial for those wishing to reinterpret the data presented here and in the more detailed reports accessible through the Reference Library at RNIB.

2.1 Questionnaire construction

2.1.1 The consultation process

We sought the widest possible consultation on the content of the questionnaire with visually impaired people, their representative organisations and those concerned with their welfare. The consultation process itself went through several steps, which we regarded as an essential part of our research strategy.

2.1.2 The information pack

As a first step, Sally Edge, who had just completed a survey of blind people in Hampshire (Edge, 1987), was commissioned to draw up a list of need headings. The list of 19 headings, produced in the 1986 *New Beacon* article (Bruce and McKennell, 1986), mostly survived the consultation process and correspond broadly with the chapter headings in this report. The list was circulated for comment to over 30 advisers, each a specialist in one or more of the areas concerned. On the basis of their comments, we prepared a rough draft of a questionnaire which would be required to do justice to the particular area. These drafts were far too long to be workable, and the next step was to condense them, at the same time producing a short prose rationale of what it was necessary to omit. The shortened, but still overlong, questionnaires, together with our commentary on each need area, were then put together as an information pack. The pack, together with the *New Beacon* article announcing the proposed survey, was circulated as a consultation document to a further list of organisations and individuals, to *New Beacon* readers who wrote in to request it, and to the steering committee guiding the research.

2.1.3 Pre-pilot qualitative interviews

Although a standardised interview schedule is essential for a quantitative survey, there is a danger that it can be prematurely standardised around its designers' preconceptions. Although we had taken the experts' views, we believed that we had not sufficiently consulted visually impaired people themselves. Before finalising the pilot schedule, therefore, one of the Survey Directors (AMK) and the Assistant Director (EW) personally carried out conversational interviews with a small but varied sample of 20 visually impaired adults. The 19 topic areas and the experts' views were a guide to issues raised in conversation, but no formal schedule was used. The interviews were non-directive, allowing scope for eliciting from respondents further issues or emphases that seemed important to them. The transcripts of the interviews (which were tape-recorded) were analysed to provide an additional source for the content and phrasing of questions in the largely standardised pilot schedule.

2.1.4 The concept of need

Although the concept of need was central to our enquiry, and to the questionnaire design, it was not possible to proceed from any abstract definition. A literature search (e.g. Bradshaw, 1972; Smith, 1980; Clayton, 1983) shows that there is no single agreed definition of 'real need'. That said, one main distinction does run through the literature, and this can be applied in turn to each of the need areas – defined pragmatically by means of the consultation process. This is the distinction between self-assessed need and comparative assessment of need. To define the former, people are asked directly if they are aware of a need or service, have tried or want to receive the service, or, if already a user, are satisfied with it. Comparative assessments, by contrast, are reached through an evaluation of statistical information on people's circumstances independent of their own perceptions. The questionnaire was designed to allow both types of assessment.

2.2 Sampling

2.2.1 Sources

Names and addresses of visually impaired people who were willing to take part in the survey were obtained from two different sources: the Office of Population Censuses and Surveys (OPCS) (wave 1) and local authority registers (wave 2).

2.2.2 The OPCS first wave sample

The OPCS master sample to which we had access was itself constructed from those who returned a short questionnaire sent (mostly) by post to 100,000 randomly drawn households. Part of the RNIB adult sample was thus a sub-sample of those who identified themselves as having visual difficulties in the OPCS screening. All respondents aged under 60 and half those aged 60 or over who recorded that they had difficulty in recognising a friend across a road, or in reading ordinary newsprint, were visited by the OPCS interviewers and given acuity tests for near and distant vision in their homes as part of a longer interview covering mainly health, social services and income. RNIB was allowed to transfer data from the OPCS questionnaires as they were returned from the field. The transfer sheets covered mainly the sight test results plus some demographic information which allowed RNIB to define its sample. Most of the original OPCS informants had agreed to a further visit by an interviewer at the time of their initial interview, but OPCS decided that they should be given a second chance to opt out by procedures, noted below, that would preserve their anonymity (section 2.2.2.3).

2.2.2.1 Home sight tests

The home sight tests used by OPCS adopted a similar procedure to those used by Cullinan (1977). Distance visual acuity was measured using a standard Snellen card (scaled down for use at 10 feet). For near vision the test type used was the standard 'N' form approved by the Faculty of Ophthalmologists. In each case the card was placed or held 'in such a position that it gets the maximum amount of illumination' (see also section 21.2.1).

2.2.2.2 The RNIB sub-sample boundaries

Only a minority of those reporting difficulties in vision in the OPCS survey are at the low acuity levels that are the concern of RNIB. At a meeting of the advisory group it was decided that the sample selected for RNIB would have a cut-off point at no better than 6/24 for distance vision and N.14 for near vision (the latter being the criterion for membership of RNIB's Talking Book Service).

2.2.2.3 Sub-sampling procedure

The transfer sheets supplied by OPCS contained 2,359 records of individuals, identifiable only by serial number, who reported difficulties with vision. Analysis by RNIB revealed 1,248 respondents who met the residual vision criterion outlined above. These were stratified by residual vision level. We selected all those reporting that they were registered and all the unregistered at the lower residual vision levels but only half those aged 60 or over at higher levels (6/36 Snellen or better).

The serial numbers of these respondents were then given to OPCS. In August 1986 OPCS wrote to these respondents on RNIB's behalf, asking if they were prepared to be re-interviewed. Only a handful refused. The remaining 524 names constituted the sampling frame for wave 1. (The response rate for this first wave fieldwork was 65%, yielding a total of 338 interviews.)

2.2.3 The second wave (top-up) sample

2.2.3.1 The further OPCS segment

The initial intention had been to achieve a target sample of 400 interviews, half aged under 60 and half 60 or over. However, even in the OPCS master sample there were only 160 people aged under 60 within the defined residual vision cut-off points, and after wave 1 fieldwork we were 90 people short in this age group. We therefore decided to 'top up' the sample with a further wave of fieldwork, and at the same time the opportunity was taken to extend the target sample to 600. There were still 67 individuals at registrable residual vision levels available in the OPCS sample, and these were selected for the second wave sampling frame. The remainder of the second wave sampling frame was taken from registers of blind and partially sighted people maintained by local authorities (LAs). This LA sample was mainly drawn with the aim of increasing the number of under-60s registered blind people available for analysis, though there was also some topping up of older registered blind people (see table in section 21.5).

2.2.3.2 The local authority component

A number of local authorities were approached, and these wrote to people registered as blind or partially sighted in their area. A total of 312 blind or partially sighted people agreed to be interviewed, from nine local authority areas – Berkshire, Dudley, Durham, Hampshire, Leeds, Nottingham, Oxford, Northumberland and Waltham Forest. The selection was not totally random, in that all the authorities were 'known' to RNIB, but they did represent a broad cross-section both geographically and in the level of service they were known (from other information) to provide. Although the LA sample cannot be portrayed as a probability sample covering Great Britain of those on the registers, the achieved sample can be re-weighted to obtain a correctly balanced sample by age groups (section 2.4.1). Together with the 'top-up' sample of 67 from the OPCS (all unregistered), the LA sample comprised the sampling frame for the second fieldwork stage. (For further details of the target sample and the response rates see section 21.5.)

2.3 Fieldwork

2.3.1 Timing

The key stages of the fieldwork were as follows:

26 September 1986	first pilot
28 October 1986	second pilot
late November/December 1986	main fieldwork (wave 1)
March/April 1987	main fieldwork (wave 2)

2.3.2 Piloting of the standardised schedule

Following construction of the questionnaire, a standardised schedule was drawn up for the pilot exercise. This, along with the main fieldwork, was carried out under contract by the British Market Research Bureau (BMRB).

Mainly because of the breadth of information to be collected, a two-stage pilot exercise took place. Eight interviews with severely visually impaired volunteers were conducted during each pilot. Care was taken to mix geographical locations and the age and residual vision levels of the interviewees. The small size of the pilot sample enabled each interview to be followed with a degree of attention that more than compensated for the small number. Very experienced BMRB interviewers, mainly fieldwork supervisors, were used and in every case a BMRB executive, or one of the RNIB Survey Directors (AMK) or the Assistant Survey Director (EW), was present. In addition, these BMRB/RNIB pilot interviews were supplemented by two further interviews conducted independently of BMRB by Sally Edge.

A period of about four weeks was allowed between the first and second pilots, and also between the second pilot and the start of the main field-work. This enabled the experiences gained from the pilot interviewing to be reviewed, and comments from RNIB senior staff who had been sent a copy of the pilot questionnaire to be incorporated. Many questions left open at the pilot stage, for the respondent to answer in their own terms, were closed in the final questionnaire. That is, either coding frames for the interviewer to check or pre-set alternatives for the respondent to choose were incorporated in the final schedule on the basis of replies obtained during the pilot.

Perhaps the most serious problem to arise from the pilot interviewing was the length of the questionnaire. During the first pilot, the interviews lasted more than two hours, which was found to be too taxing for both respondent and interviewer. After each pilot the two RNIB Survey Directors (IB and AMK) and the Assistant Director (EW) considered with BMRB executives the unavoidable deletions and other questionnaire changes. Interview times were eventually trimmed to 95 – 100 minutes for the main fieldwork stages.

2.3.3   Main fieldwork

All BMRB interviewers on the main fieldwork attended a half-day briefing session, chaired by a BMRB executive. The briefings covered: background to the survey, terminology, interviewing style, contacting procedure and a series of dummy interviews to familiarise interviewers with the questionnaire.

Interviewing on the first stage of fieldwork began in late November 1986, and was completed shortly before Christmas. In total, 338 interviews were carried out. The second stage of fieldwork was carried out in March and April 1987, when a further 257 interviews were conducted, giving a total of 595 interviews. Interviews took place in respondents' homes.

Interviewers were instructed to make at least four attempts to contact respondents. Appointments were made by telephone where possible; otherwise interviewers called on respondents personally to make appointments. The overall response rate was 66%. The outcome of all contacts was recorded, and is detailed in section 21.5.

2.3.4   Checking

In total, 52 respondents were re-contacted (either by post or telephone) to check the accuracy of the information collected.

2.4   Analysis

2.4.1   Weighting

Although resources eventually permitted interviews with 595 visually impaired people, it was particularly important that the final sample should contain sufficient numbers of respondents aged under 60 for detailed analysis. A randomly chosen 600, for example, would only have given some 10% in this age group, since most visually impaired people are elderly. The younger age group was therefore deliberately over-represented in selecting the interview sample. To restore the true proportions for tabulation purposes, the numbers of people in each age category have been multiplied by an appropriate weighting factor. More people were available at higher residual vision levels than we needed, so these too were under-sampled and the weights adjusted to restore their true proportions. The weights were finally adjusted by grossing up from the balanced sample numbers to make possible the projection from the sample to population numbers. (See section 21.3 for more detail.)

Table 2.1 illustrates some main effects of weighting. It shows the percentages and actual numbers for the three age groups in the RNIB interviewed sample (A columns), and the corresponding population proportions and projected population numbers resulting from weighting (B columns).

Table 2.1 Comparison of the age distribution in the unweighted (A) and weighted (B) RNIB sample

	(A) Age distribution of respondents in the RNIB survey (unweighted figures)		(B) Population projections from the RNIB survey (weighted figures)	
Age group	%	number	%	number
16 – 59	50	(299)	10	77K
60 – 74	21	(124)	24	180K
75 +	29	(172)	66	500K
Total interviewed	100	(595)		
Weighted population base (K = '000s)			100	757K

2.4.2 Demarcations

2.4.2.1 Actual and reported registration

The actual registration status is known for the LA sub-sample. At a number of points in the analysis, the OPCS respondents who reported that they were registered blind or partially sighted, and those who reported that they were unregistered, have been classified as if they were reporting their position correctly. The available evidence suggests that errors in classification of registration status through mistaken self-reports are likely to be small in frequency and significance (section 21.9).

2.4.2.2 Upper limit for registrable partially sighted

We call those sight testing at Snellen >6/24 but unable to read N.12 on the reading test 'N12s' for short. In the OPCS sample there were 167 N12s (see also section 21.2.1). We made a small investment in this group, drawing selectively and achieving 37 among our 595 sample. This is just enough to examine their characteristics further. We then had to decide on the treatment of the N12s with respect to their registrability classification.

Although technically these people fall outside statutory registration limits (in so far as these are determined by Snellen test results), analyses of the original data tape from the OPCS survey showed that some 17% of those reporting that they were registered partially sighted were in fact N12s (Table 21.1 and section 21.2.1). We therefore decided that some N12s should be included in our population projections of the registrable but that we would estimate their numbers conservatively. We assumed that 'at the very least' some 5% of the non-registered partially sighted would be N12s if these people had had the same opportunity/willingness to become registered as those who do. The N12s in our sample were weighted accordingly to increase the projected population numbers for the partially sighted by 5%.

2.4.2.3 The dividing line between registrable blind (B) and registrable partially sighted (PS)

The abbreviations B and PS are used in the tables in this report to stand for the registrable blind and the registrable partially sighted. This is the main division by residual vision levels used in the tabulations. The B category combines those actually registered blind and those who are non-registered but whose residual vision is at the statutory levels that render them eligible for registration as blind. The PS category similarly combines the registered and non-registered partially sighted.

For analysis purposes we have to draw a sharp line between the blind and the partially sighted, even though in reality the boundary between them is blurred. This section describes the cutting-points used, and how they were determined.

Figure 2.1 Reported registration status by Snellen categories

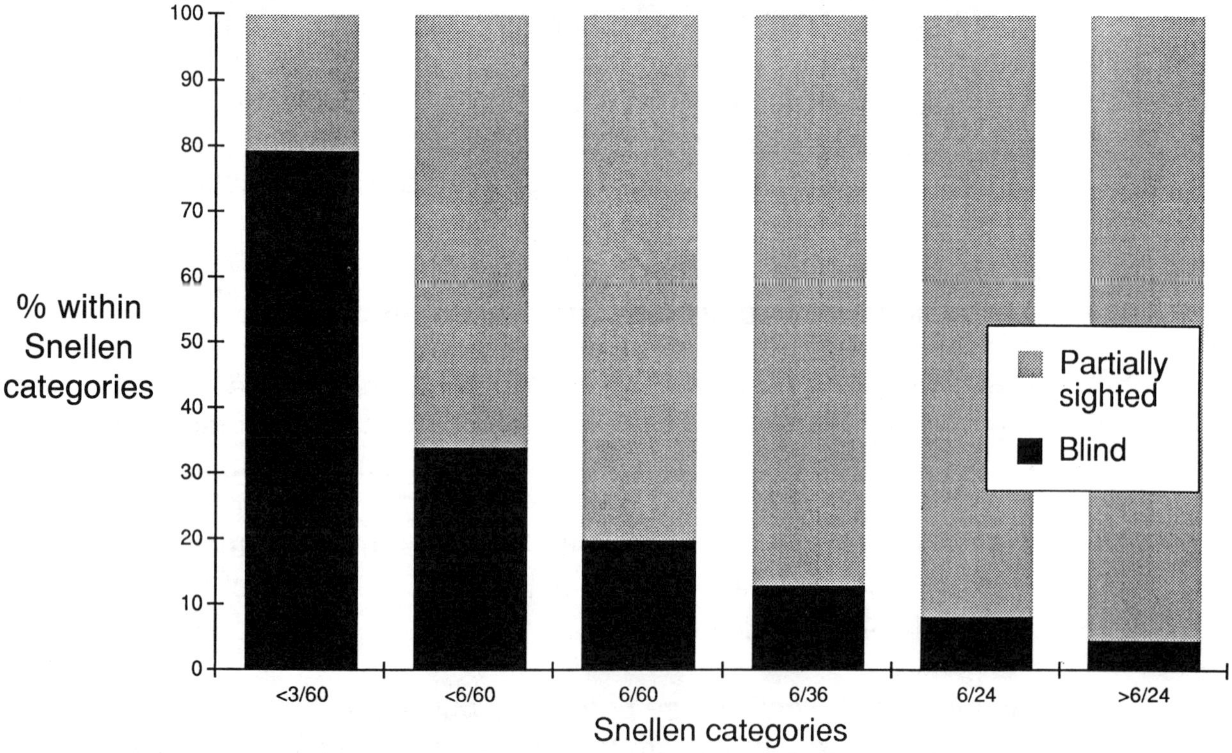

Source: OPCS master sample (section 2.2.2)

The general character of the B-PS distinction can be illustrated by the relation between registration and Snellen values. Figure 2.1 charts this relationship for the data from OPCS.

Two main points emerge from Figure 2.1. First, as we would expect, the Snellen category <3/60 is the one in which the blind predominate. Second, the blind are by no means confined to this level. They are present, albeit in diminishing proportions, at successive Snellen levels. The same holds in reverse for the partially sighted.

While more can be said about the particular set of data in Figure 2.1 (section 21.1), it serves to exemplify the fact that no single criterion other than the actual fact of registration exactly separates the blind and the partially sighted. On any other external criterion we will be dealing with two overlapping distributions. We can expect any body of data relating Snellen levels to registration status to show the same basic pattern – namely, a preponderance of blind at <3/60 with some overlap into adjacent Snellen categories.

The reason for this result is that a person with visual acuity of <3/60 is usually regarded as registrably blind. In addition, under the 1948 National Assistance Act a person is defined as registrably blind if he or she is 'so blind as to be unable to perform any work for which eyesight is essential'. Thus, over and above visual acuity, the statutory definition of blindness entails considerations of visual field along with vague, less measurable functional criteria.

In the light of the above, we made the following decisions on the criteria for separating the blind from the partially sighted for analysis purposes.

> 1   For the LA segment of the sample we used their factual registration status (209 respondents).
>
> 2   For the OPCS sample we used their reported registration status where this was available. The consideration here was that the good approximation (section 2.4.2.1) of reported with factual registration status would render the former a better criterion than any choice of Snellen cut-off values (148 respondents).
>
> 3   For the OPCS segment who reported that they were unregistered we classified those (63 respondents) with Snellen values worse than 6/60 as blind. (For further discussion, see section 21.1.)

The results (including the decisions noted at section 2.4.2.2) in terms of our tabulation is shown in Table 2.2.

Table 2.2 Classification of the registrable blind (B) and the registrable partially sighted (PS) by registration status

	Sample numbers unweighted figures		
	B	PS	Total
Registered	197	155	352
Non-registered	70	173	243
Total	267	328	595

2.4.3 The choice of classificatory variables

2.4.3.1 Strategy for an initial sift of the data

Based on a questionnaire containing more than 4,000 items of information, the survey can be considered as a rich mine of potential information. Only a limited amount can be extracted and sifted in this first report. The main strategy adopted for this initial data sift is the choice of a standard classificatory variable based on age and residual vision, against which items in each need area can be broken in one computer run, and the selection for comment of breakdowns that prove diagnostic. The shape of findings in one need area can then be related to other need areas.

2.4.3.2 Breakdowns by blind-partially sighted within three age groups

Age and residual vision were used as stratification variables at the sample design stage with a view to maximising the numbers available for analysis within these categories. Further, we were confident that age and residual vision would prove important in policy and practical considerations. The 'standard head' used for analyses within three age groups and two residual vision categories contains the data shown in Table 2.3.

Table 2.3 Blind and partially sighted respondents in age groups and the corresponding population projections

	Age								Total
	16 – 59		60 – 74		75 +		All ages		
	B	PS	B	PS	B	PS	B	PS	
Unweighted	137	162	55	69	75	97	267	328	595
Weighted (K)	30	47	65	115	205	295	300	457	757

The unweighted data are the numbers interviewed and the weighted data are the population projections (K = '000's). For definition of the B and PS categories see section 2.4.2.3

It is possible to make a more refined analysis by age and/or residual vision, but the basis for percentaging becomes rather thin unless we collapse categories for one or other of the variables. For example, we have the capability (see Chapter 6) to sub-divide the B category into those with and those with no light perception (NLP). But in the 60 – 74 group there are only 55 blind people altogether, and those with and without light perception are 31 and 24 respectively. The latter group is too small reliably to detect any but the most massive differences. Generally we only reported on more refined breakdowns of this type where differences were marked enough to be clearly reliable. Steep gradients between blind and partially sighted sub-groups, within the same age band, usually imply difference at lower levels of residual vision, i.e. between those with no light perception and others in the blind category.

2.4.3.3 Scope of the analysis

Visually impaired people are unique as individuals, and vary importantly in ways relevant to their needs in other dimensions besides age and residual vision level. Prime examples are: onset of visual loss; age (age at onset, duration of loss); presence or absence of other disabilities; living alone or with others; registered or non-registered. Breakdowns have been done on the standard basis for the registered/non-registered variable, and differences are noted accordingly in this report. But in order to complete within a finite timescale we have treated the other possible standard cross-breaks on an inference basis in the same way as for potential cross-breaks between need areas. In other words, we have examined the distributions on the primary variable and drawn inferences for findings on other variables without, as a rule, making the necessary cross-tabulation to check these.

2.5 Presentation of results

The percentages and other proportions in this report are based on weighted figures, unless otherwise stated. That is, they relate to the whole visually impaired population or to some defined section of it. To obtain an estimate of the corresponding population number, therefore, the percentage finding can be multiplied by the population numbers shown as the base figure in the tables.

For simplicity we refer to 'the percentage of respondents', though this should be understood as shorthand for a more accurate but ponderous expression such as 'the numbers of respondents weighted to represent population numbers and percentaged on the weighted population total'. The key point is that 'percentage of respondents' means, unless other-wise stated, our best estimate of the percentage of visually impaired people living in private households in Great Britain with the particular characteristic concerned.

Significance tests (section 21.4) should be based on the actual numbers interviewed (unweighted figures). Both weighted and unweighted base figures are shown in the major tables.

While data have been analysed in terms of the age/residual vision six-category standard head (section 2.4.3.2), not all tabulations show results in terms of these six categories. Separate columns of data are presented only where real differences can be noted and discussed. Adjacent age and/or residual vision categories have accordingly been collapsed where the initial tabulation showed no significant differences (section 21.4).

Most tables show the precise question wording that generated the data. The question number is always quoted, and the precise wording can be found in the questionnaire, a copy of which can be obtained from the RNIB Reference Library.

3 Demographic Characteristics and Registration

3.1 Size of the visually impaired population

Perhaps the most startling conclusion from this study relates to the number of visually impaired people in the population. An earlier report by Shankland Cox (1985), commissioned by RNIB, concluded from desk research that official registration figures underestimated 'true' figures by 30% in the case of blind people and by 20% for partially sighted people.

This study produces, for the first time, reliable estimates, based on fieldwork, of the number of visually impaired people in Great Britain. Official registration figures suggest (section 21.3.2) that there are 94,000 blind and 54,000 partially sighted people aged 16 or over in private households. Our results (Table 3.1) predict 300,000 blind people (319% above official registration figures) and 457,000 partially sighted people (846% above official registration figures) aged 16 or over in private households. When residential institutions are included (section 21.3.3), our estimate for the numbers of blind people aged 16 or over increases to 380,000, 319% higher than the official (1986 DHSS) figure of 119,000; for partially sighted people the increase is to 579,000, 839% higher than the official figure of 69,000.

The entries in Table 3.1 are population projections obtained by applying weighting procedures to the RNIB sample data as outlined in section 2.4.1 (and described more fully in section 21.3). The definitions of registrable, and the demarcation between blind (B) and partially sighted (PS), are discussed in section 2.4.2. (For a corresponding unweighted table, i.e. showing the distribution for the 595 interviews, see section 21.9.)

The policy implications of this discovery of a massive unrecognised visually impaired population are significant for both service planning and service delivery. Providers may argue, rightly, that services are *open* to the non-registered. However, results reported later (in Chapters 7 – 18 and, in particular, 19 and 20) show that in fact services only *reach* a small proportion of non-registered people. If services are to be delivered on the basis of equality of need, resources must be substantially increased to approximately three times the current level. These

Table 3.1 Estimates of the number of registrable visually impaired adults living in private households in Great Britain by age and registration status (thousands)

	Age			Total
	16 – 59	60 – 74	75 +	
* Registered				
Registered B	18	28	63	109
Registered PS	12	15	34	61
Total registered	30	43	97	170
** Non-registered				
Registrable B	12	37	142	191
Registrable PS	35	100	261	396
Total non-registered	47	137	403	587
Total registrable VI	77	180	500	757
(Number interviewed)	(299)	(124)	(172)	(595)

*DHSS published figures reduced by estimate of numbers in residential institutions (see section 21.3.3).
**Estimates derived from OPCS sample applying OPCS weighting procedures and results of home sight tests (section 21.3.2)

findings will also radically affect service planning. For example, specialist worker numbers tend to be judged on a ratio basis of the numbers of people registered blind or partially sighted (e.g. one worker to 250 or 400 registered) rather than the actual numbers who may be eligible for registration. The age distribution reported later in this chapter and elsewhere will also introduce new factors to be taken into account when planning services.

A more detailed analysis of registration status by age and residual vision levels is given in section 3.10.

3.2 Age distribution

Table 3.2 documents the well-known fact that, in comparison with the general population, the distribution of visually impaired people is enormously skewed towards older age groups. There are no significant differences between residual vision levels. Chapter 12 provides further data comparing the age distribution of visually impaired people with that of people with other disabilities and shows that visual impairment is more age-related than virtually any other disability.

Table 3.2 Distribution by age of visually impaired people in private households in Great Britain compared with the general population

	Visually impaired population (RNIB survey weighted data)	General population
	%	%
16 – 59	10	74
60 – 74	24	18
75 +	66	8
Total %	100	100
Base (population)	757K	42,903K
(Number interviewed)	(595)	

3.3 Sex and age

Tables 3.3.a, and 3.3.b, compare the sex distribution of the visually impaired population with that of the general population. In each age group there are more visually impaired women than men; the difference is greater than in the general population, and increases in the older age groups. Even in the 16 – 59 age group, where women make up half the general population, they number 57% among visually impaired people (the difference is 'statistically significant'). Women comprise 68% of visually impaired people in the 60 – 74 age group compared with 55% in the general population, and 75% of visually impaired people compared with 66% of the general population among those aged 75 + . Thus, among those aged 75 + , three out of four visually impaired people are women compared with two out of three in the general population. But because the visually impaired population is so massively skewed towards the very old, the disproportion of females overall resembles that in the oldest group. Thus 72% of the total visually impaired population are women compared with 52% in the population as a whole.

Table 3.3.a Distribution by sex within three age groups of visually impaired people in private households in Great Britain
Visually impaired population (RNIB survey)

	Age			Total
	16 – 59	60 – 74	75 +	
	%	%	%	%
Males	43	32	25	28
Females	57	68	75	72
Total %	100	100	100	100
Base (population)	77K	179K	501K	757K
(Number interviewed)	(299)	(124)	(172)	(595)

Table 3.3.b Distribution by sex within three age groups for the general population in private households in Great Britain
1981 Census Data

	Age			Total
	16 – 59	60 – 74	75 +	
	%	%	%	%
Males	50	45	34	48
Females	50	55	66	52
Total %	100	100	100	100
Base (population)	3,184K	7,797K	3,259K	42,903K

3.4   Marital status

Table 3.4 shows that even in the 16 – 59 age group fewer visually impaired people are married, 56% compared with 74% in the general population. The discrepancy widens in the 60 + age group; only 33% of visually impaired people compared with 59% of the general population are married.

Table 3.4   Marital status of visually impaired people compared with the general population (GRQ2)

	Visually impaired population (RNIB survey)		General population (GHS 1985)	
	Age		Age	
	16 – 59	60 +	16 – 59	60 +
	%	%	%	%
Single	26	10	18	8
Married	56	33	74	59
Widowed	9	55	2	30
Divorced	9	2	6	3
Total %	100	100	100	100
Base (population)	77K	680K		
(Number interviewed)	(299)	(296)	13202	5222

In line with what we know of the age skew of the visually impaired population, widowhood now becomes the main explanatory factor. Some 55% of visually impaired people aged 60 + are widowed compared with only 30% of the general population. (GHS data are for 1985, their Table 3.3; a breakdown for over 60s is not given.)

Further breakdown by age of the data shows that 61% of visually impaired people aged 75 or more are widowed (about 300,000 people). This compares with a figure of about 57% for widows in the general population in this age group (Hunt, 1978). Our figures include both sexes, but, as section 3.2 shows, three out of four visually impaired people in the 75 + age group are women.

Service planning and delivery need to take particular account of the fact that well over half of visually impaired people over 60 years are widowed and therefore lack the support and companionship they previously enjoyed.

3.5 Single person households

Equally, if not more, important than marital status for their informal support network is whether or not visually impaired people live on their own. A remarkable number, 45% or about 346,000, live on their own. Table 3.5 shows that the percentage increases incrementally with age, from 19% for the under 60s to 44% of those aged 60 – 74. Among those aged 75 and over, who carry the double burden of extreme old age and reduced vision (and in many cases of other handicaps as well – see Chapter 12), 50% (about 250,000) live on their own. However, as discussed further in section 4.1, the ability of many of these elderly visually impaired people to cope may be aided by their continuing to live in accommodation with which they have long been familiar.

Table 3.5 Visually impaired people living alone in Great Britain (GRQ3, GRQ4)

	Age			Total
	16 – 59	60 – 74	75 +	
	%	%	%	%
Years lived alone				
5 years or less	5	16	8	9
6 – 15	8	14	17	15
16 or more	6	14	25	21
Reason lives alone:				
Widowed	2	31	42	35
Other	17	13	8	10
Total living alone	19	44	50	45
Total living with others	81	56	50	55
Total %	100	100	100	100
Base (population)	77K	180K	500K	757K
(Number interviewed)	(299)	(124)	(172)	(595)

Comparative data suggest that more visually impaired people live on their own than others in similar age groups. Why this is so is not clear. Hunt's (1978) survey suggested that 25% of the general population aged 65 – 74, and 38% of those aged 75 or over, were living in one person households, compared with the 44 and 50 per cent respectively our survey finds for the same age groups.

We noted in section 3.4 that just over half visually impaired people aged 60 or over report that they are widowed. This is the primary reason people in this age group give for living alone. A comparison of Tables 3.4 and 3.5 suggests that the 17% of the 16 – 59 age group who live alone do so primarily because they have never married, and only secondarily because they are widowed, separated or divorced.

About a third of the 60 – 74 age group and half the 75 + age group who live alone say that they have done so for 16 years or more.

We found little relationship between living alone and the level of residual vision. This serves to emphasise the point that blindness is not in itself any reason to prevent a blind person of any age living alone. Far more important are other factors such as mobility (Chapter 13), the level of contact with the welfare services and the strength of the individual's social support network (Chapters 16 and 19), the age of onset of the visual handicap (Chapter 5), and the presence of other disabilities (Chapter 12).

3.6 Employment status

Table 3.6 provides a crude measure of the employment status of those people in the sample aged *under 60*. Twenty-one per cent of blind people and 29% of partially sighted people are in full- or part-time work. (About 2% of those aged 60 – 74 said that they were working full-time, but no part-time workers were found in this group; 1% of the 75 + group said that they were working part-time.) Perhaps most surprising is the similarity of the status of the blind and partially sighted respondents (the differences do not reach 'statistical significance' with these sample sizes – see section 21.4). The most significant conclusion to be drawn from Table 3.6 is that about 75% of those under 60 are not working.

Table 3.6 Employment status of visually impaired people aged under 60 (GRQ1)

	Age and residual vision	
	16 – 59	
	B	PS
	%	%
Full-time work	16	22
Part-time work	5	7
Not working	79	69
Studying	1	2
Total %	100	100
Base (population)	30K	47K
(Number interviewed)	(137)	(162)

(299 respondents: 296 aged 60 + were excluded)

This is a crude statistic because the category 'not working' includes many people who may not be available for work or who are unable to work. Chapter 17 shows that a large proportion of those 'not working' do in fact wish to work.

Nevertheless, the proportion of visually impaired people not working (approximately 75%) compares very unfavourably with the proportion of people not working in the general population of 31% (CSO, Annual Abstract of Statistics, 1990). The fact that about one quarter of visually impaired people aged under 60 are in work shows clearly that barriers to employment can be overcome. The service-planning and delivery implications in these figures are that more attention needs to be paid to enabling visually impaired people to take up paid employment.

3.7 Income and savings

Table 3.7 shows that nearly three-quarters (72%) of those aged 16 – 59 lived in households whose net weekly income was less than £139. The average weekly working wage at the time the survey was conducted was about £200. Thus, even visually impaired people of working age live at a very low standard compared with their contemporaries.

Table 3.7 Net weekly income of visually impaired people, within three groupings, living in private households in Britain

'Can you tell me how much money you have *altogether* coming in to the house, normally, after tax each week?' (GRQ8)

	Age			Total
	16 – 59	60 – 74	75 +	
	%	%	%	%
Under £50	16	38	43	39
£50 – under £70	15	11	22	18
£70 – under £139	41	46	31	36
£139 – under £200	18	4	2	4
£200 – under £400	9	2	2	3
£400 or more	2	0	0	#
Total %	100	100	100	100
Base (population)	51K	160K	330K	540K
(Number interviewed)	(214)	(99)	(120)	(433)

(433 respondents: 46 refused, 102 didn't know, 14 no information)

We should also remember that these are household incomes; we noted (section 3.4) that 81% of younger visually impaired people live with others. Some 29% of the 16 – 59 age group do have incomes above £139 (mostly between £139 and £200) compared with about 5% of those in older groups. The higher household income may be where younger visually impaired people are working or, in a large number of cases, where they are living with others. The numbers living at the extreme poverty level of under £70 per week increase from 31% in the age group 16 – 59 to 49 and 65 per cent in the 60 – 74 and 75 + groups respectively. The increment is 'statistically significant' (section 21.4) for each age step.

Breakdowns by residual vision are reported only where statistically significant differences are encountered (following the procedure in section 2.5). Table 3.8 shows that marginally more partially sighted people than blind people have incomes below £70 per week in both the 16 – 59 (36 and 22 per cent) and 60 + (67 and 49 per cent) age groups; the difference reaches 'statistical significance' (21.4) only in the latter age group.

Table 3.8 Net weekly income of visually impaired people living in private households in Britain, by two age groups and residual vision

	Age and residual vision				Total
	16 – 59		60 +		
	B	PS	B	PS	
	%	%	%	%	%
Under £50	14	17	36	45	39
£50-under £70	8	19	13	22	18
£70-under £139	46	39	45	30	36
£139-under £200	16	19	3	2	4
£200-under £400	16	4	4	1	2
£400 or more	2	2	0	0	0
Total %	100	100	100	100	100
Base (population)	19K	32K	186K	327K	565K
(Number interviewed)	(98)	(119)	(90)	(136)	(443)

(443 respondents: 46 refused to answer, 102 didn't know, 4 no information)

Table 3.9 shows that, of the visually impaired population as a whole, 53% have savings of less than £500, and a further 19% no more than £1,500. Twelve per cent have savings of more than £6,000, among whom are 16% of the 75 + group, compared with 6 – 7 per cent in the younger groups.

Thus very few visually impaired people have any substantial savings with which to cushion their meagre incomes. Since they will have to meet any extra financial costs arising out of their disability, a picture of extreme financial hardship emerges. This confirms the findings of the OPCS survey of poverty among disabled people in general, and visually impaired people in particular. However, our findings suggest greater hardship among visually impaired people than OPCS found. This gives further support to the widely held view that OPCS methodology underestimated the extent of poverty and the extra costs which disability brings. Nevertheless both surveys indicate that the vast majority of visually impaired people are poor. This is because their incomes are

Table 3.9 Savings of visually impaired people in three age groups

'And apart from this money, can I check how much money you have in savings?' (BQ9)

	Age			Total
	16 – 59	60 – 74	75 +	
	%	%	%	%
Up to £500	63	60	46	53
£501 – 1500	11	11	23	19
£1501 – 3000	13	9	10	9
£3001 – 6000	6	14	5	7
£6000 plus	7	6	16	12
Total %	100	100	100	100
Base (population)	54K	130K	343K	526K
(Number interviewed)	(221)	(88)	(117)	(426)

(426 respondents: 169 respondents did not know or refused to say)

low and in addition they have to meet extra costs resulting from their visual impairment.

3.8 Education

Table 3.10 shows the effect of raising the school-leaving age to 15 in 1947 and to 16 in 1972. The majority of the 16 – 59 age group left school at ages 14 to 16, while the majority of those in older groups finished full-time education at 14 years of age or under. As many as 27% of the 16 – 59 age group have been in full-time education beyond the statutory school leaving age. Among the older age groups there is a smaller, but still substantial, sub-group, amounting to about 12 to 21 per cent, who finished full-time education after the statutory school-leaving age.

Table 3.10 Age at which visually impaired people finished full-time education (GRQ4)

	Age			Total
	16 – 59	60 – 74	75 +	
Age finished full-time education	%	%	%	%
14 or under	33	74	74	69
15	27	5	7	10
16	13	8	5	7
17 or over	25	13	12	14
Still studying	2	0	0	#
Total %	100	100	100	100
Base (population)	77K	179K	501K	757K
(Number interviewed)	(299)	(124)	(172)	(595)

Our sample contained 138 respondents who acquired their visual impairment during or before their school years. This yields a projected figure of about 10% of the visually impaired population, that is 74,000 people (sections 5.2.2 and 5.2.3). Of this sub-group only about one-third said (at GRQ5) that they had attended a special school for the handicapped. In 60% of these cases the school was a special school for the visually handicapped.

Table 3.11 School or college examinations passed
(Comparable data for those not in full-time education aged 25 – 49 are shown for Great Britain)

'Can you tell me about any school or college examinations you have passed – have you passed...?' (GRQ6)

	Age				GB age**
	16 – 59	60 – 74	75 +	All VI	25 – 49
	%	%	%	%	%
CSE	7	–	–	1	12
O level	26	18	10	13	19
A level	10	2	3	4	9
Teaching Diploma	4	–	2	2	na
Higher education					
below degree	na	na	na	na	12
Degree	7	1	2	2	10
Foreign or other	na	na	na	na	3
Some exam passed	30	19	10	14	65
No exam passed	70	81	90	86	35
Total %	100	100	100	100	100
Base (population)	77K	179K	501K	757K	
(Number interviewed)	(299)	(124)	(172)	(595)	15,292

**Highest qualification level of those not in full-time education aged 25 – 49 in Great Britain (OPCS 1986)
'na' category for comparison not available in both surveys

For the question in Table 3.11, respondents were prompted from a list of 10 types of examination (See GRQ6). In the table, CSE grades 1 and 2 have been combined, and Scottish Low Grade and High Grade certificates have been combined with O and A levels respectively.

Levels of residual vision (B and PS) have been combined, following our routine procedure (see section 2.5), in the above tables because no systematic differences were detectable in the data.

3.9 Social status

Because a mixture of income, occupation and education and family background are involved, social grade, status or class have proved a difficult concept for social researchers to define exactly. After much consideration, BMRB decided (for routine fieldwork practice) to define the family unit's social status by the occupation of the head of the household (that is, the head of the family unit or the senior bread-winner). The social class gradings in Table 3.12 were made by the interviewer on the basis of information collected (at GRQ7) on the occupational details of the head of the household. (The BMRB handbook issued to each interviewer contained detailed instructions for coding the social grade from this information.)

On the BMRB scheme, a household is defined as a group of people who live in the same dwelling and who are catered for by the same person. Every household has a head who must be a member of the household. The head is defined as the member who owns or is responsible for the accommodation occupied by the household. It should be noted that a household does not necessarily consist only of people related by blood or by marriage, and that it can consist of only one person.

Using this classification scheme, BMRB finds that the general population falls into their grades as follows: A (upper middle) 3%, B (middle) 14%, C1 (lower middle) 23%, C2 (skilled working) 26%, D (semi-skilled and unskilled) 16%, and E (pensioners etc) 18%.

Table 3.12 Social class grouping of visually impaired people – using BMRB class gradings

| | Age | | | | GB* |
| | 16 – 59 | 60 – 74 | 75 + | All ages | House- holds |
	%	%	%	%	%
A Upper middle	1	1	2	1	3
B Middle	4	2	8	6	14
C1 Lower middle	16	22	18	19	23
C2 Skilled working	21	15	14	15	26
D Semi and unskilled	20	15	7	10	16
E Pensioners, all not working	38	45	51	49	18
Total %	100	100	100	100	100
Base (population)	77K	179K	501K	757K	22,600K
(Number interviewed)	(299)	(124)	(172)	(595)	

*Source: BMRB Target group household survey; household social grading

Of primary interest to the present study are the numbers of visually impaired people who fall into grade E. On the BMRB scheme this grade consists of old age pensioners, widows and their families, and those who, because of sickness or unemployment, depend on social security schemes. There are far more visually impaired people in this grade than in the general population at all ages. The extent of representation is quite startling taking account of the age skew, and is because of the large numbers of visually impaired people receiving social security benefits. However, if the current income and occupation of visually impaired people themselves were the only factor, we know from sections 3.5 and 3.6 that the great majority would be in grade E. Yet more than a half fall into a higher social grade. They do so because of two factors on the BMRB definitional scheme: first, respondents take the social grade of the head of the household, and, second, what counts here for the retired is their previous occupational status. For these two reasons, therefore, the social status of many visually impaired people is at a higher level than would be apparent from their low incomes.

Visually impaired people are not vastly under-represented in the A, B, C1 categories compared with the general population (26% compared with 40%). However, there is a notable under-representation among the C2, D and E categories (25% compared with 55%). This suggests that efforts made to increase the representation of visually impaired people in manual trades over the last five decades, while partially successful, have not succeeded in comparison with work placements requiring more cerebral skills.

3.10   Registration status

3.10.1   Proportion of visually impaired people registered

Table 3.13 shows that, out of the estimated visually impaired population of 757,000 living in private households, only 23% are registered as either blind or partially sighted, and 77% are unregistered. The percentage registered also declines with increasing age: from 37% of those aged 16 – 59 to 24 and 19 per cent of those aged 60 – 74 and 75 + respectively.

An important finding of this survey is the role of registration as a catalyst or trigger in the awareness and receipt of services to visually impaired people. While registration itself conveys few benefits, our survey constantly shows that it is registered blind or partially sighted people who are more likely to be aware of or in receipt of these services than the non-registered. Registration brings blind and partially sighted people into the realm of service provision for visually impaired people. Their non-registered, though registrable, counterparts are excluded from, or not made aware of, these services.

Table 3.13 Registered and non-registered (but registrable) visually impaired people in three age groups

	Age			Total
	16 – 59	60 – 74	75 +	
	%	%	%	%
Registered (B or PS)	37	24	19	23
Non-registered (B or PS)	63	76	81	77
Total %	100	100	100	100
Base (population)	77K	180K	500K	757K
(Number interviewed)	(299)	(124)	(172)	(595)

Data include all visually impaired people at registrable blind or partially sighted levels (section 2.4.2)

3.10.2 Registration status and residual vision

The last two columns of Table 3.14 show that the percentage of partially sighted people registered is lower than that of blind people: 36% of those eligible at blind (B) registrable levels are registered, compared with 13% of those at partially sighted (PS) levels. (B and PS levels are as defined in section 2.4.2.)

Table 3.14 Registered and non-registered (but registrable) visually impaired people by residual vision levels in three age groups

	Age and residual vision							
	16 – 59		60 – 74		75 +		All ages	
	B	PS	B	PS	B	PS	B	PS
	%	%	%	%	%	%	%	%
Registered	60	25	43	13	30	13	36	13
Non-registered	40	75	57	87	70	87	64	77
Total %	100	100	100	100	100	100	100	100
Base (population)	30K	47K	65K	115K	205K	295K	300K	457K
(Number interviewed)	(137)	(162)	(55)	(69)	(75)	(97)	(267)	(328)

3.10.3 Registration status, age and residual vision

Table 3.14 shows that in the three age bands (16 – 59, 60 – 74 and 75 +) 60, 43, and 30 per cent respectively of those eligible to be registered as blind are actually registered. The corresponding totals for partially sighted people are 25, 13 and 13 per cent respectively.

Thus the chances of being registered vary with both age and residual vision level. Only among registrable blind people aged 16 – 59 is a majority (60%) actually registered. At the other extreme, of those eligible for registration as partially sighted only 13% of those aged 60 or over actually are registered.

The relationship between age, residual vision level and registration status is discussed further in note 1. It may be noted, however, that there is no correlation between age and residual vision level. Young visually impaired people are no more likely to be at low levels of residual vision than the elderly. The concentration of registration among blind people aged under 60 is the result of two independent tendencies: higher registration among the young and higher registration among people with low residual vision. The coefficients of association fit a causal model in which age and residual vision have independent effects on registration. However, there is no joint effect due to any correlation between age and residual vision; by statistically testing we found that age and residual vision acted separately on the likelihood of being registered rather than together.

Concentration of registration among young people is relative. A young blind person is far more likely to be registered than an old blind person. But, in absolute terms, there are far greater numbers of elderly blind registered people. Because of the skewed nature of the age distribution of visually impaired people (section 3.2) a much smaller percentage registration generates far greater actual numbers of people aged over 60 who are registered. Table 3.1 shows that of the estimated 109,000 registered blind people living in private households, only 18,000 are aged under 60.

3.10.4   Snellen values and registration status

Although the data in Table 3.15 have been assembled from several sources, the estimates it contains can be regarded as approximately correct (see note 2). It is important to distinguish those parts of the B/PS distributions which are merely a consequence of the decisions on cutting-points adopted, as described in section 2.4.2. To recapitulate, the non-registered in our sample with Snellen values worse than 6/60 were classified as registrable blind (as discussed in section 2.4.2.3 and more fully in section 21.1). This was done because analysis showed that a lower cutting-point would have excluded many of the registered blind, and we wished to treat the non-registered on the same basis. (For example 27% of registered blind people have a Snellen acuity of better than 3/60.) The dotted line that marks this cutting-point in Table 3.15 shows that it correctly classifies all but 10% of the registered blind. By the same definition we have done the best job possible of correctly clas-sifying our unregistered but registrable blind by their Snellen values. (As noted in section 21.1, the gains here are at the necessary cost of putting some people into the registrable blind category who would have been classified registrable partially sighted with a lower cutting-point.)

Table 3.15 Snellen values, by residual vision and registration status

	Registration status and residual vision			
	R		NR	
	B	PS	B	PS
	%	%	%	%
NLP[†]	25	–	–	–
<3/60	48	17	30	–
<6/60	17	23	70	–
6/60	5	17	–	10
6/36	3	17	–	40
6/24	1	9	–	40
>6/24 <N12	1	17	–	5
Total %	100	100	100	100
Base (population)	109K	61K	192K	395K
(Number interviewed)[††]	(102)	(120)	(70)	(173)

[†]NLP. No light perception (can't see windows)
[††]Table constructed partly from original OPCS master sample.
See note 2

The difference, 17% of registered and 5% of non-registered (but registrable) partially sighted people respectively falling into the category >6/24 Snellen but less than N12 reading ability (the N12s for short), is a concomitant of our design decisions. Seventeen per cent of registered partially sighted people fall into this category even though it is beyond the statutory limit. As discussed in section 2.4.2.2, given the already very large number of the non-registered partially sighted being estimated, we deliberately aimed at a conservative assessment of the number who might fall into this category outside the statutorily defined limit.

The remaining characteristics of the distributions over Snellen levels in Table 3.15 are independent of our imposed definitions. The zero point in the questionnaire scale, marking out those with no light perception (see section 6.1.1.), can be combined with available Snellen measures to separate levels of residual vision below the <6/60 cut-off point. When this is done, as in Table 3.15, the fact emerges that, while 25% of people registered blind are without light perception, none of the non-registered falling within this boundary for blind registration have sight loss as extreme as this. In other words, those whose sight loss does place them inside the range eligible for blind registration are more likely to be registered if they are at the lower extremes of this range.

Within the partially sighted group, the same relation between registration and residual vision level can be noted. That 40% of registered partially sighted people do fall below 6/60 Snellen (i.e. lie above the dotted line) is, as just noted, a concomitant of our choice of a high inclusive cutting-point to cover most registered blind people. But even above this level, the distribution of the partially sighted tends to be skewed towards the higher Snellen values. (The exception – those >6/24 Snellen but with a reading ability of less than N12 – is another result of our design decisions as discussed above. If anything, therefore, we underestimate the extent to which non-registered partially sighted people are skewed towards higher residual vision levels.)

It is no doubt in the nature of the registration process that the more seriously visually impaired among those eligible will stand the greater chance of registration. To an extent the same process could be at work in producing a greater proportion of registered among eligible blind people compared with the eligible partially sighted people (see Tables 3.14 and 3.15).

Notes to Chapter 3

Note 1 (section 3.10.3)

Relationships between age, residual vision and registration
Dichotomising the three variables as follows:
  Age : Y = <60; O = 60+
  Residual vision : blind and partially sighted
  Registration : registered and non-registered
we have (from the data in Table 3.1) the following three 2x2 tables:

	(a) Registration within the two age groups			(b) Residual vision within age			(c) Residual vision within registration status	
	Y	O		Y	O		R	NR
R	39	20	B	39	39	B	32	64
NR	61	80	PS	61	61	PS	68	36
Total %	100	100		100	100		100	100
Base	77K	680K		77K	680K		587K	170K

Data from Table 3.1. See also section 21.10 for numbers interviewed

There is no association between age and residual vision (Table b). The relationships between registration and age (Table a) and registration and residual vision (Table c) are statistically significant (Chi Square 12.37, and 53, respectively with 1df. Approximate point correlations would be 0.15 and 0.3 taken on an N of 595).

The coefficients of association fit a causal model in which age and residual vision have independent effects on registration, but there is no effect because of any correlation between age and residual vision.

Note 2 (section 3.10.4)

Production of Table 3.15 'Snellen values and registration status' in the report

This table was constructed as follows. For registered blind and partially sighted people the distributions in Table 21.1 'Snellen categories by reported registration status' in the report were used. Partition of the <6/60 into NLP, <3/60 and 3/60 (ie <6/60) was carried out in terms of a tabulation made at an early stage in the analysis of the OPCS master sample. The tabulation showed a breakdown by Snellen level and registration status for 1,646 (older) OPCS respondents. The ratio of those at <6/60 (can't read chart) to those at <3/60 (LP but can't see chart) was used as a basis for partitioning the <6/60 in Table 21.6.a. For example there are, among the registered blind, 11 at <6/60 (strictly 3/60) compared with 32 at <3/60. The 65% registered blind respondents split in the same proportions, giving the result 17 to 48 <6/60 to <3/60, respectively. While this should ideally be done on weighted data we know that weighting these Snellen distribution data makes little difference to the distributions (working paper dated March 17, see note to Chapter 21). The distributions for the non-registered were otherwise obtained from a straightforward breakdown by Snellen values. The numbers of respondents entering into the computations in any column are shown for reference value and the purpose of testing significance; the known population totals are shown for purposes of population projection.

4 Accommodation

4.1 Length of residence

As might be expected, older visually impaired people have lived longer in their present dwelling than younger ones. However, as Table 4.1 shows, the difference is solely between people aged under 60 and 60 +. Twenty-five per cent of the former have lived at their present address for 21 years or more, compared with 40% of the latter.

Table 4.1 Years lived at present address within three age groups

'How long have you lived at this address?' (YQ1)

	Age			Total
	16 – 59	60 – 74	75 +	
	%	%	%	%
5 years and under	27	23	20	22
6 – 20 years	48	37	39	39
21 or more years	25	40	41	39
Total %	100	100	100	100
Base (population)	77K	180K	500K	757K
(Number interviewed)	(299)	(124)	(172)	(595)

The absence of differences between the two older groups, ages 60 – 74 and 75 +, shows that length of residence does not continue to increase with age. Some people in the older age groups will have moved to residential institutions whose residents are not covered in this survey, others into sheltered accommodation or to live with relatives. Two, 18 and 12 per cent respectively of those aged under 60, 60 – 74 and 75 + (data from YQ3), were living in sheltered accommodation; 6, 4 and 8 per cent respectively of the three age groups were living with friends or relatives (Table 4.2).

For those who do remain in their own home, we can anticipate that familiarity with their home environment and immediate locality, as well as neighbourhood support, will be factors in their adjustment. It was noted in section 3.5 that many elderly visually impaired people live on their own. The data in Table 4.1 suggest that most of them have lived in the same accommodation for a large part of their lives – something that they greatly value. When we asked our sample (at YQ11) if they would like to move if they could, the proportion saying 'yes' fell sharply with increasing age from 33% of the under-60s, through 23% of the 60 – 74s to 15% of those aged 75 or over. The percentage actually thinking of moving (YQ9) was about half, and again fell sharply with increasing age.

4.2 Type of tenure

Blind and partially sighted people occupied similar forms of accommodation. Age is the most significant influence on tenure, older people being more likely to occupy local authority accommodation and less likely to be owner occupiers, as shown in Table 4.2.

Table 4.2 Tenure within three age groups

'Do you own or are you renting your home?'

IF OWN 'Do you own this home outright or are you buying it with a mortgage?'

IF RENTED 'Who do you rent this house from?' (YQ2)

	Age			Total
	16 – 59	60 – 74	75 +	
	%	%	%	%
Mortgagees	25	2	2	4
Outright owners	25	30	40	36
Total owner occupiers	50	32	42	40
Local authority tenant	40	58	38	43
Private tenant	1	6	4	5
Housing Association/ charity tenant	1	0	5	4
Live with others	4	2	8	6
Other e.g. tied	4	2	3	3
Total %	100	100	100	100
Base (population)	77K	180K	497K	753K
(Number interviewed)	(299)	(124)	(171)	(594)

(594 respondents; no data from 1 respondent)

Only 4% of visually impaired people, mainly in the under 60 age group, are buying their house on a mortgage. Even in this age group, only 25% have a mortgage and another 25% are outright owners; 68% of the equivalent general population are owner occupiers. Outright ownership increases with age to 30 and 40 per cent in the 60 – 74 and 75 + age groups respectively.

A higher proportion of visually impaired people are local authority tenants than in the general population. Overall, 43% of visually impaired people are local authority tenants, although in the 60 – 74 age group the total rises to 58%. Among the under-60s, 40% of visually impaired people are local authority tenants, compared with just under a quarter of the general population (see Table 4.3). For the 60 – 74 year-olds, the figures are 58 and 37 per cent respectively, for those aged 75 +, 38 and 37 per cent.

Table 4.3. Tenure by age of household head; general population data, Great Britain 1985

	Age of household head		
	25 – 59	60 – 69	70 +
	%	%	%
Owner occupiers	68	55	48
Local authority	23	37	37
Other	9	8	15
Total %	100	100	100
Base (sample size)	5918	1677	1891

Source: GHS 1985 as quoted in Social Trends 18, page 141 (CSO, 1988)

One explanation for this pattern may be found in the generally lower income level of disabled people. While owner occupation is more common among higher income groups, disabled people in general (and visually impaired people among them) may find themselves one of the groups unable to buy their way into the private housing market.

4.3 Amenities

We asked respondents whether they had an inside toilet (YQ4), and some 5%, mainly elderly people, said that they did not. Only 2% reported that they did not have the basic amenities of a separate kitchen and bathroom (YQ5 – YQ8). This is in line with recent data for the general population (OPCS, 1985) and generally marginally better than that reported in Hunt's (1978) survey of elderly people.

5 The Onset of Visual Impairment

5.1 Reported causes of sight problem

Cullinan (1977, page 1) notes that 'To the epidemiologist falls the task of reconciling the clinician's model of disease process with the social scientist's interest in the disability it causes. The difficulty lies in getting the balance right.' He adds that 'singularly little is known of the natural history of most degenerative diseases', particularly 'in the field of failing sight'.

Precise medical description was outside the scope of our survey. We simply asked (at YQ13) 'What was the cause of your sight problem?' Medical terms were probed for and recorded when known, but were not directly mentioned by the interviewer since respondents were often vague about causes; answer categories given in Table 5.1 necessarily reflect this vagueness.

About 1 in 5 people aged 75 and over mentioned nothing more specific than 'ageing' or 'old age' or, very occasionally, 'macular degeneration'. For the most part, these respondents regarded the slow deterioration of their vision as part of the natural process of growing old. Cataracts was the specific cause mentioned most often by both those 75 and over and those aged 60 – 74.

Younger respondents mentioned a wide variety of specific eye conditions, particularly retinitis pigmentosa but also iritis, nystagmus and several other conditions, which have been grouped as 'other eye conditions' (row 5 of Table 5.1). About 1 in 5 of people under 60 fall into this composite category, which then declines sharply in the next two age groups to about 1 in 14 of the young elderly and then to a mere 1 in 50 of the very elderly. The large 'other answers' category covers replies that were too vague to be classified as a 'cause', including non-specific references to 'heredity'. (Onset at birth is examined in section 5.2.2.)

Differences in reported cause by levels of residual vision are not reported here because on the small bases available for percentaging they did not reach 'statistical significance' (section 21.4). The vagueness of the answer categories may also have been a factor.

Table 5.1 Reported cause of visual impairment, within three age groups

'What was the cause of your sight problem ?' (YQ13)

	Age			Total
	16 – 59	60 – 74	75 +	
	%	%	%	%
Cataracts	15	35	35	33
Old age	3	2	20	14
Glaucoma	3	10	11	10
General ill health	15	12	6	9
Accident	11	16	6	8
Since birth	20	8	3	6
Sudden occurrence	4	2	6	5
Diabetes	4	10	2	4
Blood vessels	3	6	1	3
Detached retina	2	3	2	2
Heart/stroke	1	4	2	2
Illness/disability	9	1	0	1
Other eye conditions	19	7	2	5
Other answers	20	21	17	19
Base (population) = 100%	76K	180K	500K	756K
(Number interviewed)	(297)	(124)	(172)	(593)

(593 respondents: no information for 2 respondents)

In so far as the categories in Table 5.1 designate disorders with a known natural history, their distribution across the age groupings reflects facts about the onset of visual impairment. We would expect to find cataracts, a disease of slow onset, most prevalent in the oldest age groups. But it is worth noting that cataracts are by no means insignificant even in the youngest age group; about 1 in 7 of those under 60 also mentioned them. The sharp decline with age in the incidence of diseases grouped under 'other eye conditions' parallels the decline with age (discussed further below) of the number of people who stated that their sight problem started at birth.

5.2 Time of onset

The length of time over which visually impaired people experience deteriorating eyesight, as well as the age at which they experience it, are both important factors in their ability to adjust and the kind of help outside agencies can provide. We distinguish sudden onset, onset at birth, and loss of sight over an extended period.

5.2.1 Sudden onset

Table 5.1 demonstrates that sudden, traumatic loss of vision (the so-called 'military model'), although featured in some literature (e.g.

Carrol, 1961), is in fact the experience of a small minority of visually impaired people. Fewer than 1 in 10 said that their condition was the result of an accident (including 'falling over'), and only 1 in 20 mentioned any other sudden occurrence ('happened suddenly/for no reason at all'). These two combined amount to 13%, but the incidence is no higher among the young than among the young elderly. The combined percentage mentions of this type of sudden onset in each of the three age groups are 15, 18 and 12 respectively.

5.2.2 Onset at birth

Much more typical of the young are people whose sight problems date from birth. They are still a minority even among the young, but they are a very substantial minority, one third. When directly questioned (at YQ14) a somewhat larger percentage (8% overall compared with the 6% unprompted mentions at YQ13) said that their eyesight problems dated from birth. The incidence was 30% among those aged under 60, and declined sharply in successive age groups, to 12% in the 60 – 74 age group and then to a diminutive 3% among the 75 and overs. The main reason for this is the massive increase in age-related visual impairment; Table 5.2 contains the results to YQ14.

Table 5.2   Reported onset of sight problem, by age

'So can I just check whether you had your eyesight problems from birth, or whether they resulted from an accident, or something else?' (YQ14)

	Age			Total
	16 – 59	60 – 74	75 +	
	%	%	%	%
From birth	30	12	3	8
Accident	8	7	3	5
Something else	60	80	91	85
Don't know	2	1	5	4
Total %	100	100	100	100
Base (population)	77K	180K	500K	757K
(Number interviewed)	(299)	(124)	(172)	(595)

Current levels of residual vision made no significant difference to the number of people (8% overall – grossing up to 60,500) mentioning impairment dating from birth (at YQ14). Of those, 73% (about 44,000) said (at YQ15) that their sight had deteriorated since birth, but once again there was no significant difference by current sight level.

5.2.3 Gradual onset

The large majority (86%) of visually impaired people do not undergo a sudden traumatic loss of vision but instead experience a progressive deterioration in their eyesight over a greater or lesser extended period.

Table 5.3 presents data relating to the duration of this period and the stage of life at which it appears.

Those whose sight had deteriorated since birth or was not the result of an accident were asked about the age at which they first realised that their vision was causing them problems in everyday life. Table 5.3 shows the variation in the pattern of onset between the three age groups.

Table 5.3 Age first noticed sight problem affecting everyday activities, by age

'How old were you when you first noticed that your sight was affecting every-day things such as reading, shopping, watching TV, or doing your job?' (YQ16)

	Age			Total
	16 – 59	60 – 74	75 +	
Age of onset	%	%	%	%
16 and under	25	16	4	8
17 – 39 years	32	13	5	9
40 – 59 years	40	40	13	22
60 – 74 years	na	28	36	30
75 +	na	na	37	26
Don't know	3	3	6	5
Total %	100	100	100	100
Base (population)	61K	162K	480K	704K
(Number interviewed)	(226)	(109)	(161)	(496)

(496 respondents; 99 respondents were not asked this question, onset from birth)

In their daily lives the majority of visually impaired people as a whole do not experience the impact of sight loss until they are at least 60; only 17% experience it before they are 40. Because of the age structure of the visually impaired population, these overall statistics chiefly reflect the onset pattern experienced by very elderly people.

Examined separately, the age groups reveal different patterns. Among visually impaired people of under normal retirement age onset is spread broadly over three periods: 25% during pre-school and school years, 32% during the first half of the working life, and 40% during the second half. Among the two older age groups, onset bunches into shorter periods. Sixty-nine per cent of the young elderly experienced serious loss of vision before they were 60, 40% between 40 and 59 years old. On the other hand, most of the 75 and over group first became aware of a disabling loss of vision after retirement; for just over a third this happened before they were 75, and the same proportion after 75.

These age patterns overshadow any effects of differences in degree of sight loss, for which the data did not throw up any significant patterns.

We also asked 'How old were you when your sight got as bad as it is now?' (YQ17). A simple breakdown by age of the answers added little to the information already obtained from the replies to YQ16. More intensive secondary analysis, comparing ages in YQ17 with ages in YQ16, may throw more light on the extent of the period over which deterioration of sight is experienced.

5.3 Medical treatment received for sight

Space did not allow an enquiry into the age at which medical treatment for sight problems was first received. However, we did ask briefly (YQ19) about treatments received; Table 5.4 contains the results.

Table 5.4 Medical treatment received for sight problems, by residual vision within three age groups

'What kind of medical treatment have you received for your eye problem?' (YQ19)

	Age and residual vision						Total
	16 – 59		60 – 74		75 +		
	B	PS	B	PS	B	PS	
	%	%	%	%	%	%	%
Seen eye specialist	87	83	99	76	78	80	81
Hospital in-patient	53	34	55	28	31	29	33
Eye operation	39	26	57	21	28	26	29
Hospital out-patient	67	63	69	69	55	52	58
Medication	57	46	66	49	51	42	49
Base = 100%	30K	47K	65K	115K	205K	295K	757K
(Number interviewed)	(137)	(162)	(55)	(69)	(75)	(97)	(595)

A large majority (81%) of visually impaired people have seen a specialist about their eye problem. A substantial but smaller majority (58%) have also attended hospital as an out-patient, 33% have attended as hospital in-patients, and 49% have received some other form of medication. (These treatment categories and proportions are not mutually exclusive.)

Although treatment varies with age differences, the variation is as great within the level of residual vision. Just over half of blind people under 75 have been hospital in-patients compared with just under a third of partially sighted people in the same age group, while 57% of blind people aged 60 – 74 have undergone an eye operation. In other age groups and among partially sighted people the figure is much lower, generally under 30%.

Our inquiry into specific forms of medical treatment for eyesight was based on evidence gained from preliminary testing of the questionnaire and was designed to cover most of the alternatives in broad terms. About 20% of younger respondents and also of blind people aged 60 – 74 stated that they had received other forms of (unspecified) medical treatment which did not appear in our check list.

Analysis by registration showed that 96% of registered people compared with 77% of non-registered (but registrable) people had seen an eye specialist. The fact that so many of the latter category had made contact with an eye specialist is important, and these data confirm anecdotal evidence that eye specialists do not always initiate the process of registration for many of their patients who are eligible, i.e. the registrable are not simply unknown to their statutory authorities. Later chapters will show the importance of registration as a trigger or catalyst for service provision, and this evidence suggests that eye specialists could do more to encourage registrable people to register.

6 Residual Vision

6.1 Distance vision

6.1.1 A questionnaire scale

The questionnaire section on residual vision contained eight carefully graded questions (YQ29 to YQ36) in which respondents were asked how much they could see in terms of everyday situations involving distance vision. After analysis of the internal consistency of the replies, six questions were selected to form a graded scale measuring seven levels of residual vision. (For more details and the distribution of interviews over the scale see section 21.8.) The six questions asked were as follows. (An abbreviation of the wording is given here; the questionnaire should be consulted for the precise wording.)

> Can you see...
>> from the light where the windows are? (YQ29)
>> the shapes of the furniture? (YQ30)
>
> Can you recognise a friend...
>> if you get close to their face? (YQ31)
>> at arms length away? (YQ32)
>> across a room? (YQ33)
>> across the road? (YQ34)

The six questions function as a scale or ladder on which respondents can be scored according to the point at which they say they can see. Table 6.1 shows the numbers who can see at each level. Those with no light perception (4% overall) receive a score of zero; the remainder (96% overall) can tell by the light where the windows are. The percentages fall as each step reaches the next level of difficulty.

The percentages in Table 6.1 should be read in the following manner. Of visually impaired people as a whole, 19, 46, 66 and 77 per cent respectively can recognise a friend across a road, across a room, at arms length and close up; 91% can see the shapes of the furniture in a room and 96% can tell from the light where the windows are, which leaves 4% with no light perception (NLP). (These figures all appear in the right hand column of the table.) Subtracting the entries from 100 gives the percentages who cannot see at each step: thus, the percentage who cannot recognise a friend across a road, across a room, at

Table 6.1 Distribution of the visually impaired population over the questionnaire scale of residual vision (QRVS7)

Scale point	Age and residual vision						Total
	16 – 59		60 +		All 16 +		
	B	PS	B	PS	B	PS	
sees:	%	%	%	%	%	%	%
0 NLP*	15	–	6	–	6	–	4
1 windows	85	100	94	100	94	100	96
2 furniture	75	100	86	95	82	94	91
Recognises friend:							
3 close up	50	94	66	85	65	87	77
4 at arms length	40	85	50	77	49	80	66
5 across room	27	59	32	57	31	58	46
6 across road	8	24	13	23	12	23	19
Base (population) = 100%	30K	47K	270K	410K	300K	457K	757K
(Number interviewed)	(137)	(162)	(130)	(166)	(267)	(328)	(595)

*NLP = no light perception (i.e. 'no' at YQ29)

arms length and close up are 81, 54, 34 and 23 respectively, while 9% cannot see the shapes of the furniture in a room.

Scores on the QRVS7 scale are strongly related to Snellen levels, though not in a one-to-one manner (section 21.8).

It is important to note the small percentage of respondents who had no light perception, 4% overall. These all fall into the blind (B) category, of whom they comprise 15% of people aged 16 – 59 and 6% of people aged 60 + . Analysis by registration (Table 3.15, section 3.10.4) shows that everyone without light perception was registered as blind. Even so, people without light perception only comprised 25% of registered blind people.

Once both lay people and professionals understand that not all registered blind people are totally blind, they ask the following question: 'How many blind people are totally blind?' This survey answers this question for the first time, but initially it is necessary to define the term 'totally blind'.

If sighted readers shut their eyes, they will, quite reasonably, think of themselves as temporarily totally blind. However, with shut eyes they can still sense 'from the light where the windows are'. Thus the definition of 'totally blind' includes people who have perception of light but nothing more. On this definition and from our data, we believe that 18% of registrably blind people are totally blind, forming 25% of the under-60s and 14% of those aged 60 and over.

While only a minority (19%) of visually impaired people (12% of blind people and 23% of the partially sighted) can recognise a friend across a road, the majority (77% – 64% of blind people, 86% of the partially sighted) can at least recognise a friend close up. However the significance of distance recognition should not be over-emphasised by sighted readers, who may not realise the extent to which visually impaired people use shape and movement for recognition purposes. In addition many blind people with some distance vision may have severe field loss.

6.1.2 Age differences

While difference in registrability levels (blind or partially sighted, see section 2.4.2) is the paramount factor in Table 6.1, consistent minor differences within age limits are also evident, particularly among blind people. Proportionally more of the younger age group (15% in comparison with 6% of the older age groups) have no light perception, and only 75% compared with 86% can see the shapes of furniture in a room. While in percentage terms a larger proportion of those in the younger age group have NLP, the age bias of the visually impaired population as a whole means that the older age group is larger in numerical terms. Approximately 4,500 people under 60 have NLP, while there are some 16,000 aged 60 and over. The corresponding numbers of people at point 1 of the scale (can tell where the windows are but cannot see the shape of furniture) are 3,000 (10%) and 20,000 (8%) respectively for the younger and older age groups.

6.2 Near vision

6.2.1 Measurements obtained

Two assessments of respondents' near vision capabilities were made, both involving visual reading ability. First, we asked about the ability to read newspapers, and, second, we administered a simplified reading test using a specimen of large print on a test card.

6.2.2 Ability to read newspapers

The ability to read newspaper print was considered a useful general benchmark of print reading ability among visually impaired people. This 'test' was also used in Gray and Todd's survey (1968), and in the OPCS disability survey (Martin et al, 1988a), therefore allowing some comparison with these two surveys; Table 6.2 shows the results.

A surprisingly large proportion (46% – 27% of blind people, 58% of the partially sighted) claim to be able to read ordinary newspaper print. Including these, as many as 75% (55 and 89 per cent of blind and partially sighted people respectively) claim to be able to read news-

71

Table 6.2   Reading newspaper print

'Can you see well enough to read ordinary newspaper print?' (YQ41)

'And can you see well enough to read newspaper headlines? (YQ42)

	Age and residual vision						Total
	16 – 59		60 +		All ages		
	B	PS	B	PS	B	PS	
	%	%	%	%	%	%	%
Read newspaper print	22	68	27	58	27	58	46
Read headlines only	30	27	28	31	28	31	29
Total able to read headlines	52	95	55	89	55	89	75
Unable to read headlines	33	5	39	11	39	11	21
NLP*	15	0	6	0	6	0	4
Total unable to read headlines	48	5	45	11	45	11	25
Total %	100	100	100	100	100	100	100
Base (population)	30K	46K	270K	409K	300K	455K	755K
(Number interviewed)	(137)	(162)	(130)	(165)	(267)	(327)	(594)

(594 respondents: no information for 1 respondent)

*NLP includes those with no light perception (i.e. 'no' at YQ29), where YQ41 and YQ42 were not asked

Interviewers were instructed to add, if necessary, 'with whatever you usually use for reading' after asking questions YQ41 and YQ42

paper headlines. There is little difference between the age groups although, as with distance vision, in percentage terms there are marginally fewer blind people under 60 because of the proportionately larger percentage of this group with NLP.

6.2.3   The reading test

Below is an actual-size reproduction of the words on the card handed to respondents. The print is 16 point bold, between N14 and N18 on the Snellen print size. Having been shown the card, respondents were asked (YQ43) 'Which of the following phrases best describes how you find reading the card?'. When answering they were requested to use their glasses or whatever else they normally used for reading.

to help you

Table 6.3 Numbers able to read the test card

'Please look at the card now. Which of the following phrases best describes how you find reading the card?' (YQ43)

	Age and residual vision						Total
	16 – 59		60 +		All ages		
	B	PS	B	PS	B	PS	
	%	%	%	%	%	%	%
Can read it comfortably	22	75	36	73	36	75	58
Can read but would find it tiring	7	13	4	5	4	6	5
Have difficulty reading it	13	9	9	8	9	8	9
All able to read card	42	97	49	86	49	89	72
I cannot read it	43	3	45	14	45	11	24
NLP*	15	0	6	0	6	0	4
All unable to read card	58	3	51	14	51	11	28
Total %	100	100	100	100	100	100	100
Base (population)	30K	46K	262K	408K	292K	454K	746K
(Number interviewed)	(136)	(160)	(125)	(164)	(261)	(324)	(585)

(585 respondents: no information for 10 respondents)

*NLP = No light perception, YQ43 not asked

Among visually impaired people generally, 72% said that they could read the card. Among blind and partially sighted people the totals are 49 and 89 per cent respectively, ignoring age differences. However, ability to read the card comfortably is probably a better guide to visual capability for sustained reading. Here the totals are 58, 36 and 75 per cent for visually impaired people generally, blind and partially sighted people. One notable age difference was among blind people who said that they could read the card comfortably: 22% of those under 60, 36% of those aged 60 and over, a statistically significant difference.

Claims to be able to read the card were put to the test of reading aloud, and the number of words read correctly was recorded. The results, not reported here, show that almost everyone who claimed to be able to read the card was in fact able to do so.

A key practical question for organisations providing services for visually impaired people is the necessity of producing documents in large print. The traditional argument runs 'since very few blind people can read, it is not necessary'. Our survey suggests otherwise and quantifies the gains of using large print. For example while only 22% of blind people under 60 can read newspaper print, 42% can read 16-point bold type; the equivalent totals for blind people 60 and over are 27 and 49 per cent, while for partially sighted people under 60 the rise is far more dramatic, from 68 to 97 per cent. Reading text of this size is still far more tiring for a visually impaired person than for a sighted person.

Nevertheless, the argument for large print seems to be proved, especially since substantial numbers of blind people are involved.

These results also point to the importance of low vision aids (LVAs) such as hand-held and stand magnifiers as well as closed-circuit television magnifiers (CCTVs). However, Tables 6.6 and 6.7 do suggest under-usage.

6.3 Field of vision

An additional crucial element in defining a person's residual vision is the completeness of his or her field of vision. To measure field of vision is a technically complicated exercise and was not feasible in our interviews. Interaction of an incomplete field of vision with poor distance vision or near vision, or both, greatly exacerbates visual impairment.

Two examples of field loss are loss of central vision and loss of peripheral vision. Loss of central vision is very common among elderly visually impaired people as a result of macular degeneration, and almost always leads to loss of ability to read or see faces. However, the remaining peripheral vision is extremely useful for mobility.

A much less common example of field loss occurs in more developed stages of retinitis pigmentosa (RP), commonly called tunnel vision. In this situation visual acuity may be good and central vision unimpaired, making reading relatively straightforward. However, the loss of peripheral vision makes mobility extremely hazardous. A person with RP can sit in a train and read a newspaper without difficulty, but on climbing out on to the platform will have to use a white cane to avoid tripping over.

In addition to these two examples of symmetrical field loss, there are many other forms of asymmetric distribution of loss, patchy distribution of loss and haphazard distribution.

6.4 Visual aids

6.4.1 Reported use of glasses or contact lenses

Table 6.4 shows that 85% of visually impaired people with some light perception wear glasses. Even among blind people the totals are high (60 and 80 per cent for the younger and older age groups respectively), while among the partially sighted the totals are 81 and 91 per cent respectively. These figures are percentages of people with light perception; however, they do not fall significantly when recast in terms of the total visually impaired population, since the percentage with NLP is so small. Of the totally visually impaired population (including people with

NLP), 82% wear glasses. In numerical terms, 620,000 blind and partially sighted people wear glasses, including 269,000 registrably blind people.

Table 6.4 Reported wearing of glasses among visually impaired people

'Do you wear glasses or contact lenses all of the time, some of the time or not at all?' (YQ37)

	Age and residual vision						Total
	16 – 59		60 +		All ages		
	B	PS	B	PS	B	PS	
	%	%	%	%	%	%	%
Wear glasses all the time	37	51	50	53	49	53	51
Wear glasses sometime	23	30	30	37	29	36	34
Not at all	40	19	20	10	22	11	15
Total %	100	100	100	100	100	100	100
Base (population)	26K	47K	255K	403K	281K	450K	730K
(Number interviewed)	(108)	(162)	(115)	(162)	(223)	(324)	(547)

(547 respondents: 48 respondents with no light perception were not asked)

Because glasses are so frequently used by sighted people, it is important to recognise that for blind and partially sighted people glasses are a prosthesis with a radically different effect. They provide some amelioration, not a total correction, just as an artificial limb does for a one-legged person.

Table 6.5 Reported use of spectacles

'What do you wear them (glasses) for?' (YQ38)

	Age and residual vision						Total
	16 – 59		60 +		All ages		
	B	PS	B	PS	B	PS	
	%	%	%	%	%	%	%
Reading	29	67	39	72	38	71	58
For close work	27	48	37	59	36	58	50
Distance vision	20	53	29	55	28	54	45
Protection	5	4	18	10	17	9	8
Other uses	22	13	14	11	13	11	13
Total wearing glasses	60	81	80	90	78	89	85
Total not wearing glasses	40	19	20	10	22	11	15
Base (population)	26K	47K	255K	403K	281K	450K	730K
(Number interviewed)	(108)	(162)	(115)	(162)	(223)	(324)	(547)

(547 respondents: 48 respondents with no light perception were not asked)

Table 6.5 shows the variety of uses to which people put their glasses. Reading, close work and distance vision were all mentioned roughly equally by about 50% of respondents. Some 13% said they use glasses for other, unspecified, reasons – this reply was most common (22%) among younger blind people. Eight per cent said spontaneously (respondents were not prompted while answering this question) that they wore their glasses merely for protection, and that their vision was not affected. This reply was most common among elderly blind people. The totals for blind and partially sighted people in the younger and older age groups were 5, 4, 18, and 10 per cent respectively.

6.4.2 Reported use of other low vision aids

Table 6.6 shows that the LVA most used after spectacles is the hand magnifier. Fifty-nine per cent of respondents used a hand magnifier. However, usage is lower among the younger age group (28 and 44 per cent for blind people and partially sighted people respectively) than among older people (60%). Usage of all other LVAs runs at under 5%; the most mentioned (4%) of these was a magnifier used as part of spectacles. However, although these percentages are low, a significant number of people are involved. For example, the 2% who use a stand magnifier amount to some 14,000 people.

Table 6.6   The possession of low vision aids among visually impaired people

'Do you have anything else (other than ordinary spectacles), for example a magnifying glass or something like that?' (YQ39)

	Age and residual vision				Total
	16 – 59		60 +		
	B	PS	B	PS	
	%	%	%	%	%
Hand magnifier	28	44	60	60	59
Magnifier as part of spectacles	4	4	5	3	4
Stand magnifier	3	2	4	1	2
Field expander	0	1	2	#	1
Hand-held telescope	2	5	2	#	1
Other LVA	7	4	5	5	5
Total who have LVAs	34	51	70	63	64
Total without LVA	66	49	30	37	36
Base (population)	26K	47K	255K	403K	730K
(Number interviewed)	(108)	(162)	(115)	(162)	(547)

(547 respondents: 48 respondents with no light perception were not asked)

6.4.3 Light fittings

At YQ46 we asked all those with at least light perception 'Have you ever had any extra light fittings or stronger light put in your home, because of your eye problems?' Only 20% answered 'yes', and there was little difference between age or residual vision groups. Of those who said 'no', only 5% gave expense as a reason. Other reasons given by those answering 'no' included not thinking it would help (42%) and never having thought about it (34%). Although extra lighting may not help in some cases, these results confirm what many experts have suspected: that visually impaired people are not aware of the generally positive results that may be gained from improved lighting levels. The large percentage (80%) who have done nothing about lighting levels present a public education opportunity to service providers.

6.4.4 Low vision aids used in the reading test

During the reading test, the interviewer was asked to code any LVAs used. The results, given in Table 6.7, confirm that glasses (59%) are the LVA predominantly used for reading, followed by hand magnifiers (13%); other types were used by no more than 2%. Fewer than half the number of blind people aged 16 – 59 used an LVA for the reading test, compared with two-thirds and three-quarters of the other sub-groups. (Although we noted in section 6.1.2 that there are marginally more younger than older blind people with NLP, this difference is discounted in Table 6.7.) More younger blind people used a hand magnifier, and fewer relied on glasses, than other groups.

Table 6.7 Interviewer coding of low vision aids used for the reading test

	Age and residual vision				Total
	16 – 59		60 +		
	B	PS	B	PS	
	%	%	%	%	%
Spectacles	31	53	56	63	59
Hand magnifier	23	6	14	13	13
Magnifier as part of spectacles	3	4	3	0	1
Contact lenses	0	1	4	0	1
Field expander	0	0	0	#	#
Stand magnifier	0	0	1	0	#
Other LVA	3	1	3	2	2
All that used LVA	46	65	74	75	73
No LVA used	54	35	26	25	27
Base (population) = 100%	26K	47K	255K	403K	730K
(Number interviewed)	(108)	(162)	(115)	(162)	(547)

(547 respondents: 48 respondents with no light perception were not asked)

These figures give some quantitative indication of the under-usage of LVAs. Table 6.6 showed that 59% of respondents have a hand magnifier, but only 13% used one in the test (Table 6.7). While the test card was printed in 16-point bold type, one can assume that the difference between the proportion of people possessing LVAs and the proportion using them in the reading test is evidence that more respondents might have been able to read the card if they had used their magnifier and if they had been trained and supported in its use.

Part B

Media Reading Habits

7 Large Print

7.1 Sight levels and the use of print

Chapter 7 deals with the amount and kind of print read by visually impaired people; visual ability to read print was discussed in section 6.2. While the sight levels of visually impaired people set the upper limit for the numbers who can read print, the total of those who in reality do read things in print depends on a variety of additional factors.

7.2 Those who normally read print

Our question 'Do you normally read anything at all in print?' (WQ1) was designed to obtain a broad assessment of the number of respondents who, while visually capable of reading print, actually did so. It was asked only of those who had been able to read the test card (section 6.2.3).

Table 7.1   Reading of print

'Do you normally read anything at all in print?' (WQ1)

	Age and residual vision						Total
	16 – 59		60 +		All ages		
	B	PS	B	PS	B	PS	
	%	%	%	%	%	%	%
NLP*	15	–	6	0	6	0	4
LP but no more*	10	–	8	3	8	3	5
Can see more but could not read card*	33	3	36	9	36	8	19
Can read large print test:							
(i) does not normally read print	2	13	8	6	7	7	7
(ii) normally reads print	40	84	42	82	43	82	65
Total %	100	100	100	100	100	100	100
Base (population)	30K	46K	262K	408K	292K	454K	746K
(Number interviewed)	(136)	(160)	(125)	(164)	(261)	(324)	(585)

(585 respondents: no information for 10 respondents)
*NLP, LP cannot/can see windows, not asked WQ1

Table 7.1 shows that 72% of visually impaired people can read the card (section 6.2.3), and that 65% claim to make use of that ability. In each age and sight band a similar proportion of those who passed our sight test claim to read print.

7.3 What is read in print

Our next question (WQ2) concerned the sort of things respondents read. This question was put first as an open question without prompting for any kind of material. However those who did not spontaneously mention large-print books at WQ2, but said (at WQ3) that they had heard of them, were specifically prompted 'Do you ever read large-print books?' (at YQ4). Table 7.2 shows the prompted and unprompted replies for large-print books, together with the unprompted replies for other items.

Table 7.2   Material visually impaired people read in print

'What sorts of things do you read?' (WQ2)

	Age and residual vision						Total
	16 – 59		60 +		All ages		
	B	PS	B	PS	B	PS	
	%	%	%	%	%	%	%
Newspapers:							
Ordinary newsprint	12	63	27	50	24	51	42
Headlines	23	60	36	39	35	40	55
Books:							
Ordinary print	17	40	20	27	20	28	25
Large-print books	5	17	8	24	8	23	17
Large-print books (WQ4)@	0	15	5	5	4	4	6
Total large-print books	5	32	13	29	12	30	23
Letters/bills	17	58	25	48	24	49	39
Other	11	13	3	3	4	4	4
All reading print*	40	84	42	80	42	82	65
Don't/can't read print+ +	40	16	58	20	58	20	35
Base (population) = 100%	30K	46K	262K	408K	292K	454K	746K
(Number interviewed)	(136)	(160)	(125)	(164)	(261)	(324)	(585)

(585 respondents: no information for 10 people)

+ +Not asked WQ2 @After prompting *(see Table 7.1)

Reading ordinary newspaper print and headlines was mentioned by 42 and 55 per cent respectively of visually impaired people generally. Among those aged 16 – 59, blind people were far less likely to read either ordinary newsprint or headlines than partially sighted people (12 and 63 per cent and 23 and 60 per cent respectively). Among those aged 60 and over, 27 and 50 per cent of blind and partially sighted people read ordinary newsprint, with similar numbers able to read head-lines (36 and 39 per cent respectively). These percentages run somewhat below those who said that they could see well enough to read these items (section 6.2.2) or were able to read 16-point bold type (section 6.2.3).

Only 17% of respondents said spontaneously that they read large-print books, but a further 6% said so after specific prompting. Some 30% of partially sighted people said that they read large-print books, compared with 5 and 13 per cent respectively of younger and older blind people. The number of people actually reading ordinary and large-print books correlates closely with those who 'comfortably' read our large print test card. (For example, 48% read ordinary or large-print books (Table 7.2), and 58% read the test card comfortably (Table 6.3). Twenty-two per cent of blind people under 60 read ordinary or large-print books.)

From the difference in proportions between those able to read large print and those who do read it, it would seem that leisure large-print reading is not undertaken by those who find it tiring or difficult (Table 6.3). Thus, while large print may reach many more blind and partially sighted people than has previously been recognised, it is only used widely for functional or necessary reasons (e.g. bills, bank statements, recipes). Similarly, ordinary print bills and letters are read by more people than ordinary print books (39 compared with 25 per cent). Indeed, bills and letters were read by virtually half of partially sighted people and 17 and 25 per cent respectively of blind people in the two age groups. (We look at this again in Chapter 15.)

Table 7.3 shows that, although a small sub-group of all visually impaired people, users of large-print books appear to be fairly regular readers. Only 7% of the sub-group said that they had read no large-print books in the last six months, and the totals reading 1 – 3, 4 – 6,

Table 7.3 Number of large-print books read in last six months by two age groups

'About how many large-print books have you read in the last six months?' (WQ6)

	Age		Total
	16 – 59	60 +	
	%	%	%
No books	25	5	7
1 – 3 books	43	28	30
4 – 6 books	10	21	20
7 – 12 books	11	16	16
13 + books	10	30	28
Total %	100	100	100
Base (population)	16K	150K	166K
(Number interviewed)	(57)	(60)	(117)

(117 respondents: 478 respondents did not read large-print books)

7 – 12, and 13 or more books were 30, 20, 16 and 28 per cent respectively. People aged 60 and over were by far the more frequent readers. Some 30% of them had read 13 or more books in the last six months, compared with 10% of the readers under 60. A quarter of the latter said that they had read no large-print books in the last six months compared with only 5% of the older group.

7.4 Why large-print books are not read

Among visually impaired people generally, 65% normally read print (Table 7.1), but only 23% read large-print books (Table 7.2). Taking into account people unable to read print at all, this means that only about a third of those able to do so actually read large-print books.

We asked (WQ3) the non-readers of large-print books in this group if they had heard of large-print books. Three-quarters, including almost all the blind people under 60, said that they had. Thus, lack of awareness does not seem to be the main reason for not using large-print books. Those non-readers who had heard of large-print books were then asked directly why they did not read them; the results appear in Table 7.4.

Table 7.4 The main reasons given for not reading large-print books

'Why don't you ever read large-print books? Is that because you don't know how to get them, you find them difficult to read, you're just not interested in reading, or some other reason?' (WQ5)

	All non-readers of large print
	%
Just not interested	31
Don't need (yet)	16
Difficult to read/follow	13
Read ordinary print	10
Read other medium	5
Too heavy/bulky	4
Don't know how to get	4
Popltn numbers (= 100%)	259K
(Number interviewed)	(203)

(203 respondents able to read test card but who did not read large-print books: 392 respondents were not asked the question)

The small number (4%) who said that they did not know how to get large-print books is consistent with the finding that lack of awareness is not a major reason for the non-use of large-print books. Lack of interest in reading (31%) is the predominant single reason given. But 13% said that they find large-print books difficult to read. We may infer that these people are among those (Table 6.4) who could read the test card but said that they would not find it comfortable to read print of this size. At the other extreme, 10% of respondents gave as a reason for not reading large-print books that they could read ordinary print.

7.5 Potentially useful large-print items

To try to gauge likely demand for large-print items, respondents were asked (WQ7) if they would find it useful to have a number of items produced in large print. These were bank statements, bills, Radio/TV Times, dictionary, and catalogues. The results are shown in Table 7.5; the percentages are of respondents who had been shown the example of large print and had been able to read it (section 6.2.3).

Table 7.5 Potentially useful large-print items

'I showed you an example of large print earlier on. Would you find any of the following items useful if they were in large print?' (WQ7)

	Age			Total
	16 – 59	60 – 74	75 +	
	%	%	%	%
Bank statements	55	52	34	41
Bills	60	54	42	47
Radio/TV Times	51	47	39	42
Dictionary	66	45	35	41
Catalogues	52	40	42	43
None useful	25	31	36	33
Base (population) = 100%	58K	136K	349K	543K
(Number interviewed)	(204)	(83)	(105)	(392)

(392 respondents able to read the test card: 48 NLP, 155 could not read test card)

The general view was that it would be useful to have all the listed items available in large print, with the figures running at 41 to 47 per cent (of those able to read large print). Only 33% said that they would not find any of the items useful in large-print; these are likely to be people who can read ordinary print (see Table 6.3). Rather surprisingly, residual vision level made no difference to the responses. Taking all the items together respondents under 60 tended to be more receptive by about 10% or so than older people; for individual items the percentage spread was greater, for example 'dictionaries' (66 and 38 per cent), 'bills' (60 and 46 per cent), 'catalogues' (52 and 42 per cent).

7.6 Comparison with Gray and Todd's 1965 results

Comparisons are only possible for a sub-set of our data. When Gray and Todd (1968) carried out the fieldwork for their major study of

Mobility and reading habits of the blind in 1965, they drew their entire sample from the local authority registers of blind people. Interviews were held with 1,044 people aged 16 – 64 and 420 aged 65 – 75. Our survey contains too few registered people in the older age group for valid comparisons. However, comparisons are possible with the 123 of our respondents who are registered blind and aged between 16 and 59. Table 7.6 compares this sub-group of 123 with Gray and Todd's results.

Table 7.6 Reading of print: comparison of RNIB results (1986) with Gray and Todd's results (1965)

'Do you normally read anything at all in print?'

	Registered blind respondents only	
	1986 RNIB survey	1965 Gray/Todd
	16 – 59	16 – 64
	%	%
NLP*	27	26
LP but no more*	17	17
Can see more but did not read card*	19	33
Read large print test: (i) does not normally read print	2	13
(ii) normally reads print	39	11
Total %	100	100
Base (population)	18K	24K
(Number interviewed)	(123)	(1044)

*NLP, LP cannot/can see windows. Not asked WQ1

Note that in this table the RNIB sample is not the same as blind people of this age group shown in Table 7.1. These groups are based on registration status rather than on residual vision, hence the somewhat different percentages

The projected population estimates for the RNIB group is 18,000; Gray and Todd suggested 24,000 based on statistics from the (then) Ministry of Health for this age group. Our smaller estimate may be a result of our narrower age range and also of the scaling down of published DHSS statistics to allow for visually impaired people who are institutionalised (section 21.3.2). However, the major similarities and differences evident in the table are unlikely to be affected by these minor discrepancies in the variables compared. We took care to retain Gray and Todd's precise question wording, and both reading tests were based on 1/8 inch lower case type. In both surveys respondents were told to use their normal spectacles or other reading aids.

The most striking difference is between the percentages of people able to read print and those who actually do so. While nearly half of the 1965 respondents (11 out of 24 per cent) who could read the large print test said that they normally did read print, in our survey nearly the entire sample (39 out of 41 per cent) who could read the print test said that they read print normally. This indicates an immense shift among young registered blind people over two decades. One cause may be improvements in general education and reading skills. However, more significant is likely to be the increased availability of large print which has proved extremely popular with the 22% of blind people who can read it easily. In 1965 large-print was not common in either libraries or bookshops.

Table 7.6 also suggests that the composition of the younger group of registered blind people may have changed in respect of residual vision levels. The percentages with NLP (who said that they could not see the windows) and those with LP but no more (steps 1 on our questionnaire scale – see section 6.1.1) were the same in each survey (44 and 43 per cent). But in 1986 41% (of the comparable registered blind sub-group) could read the test card compared with 24% in 1965. However, we cannot be certain that this is a real difference as opposed to a different definition of 'reading' here. The RNIB test card contained only three words, and almost everyone (Table 6.4) who said that they could read it read all three words correctly. Gray and Todd's report, however, mentioned that their test card contained a sentence but did not specify either the number of words or the number of words required to be correct to qualify as 'reading'. It is possible that Gray and Todd applied stricter criteria.

8 Tapes and Tape Services

8.1 Introduction

The use of tapes, especially in relation to braille as a reading medium, has long been a matter of debate. There is no doubt that there has been a major increase in the usage of commercial tape-recording and -playing machines; a major rise in the number of members of the RNIB Talking Book Service; and an increase in the number of volunteer and local tape-recording groups putting print material on to tapes at short notice. Given these changes, it is vital to understand current tape usage, for example how many blind and partially sighted people use them, and for what purpose.

Tape services are collectively one of the largest services provided by RNIB. In particular the RNIB Talking Book Service is often cited as RNIB's flagship service, and reaches a larger number of visually impaired people than any other single service. The RNIB Talking Book Service is a membership-based tape library for visually impaired people providing a wide range of fiction and non-fiction books. Other RNIB tape services are more specialised and have far fewer users, e.g. the Express Reading Service which provides a general tape-recording service for visually impaired people. Although we asked questions on most of RNIB's tape services, the design of the survey is most appropriate for comparing users and non-users of talking books and for examining the usage of tape media in general by visually impaired people; it is less suitable for examining services with only a small number of users.

We use the term tape-player in this report as a generic term to include all forms of tape-playing and recording-machines that the respondents may possess. Where it is necessary to distinguish between the RNIB Talking Book machine obtained through the RNIB Talking Book Service and other tape-players, the former is usually specifically named.

8.2 Tape-players in general

8.2.1 Possession of tape-players

Table 8.1 indicates that the main variable influencing possession of tape-players is age. In marketing terminology, the market penetration for tape-players among the under-60s has almost reached saturation-point. Over 80% of this age group have a tape-player, compared with 53% of people aged 60 to 74 and 38% of those aged 75 and over.

Table 8.1 Possession of tape-player among the visually impaired population within three age groups

'Do you have a tape-player or cassette player of any kind?' (WQ36)

	Age			Total
	16 – 59	60 – 74	75 +	
	%	%	%	%
Have tape-player	83	53	38	46
No tape-player	17	47	62	54
Total %	100	100	100	100
Base (population)	77K	180K	499K	755K
(Number interviewed)	(299)	(124)	(137)	(593)

(593 respondents: no information for 2 respondents)

There is no doubt that the percentage of older people using tape-players is growing. While 38% of those aged 75 + have a tape-player, this increases to 53% for those aged 60 to 74. It is reasonable to assume that this figure will be indicative of future ownership levels for people aged 75 and over, and that the higher ownership levels among younger elderly people will be maintained as they grow older. Nevertheless, this means that well over half of older visually impaired people do not possess a tape-player and suggests the need for a simple player to which they might be introduced in their very elderly years.

Registration status made a difference: 65% of registered blind people compared with 41% of the non-registered possessed a tape-player of some kind. Differences by residual vision level were not statistically significant (section 21.4).

8.2.2 Type of tape-player possessed

Table 8.2 shows that 12% of visually impaired people own an RNIB Talking Book machine, 33% some other type of tape-player, and 54% do not own any kind of tape-player (see note to chapter).

The breakdown of ownership of tape-players other than RNIB Talking Book machines shows that among visually impaired people as a whole, radio cassette players (26%) predominate, followed by ordinary cassette players (15%) and music centres (9%); 'other types' of cassettes (mostly small Walkman players) account for only 1%.

As a whole, younger people are more likely than the older group to possess some type of cassette-player. However, because there are many more blind and partially sighted people aged 60 +, in numerical

Table 8.2 Type of tape-player possessed by visually impaired people, by residual vision within two age groups

'What sort? Is it (tape-player) a talking book machine, a radio cassette, an ordinary cassette player or something else?' (WQ37)

	Age and residual vision						Total
	16 – 59		60 +		All ages		
	B	PS	B	PS	B	PS	
	%	%	%	%	%	%	%
Talking book machine	32	5	20	6	21	6	12
Radio cassette player	52	60	30	18	32	19	26
Ordinary cassette	28	44	12	16	14	16	15
Music centre	27	23	10	6	12	6	9
Other	12	4	0	0	1	#	1
All with non-RNIB tape-player	50	78	30	29	32	34	33
Don't know	0	0	0	2	0	2	1
No tape-player at all	18	17	50	63	47	59	54
Total %	100	100	100	100	100	100	100
Base (population)	30K	47K	270K	410K	301K	546K	757K
(Number interviewed)	(137)	(162)	(130)	(166)	(267)	(328)	(595)

(595 respondents)

terms this group possesses many more tape machines. Among the under-60s residual vision had an impact on ownership. In this age group 32% of blind people and only 5% of partially sighted people own an RNIB Talking Book machine; for ordinary cassette players the figures are 28 and 44 per cent respectively.

8.3   RNIB Talking Books

8.3.1   Profile of users

Table 8.2 shows that about 12% of visually impaired people possess an RNIB Talking Book machine. The possession-rate is higher among blind than among partially sighted people: 32 and 5 per cent among the under-60s, 20 and 6 per cent among those aged 60 and over. Our data allow us to examine the profile of the users and non-users of RNIB Talking Books simultaneously, and below we provide more detail in relation to age and registration.

The most accurate way of obtaining a user profile would be to analyse the records held on RNIB computers. For more detailed characteristics of membership of the RNIB Talking Book Service the computerised list could be treated as a sampling frame for a questionnaire enquiry. This is what Lucille Hall did in her 1981 postal survey *Who Are Britain's blind people?* (Hall, 1982). It is of interest to compare the age distribution obtained from the present survey with that found in 1981.

8.3.1.1 Age of users

Table 8.3.a. shows that the distribution of people with RNIB Talking Book machines among the three age bands is 15, 31 and 54 per cent respectively. The corresponding totals in Hall's survey, for a random sample of 1,000 people aged 16 and over selected from the complete list of RNIB members, were 21, 29 and 50 per cent respectively.

Some decrease in membership among the 16 – 59 age band seems to have taken place between the 1981 survey and ours, the fieldwork for which was done in 1986 – 87. On these sample sizes (section 21.4) the difference between 21 and 15 per cent is just statistically significant.

Membership of the scheme covers only 12% of the registrable visually impaired population. Table 8.3.b shows that membership among the three age groups is roughly level in relative terms, with a decrease from 16 to 10 per cent among the older group. Because people aged 75 and over constitute almost two-thirds of the blind population as a whole, they constitute about half the membership of the RNIB Talking Book Service.

Table 8.3.a. Age distribution of visually impaired people with and without RNIB Talking Book machines (TBs)

	With TBs	No TBs	Total VI
	%	%	%
Age group			
16 – 59	15	10	10
60 – 74	31	22	24
75 +	54	68	66
Total	100	100	100
Base (population)	90K	667K	757K
(Number interviewed)	(132)	(463)	(595)

Table 8.3.b. Prevalence of RNIB Talking Book machine ownership (TBs) within three age bands (% along rows)

Age group		With TBs	No TBs	Total %	Base	(Number interviewed)
16 – 59	%	16	84	100	77K	(299)
60 – 74	%	16	84	100	180K	(124)
75 +	%	10	90	100	500K	(172)
All ages	%	12	88	100	757K	(595)

8.3.1.2 Registration status and residual vision levels of users

Table 8.4 gives more fine detail of user characteristics defined by registration sub-groups, sub-divided again by age and residual vision levels.

Table 8.4 Prevalence of Talking Book machine ownership (TBs) by residual vision within age and registration status sub-groups (% along rows)

	With TBs	No TBs	Total %	Base for %	(Number interviewed)
Registered					
Under 60					
B %	44	56	100	18K	(123)
PS %	17	83	100	12K	(92)
60 and over					
B %	36	64	100	91K	(74)
PS %	24	76	100	49K	(63)
Non-registered					
Under 60					
B+ +%	17	83	100	12K	(14)
PS %	3	97	100	35K	(70)
60 and over					
B %	12	88	100	179K	(56)
PS %	3	98	100	361K	(103)
Total %	12	88	100	757K	(595)

+ + Small number of interviews

Registration is a much more powerful factor than age in influencing the prevalence of Talking Book usage in any of the sub-groups in Table 8.4. Every registered sub-group shows a far higher prevalence rate than the comparable non-registered (age/residual vision) sub-group. For example, among the under-60s, 44% of those registered blind use RNIB Talking Books, compared with 17% of the non-registered at blind residual vision levels (defined in 2.4.2.). Comparing registered people as a whole with all non-registered, we find that 36% of the registered but only 6% of the non-registered use RNIB Talking Books.

8.3.1.3 Information about the RNIB Talking Book Service

Table 8.5 shows that social services were the most mentioned source of information about the RNIB Talking Book Service; 33% of respondents specifically mentioned social workers for the blind, and when other social services workers are included the total increases to 43%. The other statutory service, the health service, was mentioned by 11% of respondents.

Table 8.5 Source of initial information about
the RNIB Talking Book Service

'How did you first hear about Talking Book machines?'
(WQ40)

	All Talking Book users
	%
Social worker for the blind	33
Other relative (not in household)	14
Health service	11
Social welfare worker	9
RNIB	9
Other local associations (not blind)	8
Someone in the household	5
Friend/colleague	4
Local blind association	3
Other social services	1
Others not specified	4
Base (population) = 100%	90K
(Number interviewed)	(133)

(133 respondents: only asked of current users of RNIB
Talking Books)

Someone else finding out about the service on their behalf was reported
for 22% of visually impaired people; 'other relative', 'someone in the
household' and 'friend/colleague' were mentioned by 14, 5, and 4 per
cent respectively. RNIB itself was mentioned by 9% of respondents.

The majority (61%) of users are registered, and this is the reason why
the social services appear as the most important single information
source. The various other sources listed in Table 8.5 clearly play an
important role in informing the non-registered about the service. As
social services workers are such crucial gate-keepers to RNIB Talking
Books Service, any attempts to increase membership will require their
commitment and co-operation; they are a vital target group of any
successful expansion drive.

8.3.1.4 Acquisition of RNIB Talking Book machine and onset of reading difficulty

Table 8.6 shows that about half the users acquired their Talking Book
machine as soon as they experienced difficulty reading. The
overwhelming reason given by nearly 6 in 10 of those who got one
'much later' was that they were not told about the service at the time.
Other reasons mentioned were: 'didn't want one', 'none available and
had to wait', 'waited until registered'.

Table 8.6 Time lag between onset of reading difficulty and acquisition of RNIB Talking Book machine

'Did you get one as soon as you had difficulty reading, or was it much later?' (WQ42)

	All Talking Book users
	%
Straight away	47
Much later	52
Don't know	1
Total %	100
Base (population)	90K
(Number interviewed)	(133)

(133 respondents: only asked of those who were current Talking Book users)

More of the registered than the non-registered reported that they got an RNIB Talking Book machine immediately, but the difference (13%) falls short of statistical significance on the sample numbers available. There is clear scope for providing registered and non-registered people with information about the service at an earlier stage.

8.3.1.5 Numbers of Talking Books read

Table 8.7 shows that 34% of the under-60s read fewer than one book a month, and 20% read four or more books; among those aged 60 and

Table 8.7 Reading rate of RNIB Talking Books based on books read in the previous six months by age

'How many books have you had from the Talking Book Library in the last six months?' (WQ44)

	Age		All Talking Book users
	16 – 59	60 +	
	%	%	%
None	12	2	3
Less than 1 a month	34	6	10
1 a month less than 2	11	17	16
2 a month less than 3	15	15	15
3 a month or more	3	8	7
4 or more (average 4)*	20	44	41
Don't know	4	9	8
Total %	100	100	100
Base (population)	12K	78K	90K
(Number interviewed)	(71)	(62)	(133)

(133 respondents: 462 respondents did not have TBM)
*On average, RNIB despatches four books a month to each member

over corresponding totals are 6 and 44 per cent. On average, the under-60s had read 17 books during the previous six months, those aged 60 and over 27 books, the equivalent of about three and five books per month. These figures demonstrate that older members of the service use RNIB Talking Books more heavily.

It is impressive that nearly half those aged 60 and over read four or more books a month, especially since it takes approximately twelve hours to listen to a single book. That so many elderly visually impaired people listen for so long emphasises the importance of the service.

8.3.1.6 Difficulty using the RNIB Talking Book machine

A small proportion (10%) of current users said that they found it difficult to operate the RNIB Talking Book machine (WQ45). The reasons given were 'unable to operate the machine' or 'unable to press the buttons'. Perhaps not surprisingly, almost everyone who had difficulty was aged 60 or over (most being in the 75 + age group), and were at the registrably blind residual vision level. Chapter 12 shows that very elderly blind people are more likely to experience other health and disability problems.

8.3.1.7 Announcements on RNIB Talking Book tapes

When we asked (WQ47) whether respondents ever listened to the announcements at the end of the RNIB Talking Book tapes, we found that 73% said that they 'always' or 'sometimes' did. Just under 10% of users said that they did not know about the announcements. Just under 30% of RNIB Talking Book readers said that they could remember announcements they had found particulary useful. These included information on 'sight aids' and 'books by the same author'.

8.3.1.8 Suggestions for improvements in the service

Although about two thirds of RNIB Talking Book readers suggested improvements to the service, these were so diverse that only a few ideas appeared more than once. 'Receiving tapes more frequently'; 'problems with the readers (e.g. reading too slow, not liking their voice)'; 'tapes faulty'; 'more new books' were most frequently mentioned, but in no case by more than 8% of readers.

8.3.1.9 Joint use of RNIB Talking Book machines and other tape-players

Table 8.8 shows that just under a third of RNIB Talking Book users possess only a Talking Book machine and do not have another tape-player. There is a considerable age-related variation: 8% of the under-60s but 35% of elderly people have only the RNIB Talking Book machine.

Table 8.8   Usage of Talking Book and other tape-players compared

'Do you use your Talking Book machine more or less often than your tape-players?' (WQ51)

	Age		All with a Talking Book
	16 – 59	60 +	
	%	%	%
TB more	23	44	41
Other tape-player more	40	7	12
Same usage	29	14	16
Only have TB	8	35	31
Total %	100	100	100
Base (population)	12K	78K	90K
(Number interviewed)	(72)	(61)	(133)

(133 respondents: only asked of current Talking Book users)

As already noted (section 8.2.1), the under-60s are more likely to have some kind of tape-player, and now we see that a substantial number of those who have an RNIB Talking Book machine also have another tape-player. A similar usage pattern emerges among those who possess both an RNIB Talking Book machine and another tape-player. The younger age group uses the non RNIB tape-player more intensively: 40% said that they used their tape-player more often than the RNIB Talking Book machine, compared with only 7% of those in the older age group.

Table 8.8 also demonstrates a remarkable degree of dependence on the RNIB Talking Book machine. Ninety-three per cent of elderly users either possess only an RNIB Talking Book machine or use it as often or more often than an ordinary tape-player. Even among the under-60s, who are more familiar with ordinary tape-players, the figure is 60%.

8.3.2   Lapsed RNIB Talking Book users

8.3.2.1   Profile of lapsed users

All those respondents who either did not initially say that they possessed a tape-player, or who did not mention an RNIB Talking Book machine, were asked (WQ38) if they had ever possessed one. Tables 8.9.a and 8.9.b show that, overall, 4% of visually impaired people previously had an RNIB Talking Book machine. At 12% current users are three times as great; that is, for every three current users there is one lapsed user.

Table 8.9.a. Previous and current users of Talking Books, within two age groups and two sight levels

'Have you ever had a Talking Book machine?' (WQ38)

	Age and residual vision				Total
	16 – 59		60 +		
	B	PS	B	PS	
	%	%	%	%	%
Has one now	32	5	20	6	12
Has had but not now	19	5	8	1	4
Has never had one	49	90	72	93	84
Total %	100	100	100	100	100
Base (population)	30K	47K	270K	410K	757K
(Number interviewed)	(136)	(162)	(130)	(166)	(595)

Table 8.9.b. Previous and current users of Talking Books by registration status

'Have you ever had a Talking Book machine ?' (WQ38)

	Registration status and residual vision				Total
	Registered		Non-registered		
	B	PS	B	PS	
	%	%	%	%	%
Has one now	38	22	12	3	12
Has had but not now	22	9	1	#	4
Has never had one	41	69	87	97	84
Total %	100	100	100	100	100
Base (population)	109K	61K	192K	395K	757K
(Number interviewed)	(197)	(155)	(70)	(173)	(595)

Lapsed users occur with greater relative frequency in the 16 – 59 age band and also among the registered, where their number approaches two for every three users. Since a majority of the younger age group is registered, both factors are at work. The registered older age group also has a higher than average rate of lapsed users, which indicates that registration in itself is a factor. Among the non-registered, where as we have seen (section 8.3.1.1) the uptake of Talking Books is low in relative terms (even though it amounts to 39% of the total), there are also relatively fewer lapsed users: for every six non-registered users there is only one lapsed user (average of B/PS columns in Table 8.9.b.).

In terms of absolute numbers, those aged 60 and over represent 24,000 of the estimated 32,000 people who have given up the RNIB Talking Book Service. The largest single numerical group is the registrably blind aged 60 and over, of whom 20,000 have given it up; 14,000 of these are 75 or over.

8.3.2.2 Reasons for giving up RNIB Talking Books

We asked those people (some 4% of the visually impaired population) who had given up RNIB Talking Books their reasons. Table 8.10 shows the most frequent reasons given. These cannot be divided into simple independent categories. The single most frequently mentioned reasons were 'could not be bothered', 'did not like the stories' and 'no time/too busy' (22, 18 and 14 per cent respectively). A fair proportion of respondents also mentioned some specific dissatisfaction with an aspect of the service. 'Unreliable or unsatisfactory machines' and 'stories too slow/too long' (which includes having to wait too long for the next tape continuing the text to arrive) scored 9 and 8 per cent respectively. Only 3% of respondents mentioned expense as a reason for giving up their machine, saying that they could not afford the subscriptions or, in one case, that it used up electricity. Other reasons include a variety of answers mentioned by one individual alone: 'moved district', 'deaf', 'cannot remember', 'prefer radio', 'couldn't get the hang of it', 'might still have it somewhere'.

Table 8.10   Reasons for no longer having an RNIB Talking Book

'Why do you no longer have it (Talking Book)?' WQ39

	All lapsed Talking Book readers
	%
Could not be bothered	22
Did not like stories/not a reader	18
No time/too busy/other hobbies	14
Unreliable/unsatisfactory machines	9
Stories too slow/too long to wait	8
Voices bored/ made sleepy	5
Can read/ sight improved	4
Student, want only non-fiction	3
Can't afford	3
Easier to use library tape/ own equipment	2
Other reasons	15
Base (population) = 100%	32K
(Number interviewed)	(65)

(65 respondents: 530 respondents either current users, or have never had one)

Many respondents added that they thought that they should send the Talking Book machine back for others to use, or that they had been asked to do so, if they were not using it themselves. This could explain why in relative terms there is both more uptake and more lapsed usage of Talking Books among the registered rather than the unregistered; the registered are more likely to be in touch with social services who actively 'manage' their membership. (Note that the majority of RNIB Talking Book members have their subscriptions met by their local authority social services department.)

8.3.3 Non-users of Talking Books

8.3.3.1 Non-users unaware of the service

Tables 8.11.a. and 8.11.b. show that awareness was greatest among younger respondents, of whom only about a quarter had not heard of the service. Registration is an additional factor in the 16 – 59 age group; 13% of the registered and 34% of the non-registered were unaware of the service. Among the elderly the corresponding totals were 29 and 64 per cent.

Table 8.11.a Awareness of RNIB Talking Books Service among the visually impaired population by age and residual vision

'Do you know what a Talking Book machine is?' (WQ52)					
	Age and residual vision				Total
	16 – 59		60 +		
	B	PS	B	PS	
	%	%	%	%	%
Never had a TB:					
but heard about it	29	58	16	36	30
never heard about it	21	31	56	57	54
Have or have had a TB*	51	10	28	7	16
Total %	100	100	100	100	100
Base (population)	30K	47K	270K	410K	757K
(Number interviewed)	(137)	(162)	(130)	(166)	(595)

*From WQ37 and WQ38, Tables 8.2 and 8.9

Table 8.11.b Awareness of RNIB Talking Books Service among the visually impaired population by age and registration

	Age and registration status				Total
	16 – 59		60 +		
	R	NR	R	NR	
	%	%	%	%	%
Never had a TB:					
but heard about it	33	55	22	29	30
never heard about it	13	34	29	64	54
Have or have had a TB*	54	11	49	7	16
Total %	100	100	100	100	100
Base (population)	30K	47K	140K	540K	757K
(Number interviewed)	(215)	(84)	(137)	(159)	(595)

*From WQ37 and WQ38

The 54% who did not know about RNIB Talking Books were given a brief description (WQ53) and were asked if they would be interested in having one. As Table 8.12 shows, just under one in four expressed an interest.

Table 8.12 Expressed desire for an RNIB Talking Book among those who were not aware of it before the survey

'In fact a Talking Book machine is a type of tape-player that plays specially recorded books for people with a sight problem, for example stories and technical books. If you could have one, would you be interested in having a Talking Book?' (WQ53)

	Age		Total
	16 – 59	60 +	
	%	%	%
Yes, would like one	60	22	23
No, don't want one	40	79	77
Total %	100	100	100
Base (population)	21K	377K	398K
(Number interviewed)	(67)	(127)	(194)

(194 respondents: 401 already know about Talking Books)

Answers to hypothetical questions about an unfamiliar service should be treated cautiously as a measure of potential demand. But, on the answers given, Table 8.12 shows that 23% of the 398,000 people unaware of the service would be prepared to use it if it were made accessible. In percentage terms demand is largest (60%) among those unaware of the service in the 16 – 59 age group. In absolute numbers, however, this amounts only to 12,000 people. The corresponding total (22%) among the older age group indicates a much larger sub-group of some 84,000 potential users.

8.3.3.2 Non-users aware of the service

Of the 30% of visually impaired people who knew about Talking Books but were not current or past users, fewer than 5% had made enquiries about obtaining one (WQ54). This suggests either that there was very little demand from those who knew about the product, or else that they did not know where to enquire.

Table 8.13 throws some further light on the issue. Those who knew about Talking Books but had not enquired about obtaining them, were questioned (WQ58) about whom they would ask.

The range of enquiry points indicates that many people know where to start finding out about the Service. However, four in ten said that they did not know whom they would ask. Others mentioned a variety of people. The most frequently mentioned were 'social/welfare workers'

Table 8.13 Who or where people would ask if they wanted to obtain an RNIB Talking Book

'Who would you ask if you did want a Talking Book machine?' (WQ58)

	All those who knew about TBs but had not made enquiries about getting one
	%
Social/welfare worker	14
Other social services	5
Health service	10
Friend/colleague	10
RNIB	8
Library	6
Local blind association	3
Other relative	3
Someone in the household	2
Don't know	38
Base (population) = 100 %	245K
(Number interviewed)	(247)

(247 respondents: only asked of those who knew about Talking Books but had not made any enquiries about obtaining them)

(14%), 'health service' (10%), 'friend/colleague' (10%), RNIB (8%), and the local library (6%). (Note that we were very careful not to indicate that RNIB is the supplier of Talking Books.)

These results indicate that further potential demand exists and can be stimulated by appropriate additional information, even among those who already know about the Talking Book Service.

8.4 Other tape usage

8.4.1 Frequency of use

We noted from Table 8.1 that 46% of visually impaired people possess some kind of a tape-player (including Talking Book machines) and that ownership levels are much higher among the younger age group. This section examines ordinary tape-players and compares their usage with RNIB Talking Book machines.

Interviewers were specially instructed (at WQ37) to code respondents who possessed a Talking Book machine and/or another type of tape-player. Some 42% (population projection 319,000) of the visually impaired population said that they possessed an ordinary tape-player.

Table 8.14 shows that two-thirds of them use it regularly. A third said that they used it most days, a further quarter at least weekly, while nearly a fifth said that they never used it at all. Three-quarters of those at the registrably blind vision level made frequent use of their tape-player, compared with half those at the partially sighted level. A slightly larger proportion of the registered, and of younger respondents, also made more frequent use of it.

Table 8.14 Frequency of use of ordinary tape-player by visually impaired people, by residual vision

'How often do you use your tape-player. Is it..?' (WQ61)

	Residual vision		All with a tape player (non TB)
	B	PS	
	%	%	%
Most days	44	29	36
At least weekly	31	22	26
Once a month	8	8	8
Less often	6	21	15
Never use the tape	11	21	17
Total %	100	100	100
Base (population)	133K	185K	319K
(Number interviewed)	(187)	(206)	(393)

(393 respondents: 200 without ordinary tape-player were not asked, no information for 2 respondents)

8.4.2 Use of already taped material

8.4.2.1 Type of material

Table 8.15 shows the material people listen to on tape. Music was most frequently mentioned (76%), and this probably hardly differs from the sighted population. Other than music, the main items mentioned were 'local talking newspapers'(20%), stories/books' (7%), 'national magazines' (4%), 'letters' (3%) 'religious material' (2%), and 'poetry' (1%). Of the diverse items totalling 7%, no individual item reached more than 0.5% (most other replies concerned specially recorded material which was the subject of the next question, WQ63).

Altogether, 45% of the items mentioned concerned the use of tapes for access to verbal or printed material. There was double counting here in that some individuals mentioned more than one type of item. Section 8.4.2.2 examines the count of individuals and compares it with usage of Talking Books.

The main items on which blind and partially sighted respondents differed were 'local talking newspapers' (29% and 14%), 'other national magazines' (8% and 2%), and 'letters' (6% and 1%).

Table 8.15 Material listened to on tape-players, by residual vision

'Do you listen to any of the following things on tape...?' (WQ62)

	Residual vision		All with a tape player (non TB)
	B	PS	
	%	%	%
Music	79	74	76
Local talking newspapers	29	14	20
Stories/books	7	7	7
Other national magazines	9	2	4
Letters	6	1	3
Religious material	3	1	2
Poetry	2	1	1
Radio Times	1	1	1
Other	7	7	7
Never use the tape-player*	11	21	17
Base (population) = 100%	135K	186K	321K
(Number interviewed)	(188)	(207)	(395)

(395 respondents: 200 with no ordinary tape-player were not asked)
*Never used player at WQ61

The high use of taped general-interest media, newspapers and magazines possibly illustrates the wider desire for more general interest material, and very likely its wider availability. Other usage would largely depend on the demand for specialist interests.

8.4.2.2   Comparisons with Talking Books

Table 8.16 brings together data on Talking Books and ordinary tape-players. In all, 42% of visually impaired people possess an ordinary tape-player. Even when the 7% who say that they possess one but do not use it are subtracted, the remaining 35% (row f. in Table 8.16) is considerably greater than the 12% who possess a Talking Book machine. Some 34% of all visually impaired people – 68% of those under 60, 31% of those aged 60 or over – have an ordinary tape-player but no Talking Book machine.

However, on the whole ordinary tape-players fulfil a different function from Talking Books. Table 8.16 shows that almost all those who possess an ordinary tape-player use it for listening to music (32% out of 35%). The pattern is similar in every sub-group. For example, although the percentage figure using a tape-player nearly doubles to 74% of the registrable blind in the 16 – 59 age band, 68% (of the total) use it to listen to music.

Nevertheless, some 14% of visually impaired people use their ordinary tape-players for listening to verbal material (e.g. local talking

Table 8.16 Comparison of usage of ordinary tapes and Talking Books by age and residual vision

	Age and residual vision				Total
	16 – 59		60 +		
	B	PS	B	PS	
	%	%	%	%	%
Talking Books					
a. Has only Talking Book	1	1	9	1	4
b. Has Talking Book and ordinary tape-player	30	4	11	5	8
c. Total with Talking Book	31	5	20	6	12
Ordinary tapes					
b. Has ordinary tape-player and Talking Book	30	4	11	5	8
d. Has ordinary tape-player and no Talking Book	51	79	30	31	34
e. Total with ordinary tape-player	81	83	41	36	42
f. Total using ordinary tape player	74	69	36	28	35
No tape-player at all	18	17	50	63	54
Material listened to*					
Music	68	63	32	26	32
Verbal material	42	22	17	10	14
Stories or books	7	6	3	3	3
Base (population)	30K	47K	270K	410K	757K
(Number interviewed)	(137)	(162)	(130)	(166)	(595)

Rows (a) to (e) coded at WQ37

*Count of respondents at WQ62; see Table 8.15

newspapers, other national magazines, letters on tape). At 42%, usage is markedly high among people in the 16 – 59 age group at blind registrable levels. However, as already noted in section 8.4.2.1 (Table 8.15), there is a wide range of verbal material other than fiction. A count of individuals shows that, while 14% use ordinary tape-players to listen to verbal material, only 3% use them for listening to stories or books (compare the 12% usage of Talking Books). In short, in contrast with Talking Book machines, ordinary tape-players are mostly used for listening to music and only secondarily for 'reading'. Furthermore, most of this 'reading' consists of non-fiction or information material.

8.4.3 Recording on tape

About 8% of visually impaired people as a whole, amounting to some 60,000 people, are estimated to use their tape-players for recording materials. Among those aged 16 – 59 the numbers using tape-players for this purpose reached 43% of blind people and 17% of partially sighted people. The corresponding totals for blind and partially sighted people aged 60 and over were 11% and 2%. Use of tapes for recording purposes is thus particularly prevalent among younger blind people. However, the age bias of the visually impaired population means that the one in ten of older blind people who do use tapes in this way are responsible for half of all tape usage for this purpose.

Table 8.17 contains data on the use of tapes for recording by all owners of ordinary tape-players. The number of interviews was too small to permit a breakdown by sub-groups of the types of material recorded. The various types of materials recorded were: letters, 9%; music, 6%; telephone numbers, 3%; notes for self, 3%; and shopping lists, 1%. The large 'other' category covers diverse items each below 1%; of these radio talks formed a major component (including *In Touch*, the BBC radio programme for visually impaired people), followed by addresses, recipes, study tapes and notes for meetings. Some 17% of those who owned an ordinary tape-player said that they never used it for either recording or listening.

Table 8.17 Material recorded on tape for personal use by visually impaired people with ordinary tape-players

'Do you record any of the following things?...anything else ?' (WQ63)

	All with a tape player (non TB)
	%
Letters	9
Music	6
Telephone numbers	3
Notes for self	3
Shopping list	1
Notes for meetings	#
Other	12
Never use the tape-player*	17
Base (population) = 100%	321K
(Number interviewed)	(395)

(395 respondents; 200 with no ordinary tape-player were not asked)
*From WQ61, Table 8.14

8.4.4 Difficulties experienced in operating tape-player

About 18% of those who use an ordinary tape-player reported having some difficulty in doing so. This is not very different from the percentage who reported difficulty operating the RNIB Talking Book machine. Similar sorts of reasons were given: 'finding and pressing the right button' and 'seeing how the tape goes in'. Difficulties were as likely to be expressed by younger as by older respondents and by respondents with low as with high residual vision.

8.4.5 Source of tapes

Respondents who used ordinary tape-players were asked (WQ66) where they obtained their tapes. As Table 8.18 shows, the single most frequently mentioned source was 'commercial shops' (60%), followed by 'friends and relatives' (23%), 'local talking newspapers' and 'local libraries' (13% each). The predominant use of ordinary tapes for listening to music explains the high usage of commercial shops. Likewise, the greater use of commercial shops by the non-registered reflects their less specialised use of tapes. In addition, more partially sighted people are not registered, and the tape material they use is likely to be similar to that used by sighted people.

Greater usage of specialist tape sources by the registered is not so much an indication of need but rather of a greater awareness of the material available.

Table 8.18   Sources of tapes used for ordinary tape-players by registration status

'Where do you get your tapes for your tape-player?' (WQ66)

	Registration status		Total
	R	NR	
	%	%	%
Shop	46	68	60
Friends/relatives	27	21	23
Local talking newspaper	24	6	13
Local library	24	7	13
Callbre	6	2	4
Local voluntary group	9	1	3
National talking newspaper	4	0	2
RNIB STL	2	0	1
Other	14	5	8
Base (population) = 100%	95K	171K	266K
(Number interviewed)	(256)	(93)	(349)

(349 respondents: 200 had no ordinary tape machine, 46 did not use their tape-player)

Registered respondents were more likely than non-registered to report that they obtained tapes from either the local library (24 and 7 per cent) or from local talking newspapers (24 and 6 per cent). Registered respondents also obtained more tapes from services for the blind such as Calibre, RNIB Student Tape Library (STL), now the RNIB Cassette Library, and national talking newspapers.

Age also provided some differences. Respondents under 60 were more likely that the older age group to get their tapes from shops (80 and 55 per cent), and less likely to obtain them from the local library (3 and 15 per cent). Slightly more friends and relatives provided tapes for those aged 75 and over, than for younger respondents.

Overall, the RNIB Student Tape Library Service was mentioned by only 1% of respondents. This reflects the general perception (not discouraged by RNIB) at the time the survey was carried out that this was a specialist service for students.

8.5 RNIB compact tape services

While approximately three-quarters of registered blind and partially sighted people had heard of RNIB tape services, just over half (51%) of all respondents either were not currently using an RNIB tape service or said that they had not heard of any of the RNIB tape services offered to visually impaired people.

Table 8.19 Awareness of RNIB tape services among the visually impaired population, by registration status, and two age groups

	Age and residual vision				Total
	16 – 59		60 +		
	R	NR	R	NR	
	%	%	%	%	%
Aware of RNIB tape services	87	65	71	40	49
Not aware of tape services	13	35	29	60	51
Total %	100	100	100	100	100
Base (population)	29K	48K	140K	540K	757K
(Number interviewed)	(215)	(84)	(137)	(159)	(595)

Table 8.19 brings together all the questions asked about use or knowledge of RNIB tape services. Registration and age are important factors in awareness of the RNIB tape services. Awareness among the registered was 74% compared with 42% among the non-registered, while among the under-60s and the older age groups it was 73 and 46 per cent. Table 8.19 shows that this difference is maintained within the age groups, the registered always being more aware of the services; it should be remembered that younger respondents are more likely to be registered.

Table 8.20 shows the level of awareness and use of the services. Best known was the RNIB Talking Book Service; overall 46% of respondents knew about it, including those who were current or past users. However, nearly two-thirds of those who knew about the service had not used it.

About 4% of all registrable blind and partially sighted people knew about RNIB's Student Tape Library (STL – now called the RNIB Cassette Library) and Express Reading Service (ERS). However, among people who possessed an ordinary tape-player, and who could therefore use the service, awareness increased to 12%. Among the key target group of registrable blind people under 60, awareness levels were much higher; STL and ERS were known by approximately 30 and 20 per cent respectively.

Just over 2% of the visually impaired population were actually using STL. Under 1% reported using ERS.

Table 8.20 Awareness and use of RNIB tape services among the visually impaired population, by registration status

	Registration status		Total
	R	NR	
	%	%	%
Awareness of tape services			
RNIB Talking Books	72	38	46
RNIB STL	14	1	4
RNIB ERS	6	4	4
Not aware of any of the tape services	26	58	51
Using/used tape services			
RNIB Talking Book	49	6	16
RNIB STL	4	0	1
RNIB ERS	#	0	#
Not aware of tape service and have tape-player	9	17	15
Not aware of tape service and without tape-player	16	41	36
Never use tape-player	4	8	7
Base (population) = 100%	169K	588K	757K
(Number interviewed)	(352)	(243)	(595)

(595 respondents)

These figures suggest that much could be done to raise the awareness and subsequent use of both RNIB compact tape services. However, demand for ERS may be very limited. When ERS was explained to those who had not heard of it, and they were then asked whether they might use it, fewer than 2% said that they would. Awareness of both services was greater among respondents with low residual vision. This indicates that those with useful residual vision may make more extensive use of printed materials.

Note to section 8.2.2

The 12% ownership of Talking Book machines (section 12.3.1) yields an estimated population projection of about 90,000 on a base of 757,000. There are about 70,000 (9%) known members of the Service. There are several possible reasons for this discrepancy. The 95% confidence interval for a 12% estimate on a sample of 595 is $+/-3\%$. RNIB Talking Books were not specifically mentioned in the question. In addition a response error may have occurred because many respondents may previously have had a Talking Book machine; some of these people may have responded inaccurately, saying that they still had one.

9 Readers

9.1 Visually impaired people who use a reader

9.1.1 Profile

Overall, 40% of visually impaired people said that they use a reader. That is, they obtain information from print by getting a sighted person to read aloud. The percentage varies with age, residual vision and registration status.

Two statistics demonstrate the most extreme form of this variation. Seventy-four per cent of blind people under 60 are read to, while only 28% of partially sighted people over 60 use this method of reading.

As Table 9.1.a. shows, overall more people with lower levels of residual vision use a reader: 56% of blind people, 30% of partially sighted people. Or, put the other way round, 44 and 70 per cent respectively of blind and partially sighted people do not use a reader.

Younger people are read to more than the elderly: 56 and 38 per cent respectively of those aged under 60 and 60 and over. (There is no difference between the 60 – 74 and the 75+ age groups.)

Table 9.1.a. also shows that the age difference is independent of differences in sight level. Seventy-four and 54 per cent respectively of young and elderly blind people are read to. Among partially sighted people the corresponding age group totals are 44 and 28 per cent.

Registration is an important factor: 64% of the registered compared with 32% of the non-registered have a reader. Age is related to registration in that more of the young are registered, but most of the registration effect is independent of this correlation. Table 9.1.b. shows that 74% of the registered aged under 60 have a reader compared with 44% of the non-registered in the same age group. Among those aged 60 and over, the corresponding figures are 62 and 32 per cent.

Table 9.1.a. shows that just over half of blind people (56%) and just over a quarter of partially sighted people (29%) have someone who reads to them. While the figure for blind people correlates closely with the percentage unable to read our large print card (Table 6.3), the

Table 9.1.a. Use of a reader among visually impaired people by residual vision and age

'Now, I would like to move on to reading. Do you ever have anything read to you? I mean anything at all, not just books or papers?' (WQ72)

	Age and residual vision				Total
	16 – 59		60 +		
	B	PS	B	PS	
	%	%	%	%	%
Yes, read to	74	44	54	28	40
No, not read to	26	56	47	72	60
Total %	100	100	100	100	100
Base (population)	29K	48K	270K	410K	757K
(Number interviewed)	(137)	(162)	(130)	(166)	(595)

Table 9.1.b. Use of a reader among visually impaired people by registration and age (WQ72)

	Age and registration status				Total
	16 – 59		60 +		
	N	NR	N	NR	
	%	%	%	%	%
Yes, read to	74	44	62	32	40
No, not read to	26	56	38	68	60
Total %	100	100	100	100	100
Base (population)	30K	47K	140K	540K	757K
(Number interviewed)	(215)	(84)	(137)	(159)	(595)

figure for partially sighted people seems high in relation to those unable to read our card (3% of the under-60s and 14% of those aged 60 and over).

9.1.2   Frequency of use

Residual vision is the most important factor in determining the frequency with which respondents were read to. Table 9.2 shows that 44% of blind people and 25% of partially sighted people reported being read to most days. There is a small but statistically significant tendency for people in the 75 + age group to be read to less often than younger people: 30 compared with 45 per cent of those aged 74 and under were read to on most days.

Table 9.2 Frequency read to by reader

'How often does someone read to you. Is that most days, at least once a week, once a month or less often?' (WQ74)

	Residual vision		All with a personal reader
	B	PS	
	%	%	%
Most days	44	25	35
At least weekly	27	43	34
Once a month	12	7	10
Less than monthly	17	25	21
Total %	100	100	100
Base (population)	163K	132K	296K
(Number interviewed)	(196)	(136)	(332)

(332 respondents: 256 not read to; no information for 7 respondents)

9.1.3 Items visually impaired people have read to them

Table 9.3 shows the items respondents listed as having read to them. 'Postcards/letters' (88%), 'bills' (77%), 'official forms' (76%) and 'newspapers' (53%) were the items most frequently mentioned. 'Books' and 'magazines' were mentioned by 7 and 19 per cent respectively.

The particular relevance of this list of items becomes clear in Chapter 15, which shows that 'bills and paperwork' are among the tasks that visually impaired people find most difficult and challenging.

Table 9.3 Items read to visually impaired people

'What do you have read to you? Do you have...?' (WQ77)

	All with a personal reader
	%
Postcards/letters	88
Bills	77
Official forms	76
Newspapers	53
Magazines	19
Books	7
Recipes	3
Prices/instructions	2
Bible	1
Base (population) = 100%	292K
(Number interviewed)	(335)

(335 respondents: 257 not read to; no information for 3)

The items mentioned scarcely varied in relation to residual vision and age. Books tended to be mentioned more by the under-75s than by those aged 75 or over: 30 and 12 per cent respectively. (There was no difference between the 16 – 59 and 60 – 74 age groups.) Magazines, by contrast, were mentioned more often by the under-60s than by the older age groups: 15 and 6 per cent respectively. (Here there was no difference between the 60 – 74 and the 75 + age groups.)

9.1.4 Items visually impaired people dislike having read to them

Table 9.4 shows that half the respondents did not mention any item which they particularly objected having read to them. The two items most disliked, 'private letters' (42%) and 'bills' (35%) were also among the items most read. Overall, more partially sighted people disliked being read to, 59% compared with 43% of blind people mentioning an item to which they objected being read. For specific items the corresponding percentages were 51 and 36 per cent respectively for 'private letters', and 47 and 27 per cent respectively for 'bills'.

Table 9.4 Items people with a visual impairment dislike having read to them, by two age groups and residual vision

'Some people have said that there are things which are private and they wish other people didn't have to read them out for them. Do you feel like that about anything, for instance...?' (WQ73)

	Age and residual vision				All with a personal reader
	16 – 59		60 +		
	B	PS	B	PS	
	%	%	%	%	%
Private letters	47	34	35	54	42
Bills	23	20	27	52	35
Newspapers	4	3	8	2	5
Bank statements	1	3	4	7	5
Prices and instructions	0	6	0	4	2
Other items	9	14	15	25	18
No dislikes mentioned	52	57	57	38	50
Base (population) = 100%	22K	21K	145K	113K	300K
(Number interviewed)	(117)	(74)	(84)	(63)	(338)

(338 respondents: 257 don't have anything read to them)

The major difference revealed by Table 9.4 between elderly partially sighted people and those aged under 60 is that elderly people object more to letters (54 to 34 per cent) and bills (52 to 20 per cent) being read to them. This may be because elderly people, whose visual impairment is more likely to have begun more recently (Chapter 5), find it more difficult to come to terms with being read to. Younger respondents, whose impairment has started earlier, have had a longer time to adjust. Furthermore, since elderly visually impaired people are more likely to depend on 'strangers' to read to them (section 9.1.5), they may object rather more to this intrusion on their privacy.

9.1.5   Identity of readers

Table 9.5 shows that those who read to visually impaired people are, in order of frequency, 'someone in the household' (53%), 'other relative' (27%), 'friend or colleague' (17%), and the 'home help' (9%). The pattern of readers reflects differences in the informal support network enjoyed by young and elderly visually impaired people. Among the under-60s 'someone in the household' (84%) is followed, a long way behind, by 'other relatives' (11%), 'friend or colleague' (8%) and 'home help'(2%). Among elderly people, 'someone in the household' (48%) remains the single category most frequently mentioned, but is followed far more closely by 'other relative' (30%), 'friend or colleague' (19%) and 'home help' (10%).

Table 9.5   Identity of readers to visually impaired people, by age

'Who reads to you most often?' (WQ75)

	Age		All with a personal reader
	16 – 59	60 +	
	%	%	%
Someone in the household	84	48	53
Other relative	11	30	27
Friend or colleague	8	19	17
Home help	2	10	9
Local blind association	#	#	#
Health service person	2	0	#
Other	#	2	2
Base (population) = 100%	43K	252K	295K
(Number interviewed)	(191)	(146)	(337)

(337 respondents: 257 were not read to; no information for 1)

The general pattern is that, as visually impaired people grow older, sources of help move from within to outside the household. Chapter 15 covers this in more detail, examining the way visually impaired people tackle the tasks of daily living, including 'mail' and 'paperwork', for both of which reading ability is essential.

In Section 3.4 we have already learnt that older visually impaired people are more likely to live in single households; thus any print requiring reading must wait for someone outside the household.

Perhaps the most significant point is the frequency with which the 'reading service' is offered (Table 9.2). For example, of the 56% of blind people who are read to, nearly three-quarters (71%) are read to at least once a week, and the majority of them on most days. Of the just over one-quarter (29%) of partially sighted people who need a reader service, two-thirds (68%) are read to at least weekly. Given that a reading service to visually impaired people does not form part of the statutory social services, this represents a considerable, and without doubt necessary, level of informal help.

9.2 Users and non-users of readers

9.2.1 Self-assessed need for more readers

To gauge the existence of an unmet need for more personal reading, respondents were asked whether they would like to be read to or read to more frequently. The overall demand for more reading (8%), shown in Table 9.6.a., masks differences in demand within the individual sub-groups. For example blind people, particularly in the younger age group, want more reader support; 17% of blind respondents under 60 said that they needed more help.

Table 9.6.a.   Demand for readers, by residual vision and age

'Would you like to have somebody read to you (more often?' (WQ78)

| | Age | | Residual vision | | Total |
| | 16 – 59 | 60 + | B | PS | |
	%	%	%	%	%
Yes	17	7	15	7	8
No/don't know	83	93	85	93	92
Total %	100	100	100	100	100
Base (population)	77K	680K	300K	457K	757K
(Number interviewed)	(137)	(162)	(130)	(166)	(595)

Table 9.6.b. shows that once visually impaired people have experienced the benefits of reader support they are significantly more likely to want more of such help than those who have not experienced it. For example, as many as 20% of visually impaired people under 60 currently using a reader say that they would like to be read to more often.

Table 9.6.b. Demand for readers from people with and without readers

'Would you like to have somebody read to you /more often?' (WQ78)

	Those with existing readers			Those without readers		
	16 – 59	60 +	All	16 – 59	60 +	All
	%	%	%	%	%	%
Yes	20	11	12	13	4	4
No	80	89	88	87	96	96
Total %	100	100	100	100	100	100
Base (population)	43K	257K	301K	34K	422K	456K
(Number interviewed)	(191)	(147)	(339)	(107)	(148)	(256)

9.2.2 Reasons for not wanting a reader

Table 9.7 shows that the single most mentioned reason, reported by 37% of respondents, for not wanting to increase the use of readers was simply that people preferred to manage for themselves. The totals, 44 and 26 per cent for partially sighted and blind people respectively, vary with residual vision. Section 9.2.3 examines how far these figures correspond with respondents' actual ability to read print for themselves. The reason that no help was needed as yet also varied with residual vision, being given by 12% of partially sighted and 3% of blind respondents. Fourteen per cent of blind people and 8% of partially sighted people said that they were read to when they needed it. The responses 'too old/forgetful' and 'too deaf', amounting to 5% in total, were mentioned solely by those aged 60 or over.

Table 9.7 Reasons for not wanting to increase use of readers

Respondents who would not like to be read to more often were asked: 'Why is that?' (WQ79)

	Residual vision		Total
	B	PS	
	%	%	%
Prefer to manage by myself	26	44	37
Relatives read when needed	14	8	10
Don't need help yet	3	12	8
Prefer/like radio/television	14	3	7
Don't like reading	4	5	5
Can't take things in	3	5	4
Too old/forgetful	8	2	4
Not same as reading for self	4	2	3
Too deaf	2	6	1
Other	42	23	30
Base (population) = 100%	268K	432K	700K
(Number interviewed)	(228)	(305)	(533)

(533 respondents: 62 respondents were not asked WQ79)

9.2.3 Use and non-use of readers and print reading

In Chapter 7 it was noted that 65% of visually impaired people could read the large print test and said that they normally do read print (section 7.2.). This overall figure of those able to read print by themselves compares fairly closely with the 60% who do not use a reader (section 9.1.1). About 80% of partially sighted and 40% of blind people read the test and said that they normally read print (section 7.2). Again, this accords fairly well with the 70% of partially sighted and the 44% of blind people who said that they did not use a reader (section 9.1.1).

Forty two per cent said that they could read ordinary newspaper print; 51% of partially sighted people and 25% of blind people (section 7.3). These figures again correspond quite closely with the totals (44 and 26 per cent respectively) noted in section 9.2.2 saying that they could manage for themselves.

From this evidence alone and without more detailed analysis, there does appear to be a broad correspondence between the use and demand for readers and the print-reading ability of visually impaired people.

10 Braille

10.1 Introduction

This chapter examines braille and Moon, the other embossed reading method for visually impaired people. In addition, comparisons in section 10.9 are made with the last major national survey of braille and Moon usage made for the (then) Ministry of Health by Gray and Todd (1968). (The survey was carried out in 1965 and the report published in 1968.) The present survey has been designed primarily to set the role of braille in the wider context of the reading habits of visually impaired people, and is therefore less appropriate for an analysis of the reading habits of braille readers. Caution is necessary in drawing inferences where the percentages quoted are based on a small number of braille readers (section 21.4).

10.2 Establishing braille usage

Respondents who said that they knew what braille was were asked the following question: 'Have you ever had any lessons, or tried to teach yourself to read braille?' (WQ9) Those who answered 'yes' to this question were then asked the following supplementary question: 'Did you become good enough to understand a braille book or magazine?' (WQ15)

10.3 The braille user group

These two questions, WQ9 and WQ15, were deliberately given the identical wording used by Gray and Todd. Following their example, the two questions together allow visually impaired users and non-users of braille to be placed into one of three categories, as Table 10.1 shows.

We use the term 'braille reader' to describe those who have become sufficiently fluent in braille to read a book or magazine. These respondents were later asked a series of questions about their use of braille (sections 10.5, 10.7).

Table 10.1 shows that only 3% (2.51% rounded up) of visually impaired people are braille readers as defined above (84 respondents in our sample). On a base population of 757,000 visually impaired people, our estimate is that there are some 19,000 braille readers. Of these, about

Table 10.1 Braille readership in relation to age

'Have you ever had any lessons, or tried to teach yourself to read braille?' (WQ9)

'Did you become good enough to understand a braille book or magazine?' (WQ15)

	Age		Total
	16 – 59	60 +	
	%	%	%
Never learned braille (WQ9)*	73	98	95
Learned but not good enough to read (WQ15)	13	1	2
Learned and got good enough to read (WQ15)	14	1	3
Total %	100	100	100
Base (population)	77K	680K	757K
(Number interviewed)	(229)	(296)	(595)

*includes no/don't know from WQ8

70%, some 13,000 people, are still active readers, and some 10,000 write in braille as well (section 10.7).

Gray and Todd's survey of braille reading was confined to registered blind people under 80 years old. Before the two surveys' estimates of the number of braille readers can be compared, it is necessary to examine the specific characteristics of braille readers and non-readers.

10.4 Characteristics of braille readers

10.4.1 Age of braille readers

Table 10.1 shows the extreme extent to which braille usage is concentrated among younger visually impaired people. Some 27% of those aged 16 – 59 had learnt some braille, 14% well enough to read a book or a magazine. The corresponding proportion of those aged 60 or over is 1% in each category. It is important to remember that in numerical terms most visually impaired people are aged 60 or over. Thus 1% (1.2% rounded) of elderly braille readers represents a population projection of about 8,000 on a base of 680,000. Fourteen per cent of younger readers represents 11,000 readers on a base of 77,000.

10.4.2 Registration status

Table 10.2.a. shows that 81% of registered blind people under 60 were taught braille. Given that braille is inappropriate for a few people (e.g.

some multi-handicapped blind people), this represents a high penetration of braille teaching. However the fact that 30% learnt braille but failed to master it sufficiently to read a magazine or book is of concern.

Table 10.2.a. Braille readership, by residual vision and registration status among visually impaired people aged 16 – 59 (WQ9 and WQ15)

	Registered		Non-registered		Total
	Residual vision		Residual vision		
	B	PS	B	PS	
	%	%	%	%	%
Never learned braille	19	66	95	96	73
Learned but not good enough to read	30	25	0	5	13
Learned and got good enough to read	51	9	6	0	14
Total %	100	100	100	100	100
Base (population)	17K	12K	12K	36K	77K
(Number interviewed)	(123)	(92)	(14)	(70)	(299)

Table 10.2.b. Braille readership, by residual vision and registration status among visually impaired people aged 60 + (WQ9 and WQ15)

	Registered		Non-registered		Total
	Residual vision		Residual vision		
	B	PS	B	PS	
	%	%	%	%	%
Never learned braille	84	99	98	100	97
Learned but not good enough to read	7	#	2	0	1
Learned and got good enough to read	9	0	0	0	1
Total %	100	100	100	100	100
Base (population)	91K	49K	180K	361K	680K
(Number interviewed)	(74)	(63)	(56)	(103)	(296)

Tables 10.2.a. and 10.2.b. not only confirm the concentration of braille readers among younger visually impaired people but also indicate a further concentration among those people registered as blind. Among

registrable blind people aged 16 – 59, 51 and 6 per cent of registered and non-registered respectively are braille readers. Our sample contained only fourteen younger non-registered blind people (section 21.9), and so caution is required when conclusions are made from percentages and population projections on such a small base. Nevertheless, the difference between 51 and 6 per cent far exceeds any possible random sampling error, even on such a small base. Moreover, the findings for those aged 60 + , and for partially sighted people, increase confidence in the conclusion that registration, far more than age and residual vision level, is the crucial factor. Although only 1% of older visually impaired people can read a book or magazine in braille, all these are registered blind, and none at all are unregistered blind or partially sighted. Among the younger respondents, 9% of the registered partially sighted, and none of the non-registered partially sighted, said that they could read braille.

10.4.3   Age of onset of visual impairment

Table 10.3.a. confirms that the ability to read braille is closely related to the age of onset of the visual impairment. People who lost their vision at birth or before the age of 17 are most likely to become braille readers. Thirteen per cent of these did so, compared with 4% of those aged 17 – 59 and less than 0.5% of those aged 60 or over.

As so many more visually impaired people lose their sight between the ages of 17 and 59 than before the age of 17, the 4% (4.4% rounded) of this group who become braille readers represents, in numerical terms, a substantial part of the total. As Table 10.3.b. shows, almost all of them are registrable blind rather than partially sighted. Population projections indicate that about 8,000 braille readers (4.4% of 182,000) lost their sight in their post-school years, compared with about 10,000 (13% of 78,000) who lost their sight at an earlier age.

Assuming that the age at which braille is learned is closely related to age of onset of vision loss, the data in Table 10.3.a. do not suggest that those who learn braille in childhood are more likely in relative terms to become good enough to read than those who study it between the ages of 17 and 59. Ten per cent of the former group learned braille but did not become good enough to read, while 13% did, which produces a 56% success rate (13/23). Among the older group, the corresponding percentages are 4 and 4, producing a 50% success rate. This difference in success rate is well short of statistical significance.

Given these comparable success rates, and knowing that a significant number of the successful adult learners are at the older end of the age range, two conclusions are suggested. First, more extensive teaching of braille to adults under 60 would be likely to produce a fair degree of success. Second, given that, according to our findings, only 1% of

Table 10.3.a. Braille readership and age of onset of visual impairment among all visually impaired people (WQ9, WQ15)

	Age of onset			Total
	Birth to 16	17 – 59	60 +	
	%	%	%	%
Never learned braille	77	92	99	95
Learned but not good enough to read	10	4	#	2
Learned and got good enough to read	13	4	0	3
Total %	100	100	100	100
Base (population)	78K	182K	456K	716K
(Number interviewed)	(151)	(263)	(156)	(570)

(570 respondents: no age of onset given for 23; no information on the understanding of braille for 2)

\# less than 0.5% (only 1 respondent over 60 reported learning any braille)

Table 10.3.b. Braille readership related to age of onset of visual impairment and current residual vision levels (WQ9, WQ15)

	Age of onset and residual vision				Residual vision		Total
	Birth to 16		17 +				
	B	PS	B	PS	B	PS	
	%	%	%	%	%	%	%
Never learned braille	61	90	95	99	77	98	95
Learned but not good enough to read	12	8	3	#	10	1	2
Learned and got good enough to read	27	2	3	#	13	1	3
Total %	100	100	100	100	100	100	100
Base (population)	36K	42K	251K	386K	78K	638K	716K
(Number interviewed)	(73)	(78)	(184)	(235)	(151)	(419)	(570)

(570 respondents: no age of onset given for 23; no information on the understanding of braille for 2)

elderly visually impaired people are taught braille, an opportunity exists to develop braille teaching among this age group. One possible argument against expanding braille readership among the over-60s is that Moon may be 'more appropriate' for this age group. However, section 10.6.2 shows that penetration of Moon is extremely low, and so in practice it does not provide an alternative.

10.4.4 Residual vision level

Table 10.4 shows the extent to which braille reading is related to residual vision levels required for reading print. Three residual vision levels are distinguished: NLP (no light perception), LP (light perception) but unable to read large print, and able to read large print. These three levels correspond to QRVS7 scale point zero, with the remainder divided by the results of the reading test (sections 6.1 and 6.2.3). The total of braille readers in these three categories is 18, 5 and 1 per cent respectively. The corresponding totals in the same three categories of all those who learnt braille, whether or not they got good enough to read, are 26, 10 and 3 per cent.

Table 10.4   Residual vision level and learning of braille (WQ9 and WQ15)

	Residual vision			Total
	NLP	Light perception and reading large print*		
		Not read	Read	
	%	%	%	%
Never learned braille	74	90	97	95
Learned but not good enough to read	8	5	2	2
Learned and got good enough to read	18	5	1	3
Total %	100	100	100	100
Base (population)	27K	195K	535K	757K
(Number interviewed)	(48)	(164)	(383)	(595)

*Large print refers to the sample print respondents were asked to read (section 6.2.3)

Thus Table 10.4 reveals a very strong correlation between braille readership and residual vision, and this may well be produced by more than one factor. The threefold difference between those with NLP and the next category (LP but unable to read large print) is large enough to be statistically significant (despite the small base of 48, see section 21.4). Since neither of these two groups can see well enough to read large print, they can be deemed to have the same incentive to succeed at learning braille. This therefore suggests a difference in the opportunity to learn. We noted in section 3.9.4 (see also Table 3.14) that those with NLP are all registered blind, while the non-registered but registrable blind, though still less than our 6/60 cut-off point, are skewed towards those with some light perception. The inference is that the very high incidence of braille readership among people with NLP, and so in the extreme residual vision stratum, is an indirect consequence of the increased likelihood that people with NLP will be registered and so form part of the welfare system catering for blind people.

10.5   Learning braille

10.5.1   Lessons and self-tuition

Those who responded positively to WQ9, 'Have you ever had any lessons, or tried to teach yourself to read braille?' (151 respondents, population projection 39,000) were then asked the following supplementary question: 'Is that lessons from other people, self-taught or both?' The responses to these three alternatives, as shown in Table 10.5.a., were 74, 8, and 18 per cent respectively. Thus for most people, learning braille is through formal lessons.

Table 10.5.a.   Methods of learning braille

'Have you ever had any lessons, or tried to teach yourself to read braille?' If 'Yes', PROBE: 'Is that lessons from other people, self-taught or both?' (WQ9)

	All who have tried to learn braille
	%
Formal lessons only	74
Self-taught and lessons	18
Self-taught only	8
Total %	100
Base (population)	39K
(Number interviewed)	(151)

(151 respondents who said that they had tried to learn braille; 444 did not learn braille)

We already know (Table 10.1) that only 3 out of 5 (60%) of those who try to learn braille become good enough to read a braille book or magazine. Table 10.5.b. provides clear evidence that self-tuition is an inadequate basis for learning braille. No one who attempted to learn braille on his or her own, without formal tuition, became good enough to read a book.

Table 10.5.b. Proficiency in braille through different forms of learning (WQ9 and WQ15)

	Able to read book	Not able to read book	All who learnt braille
	%	%	%
Formal lessons only	81	65	74
Self-taught and lessons	19	19	19
Self-taught only	0	16	8
Total %	100	100	100
Base (population)	19K	17K	36K
(Number interviewed)	(84)	(65)	(149)

(149 respondents: no information on level of braille proficiency for 2 respondents; 444 did not learn braille)

10.5.2 Source of braille lessons

Respondents who had received lessons in braille were asked (at WQ13) who provided them. The results, given in Table 10.6, show that the chief sources were welfare services (36%), schools (28%), RNIB (12%), and local blind associations (7%).

Table 10.6 Source of braille lessons

'Who gave you the (braille) lessons?' (WQ13)

	Age		Total
	16 – 59	60 +	
	%	%	%
Welfare services*	38	35	36
School	34	24	28
RNIB	23	0	12
Local blind association	2	12	7
Other	3	29	17
Base (population) = 100%	19K	17K	36K
(Number interviewed)	(120)	(22)	(142)

(142 respondents: 9 respondents were self-taught; 444 had not learnt braille)
*Includes all services under this broad heading, e.g. mobility officer, social worker for the blind

The composite 'other' category (17%) is almost entirely confined to people aged 60 and over, many of whom could not say who gave them braille lessons. The single category of provider mentioned most often was 'friend or neighbour'. Likewise, mentions of local blind associations were almost entirely confined to elderly people. The welfare agent most frequently named was 'social worker for the blind' (by 23% of this age group), the others being mainly 'technical officers'.

RNIB is a very significant provider of tuition to the younger age group, where by far the greatest concentration of braille readers lies (Table 10.6). Twenty-three per cent of 16 – 59 year olds, but no one in the older age group, mentioned RNIB directly. Most of this RNIB tuition is likely to have taken place at an RNIB rehabilitation centre, but a number of respondents may have attended an RNIB school. In addition, many respondents answering 'school' may have learnt braille at an RNIB school.

Although the other composite categories, school and welfare services, show slightly higher percentages (34 and 38) than RNIB in the younger age group, the small size of the sample should be taken into account. Only 120 respondents in this age band said that they had learnt braille, and on this base the differences between the various categories are not statistically significant.

10.6 Moon

10.6.1 Numbers learning Moon

Moon, which was invented in 1847, eighteen years after braille, is promoted as simpler to learn than braille, and also as requiring less sensitivity in the fingers to read; for these reasons it has largely been considered more suitable for older blind people. However, it has been developed far less than braille, and until recently a Moon writer has not been readily available, which has limited its everyday use.

The series of questions we asked about Moon readership paralleled those asked about braille. However, the low number of respondents made detailed analysis impossible. Our sample contained 37 people who claimed to have learned Moon, but only four of these said that they had become good enough to read a book or magazine, and only one was a current user.

The next section provides detailed evidence of the lack of knowledge of Moon and the low learning success rate. At 11%, this compares very unfavourably with braille success rates. Furthermore, only one person of the four has sustained the reading habit, which also compares very unfavourably with braille.

10.6.2 Awareness

Respondents were asked (WQ24) about their awareness of Moon, in a parallel question to that asked about braille. While braille was widely known, by more than 8 in 10 respondents, fewer than 1 in 10 had heard of Moon (Table 10.7). Unlike braille, awareness of which was spread across age and sight level groups, Moon was mainly known among younger respondents with low residual vision; the highest awareness level (48%) was among registrable blind respondents under 60. Twenty-seven, 13 and 2 per cent respectively of the under-60s, 60 – 74 year olds and those aged 75 + knew what Moon was (Table 10.7).

Table 10.7 Awareness of Moon and braille, by residual vision within three age groups

'Do you know what Moon is?' (WQ24)

'Can I just check, do you know what braille is?' (WQ8)

	Age and residual vision						Total
	16 – 59		60 – 74		75 +		
	B	PS	B	PS	B	PS	
	%	%	%	%	%	%	%
Moon awareness							
Know what Moon is	48	13	25	6	4	1	7
Not know what Moon is	52	87	75	94	96	98	93
Braille awareness							
Know what braille is	94	96	86	94	84	83	87
Not know braille	6	4	14	6	16	17	13
Total %	100	100	100	100	100	100	100
Base (population)	30K	47K	65K	115K	205K	295K	757K
(Number interviewed)	(137)	(162)	(55)	(69)	(75)	(97)	(595)

While 48% of blind people under 60 know of Moon, the figures are only 25% of those aged between 60 and 74 years and 4% of those aged 75 and over. Since one of Moon's benefits is considered to be ease of learning in comparison with braille, particularly for older visually impaired people, this low level of awareness should give cause for concern. Awareness of Moon is concentrated among registered people, in contrast with braille, awareness of which cuts across the registered/non-registered dichotomy. Perhaps awareness of any 'new' product or service for visually impaired people will only be diffused among those who are part of the visually impaired 'system'. Those outside the 'system' may need to make considerable efforts to find out what is available.

10.7 Use of braille

10.7.1 Current braille users

Those 84 respondents who said that they had become proficient enough to read a book or magazine represent 3% of visually impaired people, giving a population projection of 19,000. When asked an additional question – 'Do you ever use braille nowadays?' (WQ16) – approximately 1 in 3 answered in the negative. The 56 individuals who said 'yes' constitute the currently active braille readers in our sample, producing a population projection of 13,000. Further questions on the use made of braille were put only to this sub-group of currently active readers in the sample.

10.7.2   Use for reading

10.7.2.1   Material in braille

Table 10.8 shows the replies given by currently active readers of braille to the question 'Do you read any of the following in braille?' (WQ19). The first six items – magazines, private letters, books, *Radio Times*, bank statements and newspapers – were prompted from a check list.

Table 10.8   Material read in braille

'Do you read any of the following in braille?' WQ19

	Current braille readers
	%
Magazines	75
Private letters	72
Books	70
Radio Times	42
Bank statements	25
Newspapers	9
Calendars +	2
Technical special books +	1
Knitting/sewing instructions +	1
Other things +	27
Base (population) = 100%	13K
(Number interviewed)	(56)

(56 respondents: only asked of braille readers)
+ Items mentioned without prompting

A wide variety of other items was mentioned spontaneously, but only calendars (2%), technical special books and knitting and sewing instructions amounted individually to more than 1%. The 42% who read the braille *Radio Times* (produced by RNIB) gives an estimated readership of 5,000. RNIB has 4,000 subscribers which would suggest a larger number of readers. However, the two figures represent good agreement within the limits of sampling error, given that they are projected from a small base of only 56 respondents. About three-quarters of currently active readers said that they read 'books', 'magazines' and 'private letters' in braille, while 'bank statements' were mentioned by a quarter. Nine per cent of respondents mentioned braille newspapers, and other items such as 'knitting/sewing patterns', 'crossword puzzles' and 'calendars' were mentioned by one or two people.

When asked (at WQ20), only three respondents mentioned an item they would like to read that was currently unavailable in braille.

10.7.2.2   Access to braille and Moon books

The data discussed in this section are based on the 29 out of 56 current active readers who said (at WQ30) that they borrowed books in braille or (one person) Moon. Such low numbers provide only a thin basis for generalisation (section 21.4), and so findings must be interpreted cautiously. Note also that most respondents read braille, not Moon, books. Table 10.9 lists the various sources for borrowing.

Table 10.9   Main borrowing sources of braille and Moon books

'Where do you borrow braille/Moon books from?' (WQ31).

	Those who borrow braille or Moon books
	%
National Library for the Blind	73
RNIB (general, no specific service)	29
RNIB Braille Library	11
Local blind association	2
Social services	2
Monument Trust	2
Other lenders	12
Base (population) = 100%	6K
(Number interviewed)	(29)

(29 respondents: only those who borrow braille or Moon books)

Current readers are equally likely to buy or borrow books; only a small number said that they only bought them. The main source for borrowing books was the National Library for the Blind, mentioned by 73% of borrowers. Next most frequently mentioned was RNIB generally (29%), while the RNIB Braille Library was specifically reported by 11%. A number of other sources were named, including local blind associations, social services and the Monument Trust.

Two sources received significant mentions as sources for buying books (WQ32). Thirteen of the 22 respondents who said that they bought books mentioned RNIB, 9 the social services.

Of those respondents who were currently borrowing or buying books, 3 in 10 had not read any or had read 1 to 3 in the previous 6 months, while 4 in 10 had read 4 or more books in the same period (WQ33).

The vast majority of current buyers or borrowers were satisfied with the provision of braille and Moon books.

10.7.3 Use for writing

Braille readers (section 10.3) were asked (at WQ16) whether they used braille for writing. Their replies indicate that about 10,000 do, of whom 7,000 were aged under 60. A negligible fraction of the 7,000 were registered as partially sighted, or registrable as blind. About a third use a writing-frame, over half use a writing-machine, and about 1 in 5 use both. These fractions should be regarded as approximate because of the small base. The most frequently mentioned brand of machine was the Perkins brailler, which was named twice as often as the Stainsby (WQ18).

10.7.4 Braille and work

We estimate that about 3,000 people use braille at work (WQ21). This represents 10% of blind people of working age, or nearly half the registrable blind people currently at work. When these respondents were asked (at WQ23) if work would be easier if they could use braille more, they all responded negatively. There are several possible reasons for this response. The first is that the finding is completely accurate. The second is that respondents cannot visualise how their working situation might be improved with increased provision of braille. The third reason could be that they do not foresee that their employer would increase the amount of braille and therefore rationalise the situation as making the maximum current use of braille.

Perhaps not surprisingly, all those who reported using braille at work were registered.

10.8 Non-users of braille (or Moon)

10.8.1 Awareness

Overall, a high proportion of respondents (87%) reported awareness of braille (Table 10.7). The percentage was somewhat greater among younger respondents than that reported among elderly people (95 and 86 per cent respectively). Neither residual vision nor registration status had any impact on these figures.

10.8.2 Reasons for not learning braille

While lack of awareness may have something to do with why few people learn Moon, this is clearly not the case with braille. Those respondents who were aware of braille but had not received lessons (a large majority of the sample) were asked 'Would you like to learn braille if given the opportunity?' (WQ10). Eleven per cent answered 'yes', with blind and partially sighted respondents represented equally. Age was the main determinant in these responses, 31 and 9 per cent of the younger and older age groups respectively saying that they would like to learn braille.

The 11% who answered 'yes' were then asked 'Why haven't you tried to learn braille?' (WQ11). The two reasons most frequently given were that they did not think that they needed to yet and that they could manage without it; the latter answer was more common among partially sighted respondents. A small number, running across residual vision levels, said that they were 'too old' or 'physically not able to'. One-third of respondents gave answers such as 'don't know how to' (13%); 'nobody suggested it' (11%); 'no opportunity' (6%); 'never thought of it' (5%).

Those who responded 'no', i.e. they did not want to learn braille if given the opportunity, were asked 'Why is that?' (WQ12), with the results shown in Table 10.10. The reasons respondents most frequently gave were that they were too old (31%) or that they could see well enough to read (17%); a further 21% said that they did not need braille or didn't need it yet, which suggests either that they could read print or that they managed in some other way. Only 10% said that braille was too difficult.

Table 10.10 Reasons for not wanting to learn braille shown by residual vision (WQ12)

Those who do not want to learn braille			
	Residual vision		Total
	B	PS	
	%	%	%
Too old	40	26	31
See well enough to read	18	17	17
Don't need to	6	14	11
Hope sight will improve	6	15	11
Don't need to yet	9	10	10
Too difficult to learn	12	8	10
May if sight gets worse	2	8	5
Lack of feeling in fingers	4	4	4
Not interested in reading	4	4	4
Base (population) = 100%	198K	348K	546K
(Number interviewed)	(104)	(207)	(311)

(311 respondents: 151 learnt braille; 56 not aware of braille; 75 want to learn braille; 2 no data)

These replies reveal systematic differences between blind and partially sighted people. Some 40% of blind respondents, but only 26% of partially sighted respondents, gave being 'too old' as their main reason for not wanting to learn braille. No difference between blind and partially sighted respondents was revealed in the answer 'see well enough to read'. However, partially sighted respondents consistently produced more replies reflecting their better vision, e.g. 'don't need to', 'don't need to yet' and 'hope sight will improve'.

10.9 Comparison with Gray and Todd's 1965 survey

Tables 10.11.a. and 10.11.b. compare the findings on braille readership among registered blind people revealed in the RNIB and the Gray and Todd survey carried out in 1965. Gray and Todd's report does not contain population estimates, but the information provided allows others to do so (their section 2.10).

Although there are some discrepancies in the age bands compared, the broad comparisons that can be made between the two surveys are valid.

Table 10.11.a. Comparison of braille readership among registered blind people as shown in RNIB and Gray and Todd surveys

	1986 RNIB survey		1965, Gray and Todd survey	
	Age		Age	
	16 – 59	60 +	16 – 64	65 – 79
	%	%	%	%
Never learned braille	19	84	33	76
Learned but not good enough to read	30	7	27	13
Learned and got good enough to read	51	9	40	11
Total %	100	100	100	100
Base (population *)	17K	91K	24K	32K
(Number interviewed)	(123)	(74)	(1044)	(420)

(* Weighted data here applies only to RNIB data)
Source: Mobility and reading habits of the blind, Gray and Todd (1968)

Table 10.11.a. shows that in 1965, 33% of registered blind people aged 16–14 had never learned braille, compared with only 19% in 1986. This statistically significant difference suggests that during the two decades a notable increase in the teaching of braille to young registered blind people has occurred. From Table 10.11.b. we can see that in 1986 there were about 16,400 braille readers compared with about 13,000 in 1965. Only one of the 84 braille readers in our sample was over 75, and it is unlikely that Gray and Todd missed many braille readers by excluding people of 80 and over. Thus Table 10.11.b. implies that most of the growth in braille readers is among people aged about 60 to 74. We estimate that there are about 27,000 registered people in this age band (private households, 1986); the 8,000 braille readers shown in Table 10.11.b. represent about 30%, compared with 11% of the roughly

Table 10.11.b. Comparison of braille readership among registered blind people as shown in RNIB and Gray and Todd surveys – population estimates

	1986 RNIB survey		1965, Gray and Todd survey	
	Age		Age	
	16 – 59	60 +	16 – 64	65 – 79
	(000)	(000)	(000)	(000)
Never learned braille	3.4	76.4	7.9	24.3
Learned but not good enough to read	5.4	6.3	6.5	4.2
Learned and got good enough to read	8.2	8.2	9.6	3.5
Base (population *)	17.0K	91.0K	24.0K	32.0K

(* Weighted data here applies only to RNIB data)
Source: Mobility and reading habits of the blind, Gray and Todd (1968)

comparable age group in 1965. Since a difference of some 20% is statistically significant, we can be confident that this represents a real change.

These two findings – an increase in teaching of braille to the under-60s and over the years an increase in the number of braille readers over 60 – fit together, since cohorts of the former age group have moved into the latter age group.

Gray and Todd's results did not include partially sighted or non-registered braille readers, since these were not sampled. We estimate that there are about 1,000 additional registered partially sighted braille readers, and rather less than a further 1,000 non-registered blind readers in the 16 – 59 age group. (See Table 10.3.a., but note that the latter figure is based on only 14 respondents.) However, we also found that only about two-thirds of braille readers, those who learnt braille well enough to read a book or magazine, actually make use of their ability (section 10.7.1, WQ16). Gray and Todd did not ask this question, but both their and our estimates of active braille readers must be reduced accordingly.

We repeated a few of Gray and Todd's many detailed questions on braille readers' choice of material. Their sample of 1,044 and 420 registered respondents aged 16 – 64 and 65 – 79 respectively produced some 457 braille-reading respondents for more detailed analysis, while we had only 84. The small numbers in the RNIB sample therefore preclude close comparisons that rely solely on breakdowns confined to the braille reader sub-group.

Our survey estimates that there are 18,000 registered blind people aged 16 – 59, while Gray and Todd estimated 24,000 aged 16 – 64. The difference in age band and any real changes over the 20-year interval may not be the only reasons for the discrepancy. Our estimates are for private households, whereas Gray and Todd surveyed all the registered, which includes people living in communal establishments. (We estimated that a surprising proportion, 22%, of people aged 16 – 59 likely to be registered blind live in communal establishments; see Chapter 21.) Gray and Todd excluded from their sample anyone classified by the local authority as mentally sub-normal, mentally ill, or deaf, which may have covered many people living in communal establishments.

11 Overview of Reading Habits and Communications Media

11.1 Reading habits

11.1.1 Introduction

Chapters 7 – 10 (on large print, tapes, personal readers and braille) provide detailed information on each of these separate reading methods, but do not discuss their use in combination. While most visually impaired people read in more than one way, they generally prefer a particular method. This chapter examines the choice of media and also reviews data collected on writing habits.

11.1.2 The extent of reading

Respondents were asked to consider all the media together in the following terms: 'I would like you to think about all the different ways in which people can read, whether ordinary print, braille, Moon or tapes or having a sighted person read to you...'.

Following this introduction, respondents were asked: 'Would you say that you read now more, or less or about the same amount as before your sight problem began?' (WQ82) Overall, 9% said that they read more, 21% the same and 69% less. Interestingly the responses were similar across the three age groups, except that 77% of blind people aged over 75 said that they read less. The finding that almost one-third (30%) of blind and partially sighted people read as much or more than before the onset of their vision problems is quite startling. Indeed just over one-third (35%) of blind people under 60 said that they read more than before. While we should not be complacent about the 69% who read less, this increase in reading represents a substantial tribute to the individuals concerned and to the various organisations that supply their needs.

11.1.3 The media used

Following the introductory question (WQ82), respondents were asked (WQ83) about the media they employed most frequently. The results, shown in Table 11.1, reveal that the reading habits of blind people are quite different from those of partially sighted people. Personal readers

(33%), ordinary print (29%) and tapes (24%) are the media most frequently used by blind people in each of the three age groups.

Two perhaps surprising aspects of the data are that, for 29% of blind people, ordinary print is the most popular medium, and, second, that individual readers are used so frequently. Statutory and voluntary organisations should note this second conclusion, for this most frequent form of reading receives little or no outside support and encouragement and is almost always left to the individual's initiative. While such initiative should not be discouraged, it would seem important for both the statutory social services and the voluntary sector to expand their work in this area, particularly given the evidence of unmet need among younger blind people (Chapter 9).

Table 11.1   Use of reading methods by residual vision

'Still thinking about all the different ways of reading, which do you use most often...?' (WQ83)

	Residual vision		Total
	B	PS	
	%	%	%
Ordinary print	29	60	48
Large print	14	30	24
Personal reader	33	12	21
Tapes (including Talking Books)	24	6	13
Braille	2	0	1
Moon	0	0	0
Don't know	10	5	7
Nothing reported	#	2	1
Base (population) = 100%	301K	456K	757K
(Number interviewed)	(267)	(328)	(595)

Overall, 2% of registrably blind people used braille most frequently; 12% of under-60s and 3% of 60 – 74 year-olds did so. There are two reasons why braille cannot be expected to be the most frequently used form, even among younger people. First, as Chapter 10 shows, braille is only used by a minority of blind people; second, insufficient material is produced in braille to make it a dominant reading medium.

As Table 11.1 shows, for partially sighted people ordinary print (60%) is the dominant reading form by far, followed by large print (30%). The popularity of these two media varied very little across the different age groups, although people over 75 showed a greater preference (34%) for large print compared with those aged 16 to 74 (22%). Personal readers and tapes trailed at 12 and 6 per cent respectively.

It is worth noting that so many partially sighted people make use of large print, and that 12% use sighted readers.

11.1.4 Overlap between media

We did not enquire specifically whether respondents used one preferred medium more than others or whether they used two or more equally. However, Table 11.1 provides indirect evidence that most did have a preferred medium. At WQ83 interviewers were instructed to code more than one medium if the respondent was at all uncertain about which was the most frequently used. The amount by which the items listed in Table 11.1 total more than 100% therefore indicates how many respondents mentioned more than one medium. Very few did. The overlap amounted to only 15%, and this varies little between sight levels. Even if we assume that the 'don't knows' (7%) include people who could not decide between different media they use equally frequently, the total is still not large.

11.1.5 Customary, temporary and occasional use

Evidence of the occasional use of a particular medium can be obtained by using answers to questions in earlier chapters that focused on any use at all rather than on most frequent use. Table 11.2 brings together the relevant data.

Table 11.2 Reading methods used most often and occasionally

'Still thinking about all the different ways of reading, which do you use most often?' (WQ83)

	Use*	Use most often
	%	%
Ordinary print	–	48
Large print	–	24
Normally reads print	65	–
Braille	2	1
Moon	#	0
Tapes (including Talking Books)	–	13
Talking Books	12	–
Ordinary tapes	12	–
Personal reader	40	21
Base (population) (= 100%)	757K	757K
(Number interviewed)	(595)	(595)

*Data from Chapters 7, 8, 9, 10

Braille The data on braille reveal that while some 2% of respondents (corresponding to 13,000 visually impaired people) said that they currently used braille (section 10.3), only 1% (approximately 7,000 people) used braille most often.

Print   According to Table 11.2, 48 and 24 per cent respectively said that they used ordinary print and large print most frequently. (These figures may overlap, since some of the 48% may also have said that they used large print.) This percentage, and the 65% who use print (see section 7.2), make it clear that a large proportion of visually impaired people use print regularly rather than merely occasionally.

Personal readers   While 40% of respondents said that they used readers, second only to print, only 21% said that this was their most frequent reading method. Thus, for 19% of visually impaired people, readers provide a vital back-up to other more frequently used media. However, the unique role of an individual reader means that the description 'back-up' probably undervalues this essential contribution. Depending upon circumstances, a reader is often instantly available to read print material that would take a long time to be transcribed into braille or to be taped by one of the volunteer taping groups. Also, personal readers are preferable for certain kinds of material. For instance, when large quantities of information have to be scanned, but only certain parts need be read carefully, the individual reader can be selective according to the brief given, something that is impossible for taping and transcription services.

Tapes   The wording of WQ83 allows no distinction to be made as to whether the respondent was referring to ordinary tapes or to Talking Books. Only 13% mentioned tapes as their most frequent medium in response to this question. In section 8.2, we saw that 12% use Talking Books, and use of ordinary tapes for reading was estimated at approximately the same percentage, though with an emphasis on non-fiction information material (section 8.4.2). If 'tapes', using the term to cover both Talking Books and ordinary tapes, were the most frequently used medium, we would expect mentions of tapes to exceed that of Talking Books alone. That it does not suggests that tapes have an occasional, back-up function, and that many who use tapes rely on other media for regular access to printed material.

Moon   As noted, our sample contained only one individual – a registered blind person aged between 16 and 59 – who currently uses Moon, and hence the data do not allow any generalisation about Moon readers as a group. For what it is worth, this one individual not only used Moon but also said that Moon was the most frequently used medium.

11.2   Communications media

11.2.1   Introduction

Large print books, tapes, personal readers and braille (discussed in detail in Chapters 7 to 10 and reviewed collectively in section 11.2) are of course not the only communication channels available to blind and partially sighted people. Writing media and telephones are considered in sections 11.2.2 and 11.2.3. Section 11.3 discusses the relative importance of all these media, together with personal contact and broadcast media, as sources of information for visually impaired people, and in section 11.4 the relationship between information needs and communication media is considered.

11.2.2 Writing media

An estimated 10,000 registered blind people write in braille, of whom nearly 7,000 are aged under 60 (section 10.7.3). These constitute 39% of registered and 23% of registrable blind people under 60, and 1% of the registrable blind aged over 60. (Braille writing and braille reading was almost exclusively confined to people registered blind.)

Ability to use a typewriter is crucial for blind people who cannot write, and also for partially sighted people who need to write formal material and believe that their handwriting is not good enough. At WQ84 we asked 'How often do you use a typewriter nowadays?'

The answers revealed that, while less than 5% (population estimate 32,000) ever use a typewriter, the distribution between age levels is uneven. For example, among the under-60s, 25% of blind people (population estimate 7,000) and 21% of partially sighted people (population estimate 10,000) use one, the majority doing so either 'most days' or 'at least once a week'. Almost all registered blind people who write in braille also use a typewriter.

Although we did not ask specific questions about writing by hand, we know that 58% of blind people under 60 (Table 6.3) were unable to read our large-print card. This figure suggests an approximate proportion of blind people in this age group who either cannot write at all or who find writing legibly extremely difficult. Since only 25% of the same group use a typewriter, this suggests a major unmet need, in a world so dependent on written communications, for training in keyboard skills.

11.2.3 Telephones

11.2.3.1 Possession of a telephone

According to the 1985 General Household Survey (OPCS, 1985), 81% of private households in Britain possess a telephone. Among visually impaired people overall the figure is 72% (Table 11.3). However, this statistic conceals a significant difference. Eighty-seven per cent of the registered possess a telephone, above the national average, but only 67% of the non-registered. Age makes no difference among the registered. Among the non-registered, 77% of people aged 16 – 59, and

66% of those aged 60 or over, possessed a telephone. GHS found that nationally 66% of households with a gross weekly income of £60 – 80 had a telephone (GHS, 1985, Table 5.29).

For blind and partially sighted people, telephones form an important means of obtaining information. As is shown in section 11.3.1, 16% of respondents said the telephone was the most important way they discovered things they needed to know, and a further 20% listed it as the second most important.

11.2.3.2   Subsidies for telephones

According to the BBC *In Touch Handbook* (Broadcasting Support Services, 1991)

> Local authorities tend to follow nationally agreed guidelines to decide whether a telephone is a necessity. The applicant must live alone, or be frequently left alone, or be housebound and be able to show that a telephone is needed for medical and social reasons. Only when all these conditions have been met, and the client has also been assessed as needing financial help, will most local authorities... consider a telephone to be a necessity, and therefore something that they have a duty to provide. Some local authorities, however, interpret 'need' more generously than this.

The *In Touch Handbook* for 1982 noted that in 1978/79 the amount spent by local authorities on telephone rental and installation in England and Wales ranged from £16 per 1,000 population to £616.

In Touch also discusses help from voluntary sources through the Telephones for the Blind Fund.

> This Fund will help meet part of the cost of installation and rental of telephones for blind people of limited means who live alone, or are often alone especially at night, or whose partner is also disabled by infirmity or age. The Fund needs to be satisfied that the applicant has been refused help from his or her local authority under the... Chronically Sick and Disabled Persons Act.

Our data (Table 11.3) indicate that the total contribution of local authorities and the voluntary sector to telephone possession among visually impaired people amounts only to about 11%. Although proportionately small, this corresponds in absolute numbers to about 60,000 telephones. However, some 89% of telephones possessed by visually impaired people (about 475,000) are paid for entirely out of their own incomes. Given the low income of visually impaired people (section 3.6), telephone costs necessarily consume a disproportionately large part of their income compared with the general population, which indicates how essential the telephone is seen to be. Where a subsidy is received, it usually covers the total cost, approximately equal between installation and rental. Only 2% out of the 11% received a partial contribution.

Table 11.3 Telephone possession and assistance with installation and rental costs, by registration and age

'I'd now like to check with you about how you find out things that affect your daily life. Do you have a telephone of your own?' (CQ37)

'Did anyone help you with the cost of installing your telephone or paying the rental?...did they pay part or all of the cost?' (CQ38)

	Registration status and age				
	Registered		Non-registered		
	16 – 59	60 +	16 – 59	60 +	Total
	%	%	%	%	%
Installation:					
All of cost	2	9	6	2	4
Part of cost	#	2	3	#	1
Rental:					
All of cost	5	9	4	3	4
Part of cost	#	2	1	0	#
No, no one helps with cost	78	70	63	60	63
All with a phone	86	86	77	66	72
Those without a phone	15	14	23	34	29
Total %	100	100	100	100	100
Base (population)	30K	140K	47K	538K	757K
(Number interviewed)	(215)	(137)	(84)	(159)	(595)

11.3 Relative importance of different sources of information

11.3.1 Prompted replies

Respondents were read a list of the different media or communication channels and asked to compare their importance. They were asked to say which were important (CQ41); which was most important (CQ42); and which was second most important (CQ43). Tables 11.4, 11.5.a. and 11.5.b. show the precise wording of the questions (see note 1) and the data obtained.

When asked (CQ41) to choose between saying a medium was important or unimportant, respondents gave 'asking people' most votes (85%) for being important; radio received 64%; television 63%; telephoning people 54%; local magazines and newspapers 41%; tapes and Talking Books 13%; talking newspapers 7% and braille books 1%. These figures mean that, for example, 41% of visually impaired people said that they found printed media in the form of local magazines and newspapers an important information source. This percentage did not change drastically among different age groups, or between registered and non-registered people, or between blind and partially sighted people. It is perhaps a surprisingly high figure, but it is not inconsistent with data noted earlier (section 7.2) about the numbers of visually impaired people who can read print. Nor is it surprising when one considers how many visually impaired people have sighted people who can read to them.

The percentage of respondents mentioning other print-substitute media did vary according to registration status. Very few of the non-registered mentioned either Talking Books or talking newspapers (3 and 8 per cent respectively), whereas 23 and 30 per cent respectively of the registered named them. All mentions of braille books came from registered blind people: 25% of the 16 – 59 age group and 4% of those aged 60 and over (data mostly from Table 11.5.a.).

When we asked respondents (at CQ42) to say which of these media were most important, 'asking people' predominated at 48%. 'Phoning people' received 16%, radio 11%, television 9%, local magazines and

Table 11.4   Important sources of information for visually impaired people: prompted replies

'I am going to read out a list and I want you to tell me which of these are important for you for finding out things you want to know. Would you say that ... was important or not?' (CQ41)

'Which of these would you say is the most important way for you to find out about things? And which would you say is the second?' (CQ42 and CQ43)

	Important sources	Most important	2nd most important
	%	%	%
Asking people	85	48	18
Telephoning people	54	16	20
Broadcast media:			
Television	64	9	16
Radio	63	11	13
Print/print substitutes:			
Tapes or Talking Books	13	#	2
Braille books	1	#	#
Talking newspapers	7	1	1
Local magazines/newspapers	41	7	7
None mentioned	4	1	8
Don't know	–	3	5
No information	–	7	9
Base (population) = 100%	757K	757K	757K
(Number interviewed)	(595)	(595)	(595)

(595 respondents)

Table 11.5.a. Important sources of information for visually impaired people by registration status and age: prompted replies (CQ41)

	Registration status and age				
	Registered		Non-registered		
	16 – 59	60 +	16 – 59	60 +	Total
	%	%	%	%	%
Asking people	96	90	88	83	85
Telephoning people	82	60	70	50	54
Broadcast media:					
Television	63	47	63	63	60
Radio	78	63	70	59	62
Print/print substitutes:					
Tapes or Talking Books	33	29	6	8	13
Braille books	16	3	0	0	1
Talking newspapers	26	22	3	3	7
Local magazines and newspapers	46	31	52	42	41
None mentioned	1	4	1	4	4
Base (population) = 100%	30K	140K	47K	540K	757K
(Number interviewed)	(215)	(137)	(84)	(159)	(595)

(595 respondents)

newspapers 7% and talking newspapers 1%. Tapes and Talking Books and braille books did not reach 0.5% overall, and even among registered blind people aged 16 – 59 only received 2% each. The question (CQ43) concerning second most important of the prompted items did not produce any new findings (Table 11.4).

The tables do reveal significant differences between blind and partially sighted people, especially among those under 60. In this group, blind people were more likely to rely on asking and telephoning people, and on the radio, Talking Books, talking newspapers, and braille books. While partially sighted people use all these media, they do so to a lesser extent and rely on television and local newspapers more (Table 11.5.b.).

Table 11.5.b. Important sources of information for visually impaired people by age and residual vision: prompted replies (CQ41)

	Age and residual vision				Residual vision		Age		Total
	16 – 59		60 +		All ages		16 – 59	60 +	
	B	PS	B	PS	B	PS			
	%	%	%	%	%	%	%	%	%
Asking people	96	88	86	84	87	84	91	85	85
Telephoning people	83	70	49	54	52	55	75	52	54
Broadcast media:									
Television	56	67	54	64	54	64	63	60	60
Radio	83	66	60	61	62	62	73	60	62
Print/print substitutes:									
Tapes or Talking Books	31	7	24	5	24	5	16	13	13
Braille books	15	1	1	0	3	#	6	1	1
Talking newspapers	24	4	10	5	11	5	12	7	7
Local magazines and newspapers	39	56	40	40	40	42	50	40	41
None mentioned	1	2	4	4	4	4	1	4	4
Base (population) = 100%	30K	47K	270K	410K	301K	456K	77K	680K	757K
(Number interviewed)	(137)	(162)	(130)	(166)	(267)	(328)	(299)	(296)	(595)

(595 respondents)

11.3.2 Unprompted replies

Before presenting respondents (at CQ41, CQ42 and CQ43) with a pre-determined check list of items, we asked them the following open question: 'How do you find out about things you want to know about?' (CQ39) This is an alternative way of capturing relative importance, since a spontaneous mention of an item is an indication of its significance to the respondent rather than to the investigator. However, since our own check list was drawn up as the result of pilot work, we expected that the two approaches would show broad agreement, and the data shown in Table 11.6 confirm this. The open responses to CQ39 have been coded into categories similar to those used for the check list. Again, personal contact (i.e. 'asking people') predominates across the various age and registration categories. The other categories retain their previous importance, with similar differences between sub-groups.

Table 11.6 throws additional light on the detailed content of each category. Personal communication divides into informal and formal contacts, and informal contacts, themselves mentioned about four times as frequently as formal contacts, divide further into 'someone in the household' and 'other relative' (each 32%) and 'friend or colleague' (21%).

Our results confirm those of the major survey (Epstein, 1980) carried out by the Research Institute for Consumer Affairs (RICA) into the information needs of elderly people. Elderly visually impaired people, no less than elderly people in general, largely rely on personal contact sources such as family and friends (the informal care network) for information. In addition, this finding also applies to younger visually impaired people. Within this high level of reliance on informal contacts, marked age-related trends are noticeable. In particular, elderly people rely less on 'someone in the household' and more on 'other relatives'. Among 16 – 59 year-olds, 50 and 19 per cent respectively mentioned 'someone in the household' and 'other relative', while among those aged 60 to 74 the corresponding proportions were 36 and 24 per cent, and among old elderly people 28 and 37 per cent (data not shown in the tables).

Among various social services field-workers (the formal care network) mentioned as sources of information were 'home help' (9%), 'social worker' (5%) and 'social worker for the blind' (1%). 'Home help' was mentioned by 10% of those aged 60 or over and by 1% of those aged 16 – 59. Mentions of both types of social worker were more closely related to registration than to age: they were mentioned by 15% of the registered, but by only 4% of the non-registered.

Mentions of the voluntary sector were small (5% overall) and came mostly from registered respondents. Although the differences are too small to reach statistical significance, the data do suggest that local

Table 11.6 Sources of information for visually impaired people by registration status and age: unprompted replies

'How do you find out about things you want to know about?' (CQ39)

	Registration status and age				
	Registered		Non-registered		
	16 – 59	60 +	15 – 59	60 +	Total
	%	%	%	%	%
Personal contact:					
Someone in the household	54	39	47	28	32
Other relative	19	26	20	35	32
Friend or colleague	31	22	20	20	21
Social services:					
Home help	2	9	1	10	9
Social worker	9	10	2	4	5
Social worker for blind	6	4	2	0	1
Mobility Officer	1	#	0	0	#
Department of Social Security	3	6	6	4	6
Voluntary sector:					
Other local association (non visual handicap)	0	1	2	4	3
Local blind society	3	7	0	0	1
RNIB	6	2	2	0	1
Broadcast media:					
Radio	33	13	18	18	18
Television	24	5	16	19	16
Health service	2	6	15	4	5
Telephone	15	12	13	12	12
Print/print substitutes					
Local magazine/newspaper	10	3	9	8	7
Talking newspapers	6	6	0	0	1
Talking books/cassettes	2	2	1	1	1
Braille books	1	0	0	0	#
Base (population) = 100%	30K	140K	47K	538K	757K
(Number interviewed)	(215)	(137)	(84)	(159)	(595)

blind societies reach elderly people more often, while RNIB reaches younger registered people. Among registered people aged 16 – 59 and 60 or over, local blind societies were mentioned by 3 and 7 per cent respectively, while RNIB was mentioned by 6 and 2 per cent. Some 2% of the non-registered aged under 60 mentioned RNIB, while none of the non-registered of any age mentioned local blind societies.

Radio and television were mentioned more often by the younger registered than by other sub-groups. The telephone was mentioned by 12% overall, with little variation across sub-groups.

11.4 Communications media and information needs

The information needs of blind and partially sighted people relate to the knowledge and awareness that they have of both services and sources of information about services. The RICA survey found that as a whole elderly people are not knowledgeable about the various services and programmes available, relying largely for information on informal sources such as family and friends. The survey also showed that very few information providers use non-print communications media. Perhaps not surprisingly, elderly visually impaired people were found to be even less well informed than others, including deaf people, without vision problems (Epstein, 1980).

Our results confirm that elderly visually impaired people obtain information largely from these informal sources and also show that this applies to the younger age group as well.

Although no single chapter in this report covers knowledge and information as such, relevant data appear in several different places. As far as possible, we included questions on awareness of services and sources of information on each need area in each section of the interview. The results obtained have been reported in the appropriate section. Thus awareness of braille, Moon, large-print books, tapes and talking book services and of sources of information about them are discussed in Chapters 7 to 10. Chapter 13 deals with mobility, Chapter 15 with household aids and gadgets, and Chapter 18 with benefits and allowances, reporting on awareness of related services and the possibility of obtaining training and advice. Chapter 20 reports on knowledge of voluntary organisations and RNIB in particular. A common feature in all these sections is the higher information level of the registered compared with the non-registered. Chapter 19 deals specifically with knowledge about and attitudes towards being registered and the social services as a whole.

It remains a considerable task for further analysis to bring together all the data on awareness and information spread throughout this report. Factors relating to information needs in specific areas should be distinguished from those factors making for awareness or lack of awareness that are common across all need areas. Correlations can then be sought between awareness and lack of awareness and the use of communication sources. These correlations should be examined both within and across need areas. Differences in circumstances and lifestyles between sub-groups, e.g. blind and partially sighted people will also have to be taken into account. (See note 2 for further discussion of information needs and suggestions for secondary analysis.)

Notes to Chapter 11

Note 1

The wording of questions CQ39, CQ41, CQ42 and CQ43 – 'things you want to know about' – does not specify the type of information source the respondent is being asked to think about. However, it is well known that questions left as open as this are subject to frame of reference effects set by previous questioning. Since these questions came at the end of almost an hour of questioning on needs and services, it can be assumed that this will be the context within which the questions are answered.

Note 2

A survey focusing specifically and comprehensively on the information needs of visually impaired people would require a questionnaire as long as the one in the RICA survey, which itself was about as long as the questionnaire we developed in this survey to cover the entire range of needs. Many questions we would have liked to have asked specifically on information needs had to be cut out at the pilot stage (Chapter 2). Nevertheless some remain. As noted in section 11.4, the considerable data on awareness and information are spread throughout the report, and available for secondary analysis. Possible topics for study include information common to the profiles of those aware and unaware among the non-users of services, or clusters of services, in general; and construction of a knowledge or awareness index in order to examine common factors in the transmission of knowledge, or the failure to do so, across a range of need areas. The standardised coding frame used to categorise sources of information in several need areas – family, friends, neighbours, voluntary organisations, social service field-workers, radio and other media – should make possible analyses in terms of common communication channels.

Part C

Other Disabilities

12 Visual Impairment and Other Disabilities

12.1 Background

In order to leave room for the many aspects of visual disability that were our special concern, our questioning on other disabilities was limited to the objective of complementing the information obtained in the OPCS disability survey (Martin et al, 1988a, 1988b, 1989). Because of the unprecedented range of disabilities this survey encompassed, coverage of visual disability as such was necessarily limited. Only secondary analysis of the archived OPCS data will provide a complete and accurate account of the overlap between registrable visual impairment and other types of disability. However, the OPCS prevalence data on disabilities in general, and particularly on age trends, do serve as a frame of reference for our own findings. This chapter also draws on other major government surveys of general disability, notably the General Household Survey (OPCS, 1985 and 1986) and the survey by Harris (1971).

12.2 OPCS data

12.2.1 Prevalence in the general population

The OPCS survey, which contained detailed questions on a range of disabilities including vision, estimates that 1,384,000 people aged 16 or over with a 'seeing disability' are living in private households in Great Britain. At 757,000, our own estimate, given in section 3.1, of the numbers of registrable visually impaired people in the same age group was much smaller. The reason for the difference is that our sample consisted solely of people at registrable levels of visual impairment. OPCS included some 600,000 people whose sight level was above that needed for registration as partially sighted. The comparisons shown between visual impairment and other disabilities in Table 12.1 are nevertheless useful since in its report OPCS established a common scale of severity across all areas. However, it must be remembered that the OPCS threshold for inclusion was not as high as ours, and any comparisons will include many people with relatively moderate loss of vision.

With this proviso, we can note from Table 12.1 that seeing disability ranks fifth among the 13 types of disability OPCS considered, preceded by disabilities associated with locomotion, hearing, personal care and dexterity. (The types follow the World Health Organisation's classification, International Classification of Impairments, Disabilities and Handicaps – ICIDH.)

Table 12.1 OPCS estimates of prevalence of disability among adults in private households in Great Britain by type of disability and age

	Age and prevalence			All ages	Ratio (c/a)
	(a) 16 – 59	(b) 60 – 74	(c) 75 +		
	Prevalence rate per 1,000				
Locomotion	31	195	464	93	15
Hearing	16	108	307	55	19
Personal care	17	93	263	50	16
Dexterity	12	76	180	37	15
Seeing	8	52	225	32	28
Intellectual	17	37	107	28	6
Behaviour	19	36	88	27	5
Reaching and stretching	8	52	129	25	16
Communication	10	38	112	23	11
Continence	8	38	120	22	15
Disfigurement	5	18	27	9	5
Eating, drinking	2	11	18	6	9
Consciousness	4	4	6	4	2
All disabilities	58	267	564	135	10
Base* (for per 1,000)	31846	7797	3259	42902	

*Total population (thousands)
Source: OPCS Report 1 reproduced from Tables 3.12 and 3.14 (Martin et al, 1988a)

12.2.2 Age trends in visual impairment and other disabilities

The final column (ratio c/a) of Table 12.1 provides a rough but telling index of the steepness with which prevalence rates rise with age. For vision, the ratio of the 16 – 59 to the 75 + age group is 28. In other words, people over 74 are 28 times more likely to suffer a seeing disability than people aged 16 to 59. The likelihood of a disability occurring increases with age. However, the ratio for vision is by far the highest of all the disabilities listed in Table 12.1, and is nearly three times greater than the average. The ratios for the other types of disability are: hearing (19), reaching and stretching, personal care (16 each), locomotion, continence, dexterity (15 each), communication (11), eating, drinking (9), intellectual (6), behaviour, disfigurement (5 each) and consciousness (2). Seeing disability also produces the greatest increase between the two older age groups, 60 – 74 and 75 + ; the ratio of these two groups is 4, compared with an overall average of about 2.

The extra-steep rise in age-specific prevalence rates for seeing disability means that the visually impaired population contains relatively more old people in comparison with other disabled populations. Table 12.2.a. compares the age distribution for seeing disability with that of other disabilities. Thirty-one per cent of all disabled people are aged 16 – 59, 37% 60 – 74 and 32% 75 or over. The corresponding figures for people with a seeing disability are 18, 29 and 53 per cent respectively. Thus, half of all people with a seeing disability are aged 75 or over compared with only one-third of people with disabilities in general.

Table 12.2.a. Distribution of disabilities over age groups in private households

	All disabilities	Seeing disability
	%	%
Age		
16 – 59	31	18
60 – 74	37	29
75 +	32	53
Total %	100	100
(Base 000s)	(5780)	(1384)

Source: OPCS Report 1 (Martin et al, 1988a)

12.2.3 Relative incidence of registrable and non-registrable visual impairment over age groups

The data for seeing and other disabilities in Tables 12.1 and 12.2.a. have been equated for level of severity by the methods used in the OPCS survey. The data included cover all levels of severity above the lower threshold in the OPCS survey. Using the data on registrable visual impairment obtained in the RNIB survey (as defined in 2.4.2.2),

Table 12.2.b. Age distribution in moderate and registrably visually impaired adults in private households

	(a) Seeing disability	(b) Registrably visually impaired	(c) Moderate i.e. non-registrably visually impaired
	%	%	%
Age group			
16 – 59	18	10	27
60 – 74	29	24	36
75 +	53	66	37
Total %	100	100	100
Base (population)	1384K	757K	627K
(Number interviewed RNIB survey)	(595)		

(a) OPCS data   (b) RNIB data   (c) Obtained by subtracting (b) from (a)

153

we are able to separate non-registrable and registrable and examine the age trends in each group (Table 12.2.b.).

Table 12.2.b. reveals that in percentage terms the incidence of 'moderate' visual impairment (i.e. people at non-registrable (section 2.4.2) residual vision levels) changes little with age. The totals for the three age groups are 27, 36 and 37 per cent respectively. By contrast, the number of people with registrable loss of vision rises dramatically through each age band. In each of the three age groups the totals of people with a registrable visual impairment are 10, 24 and 66 per cent. In other words, the huge rise in visual impairment (column (a)) does not take place uniformly over the residual vision range. What increases so dramatically with age is the onset of severe, registrable visual impairment.

Table 12.2.c. expresses the data given in Table 12.2.b. as proportions of the total population. Analysis by age groups produces the age-specific prevalence rates (see also Table 12.1).

Table 12.2.c.   Prevalence of moderate and registrable visual impairment among adults in private households

	Age and prevalence			All ages	Ratio (c/a)
	(a)	(b)	(c)		
	16 – 59	60 – 74	75 +		
	Prevalence rate per 1,000				
Seeing disability (OPCS)[1]	8	52	225	32	28
Registrable VI[2]	3	23	152	18	51
Non-registrable VI[3]	5	29	73	14	15
Base (population*)	31846K	7797K	3259K	42902K	

*population base for prevalence rate per 1,000
(1) OPCS data   (2) RNIB data   (3) Obtained by subtracting (2) from (1)

A comparison between non-registrable and registrable (section 2.4.2) visual impairment can now be made in terms of the ratios for age-specific prevalence rates. The first line of Table 12.2.c., which repeats the data for seeing disability given in Table 12.1, shows that the ratio for the growth of age-specific prevalence rates for seeing disability as a whole is 28. This figure is composed of two parts: first, a relatively slow rate of growth, indicated by a ratio of 15 among non-registrable visually impaired people and, second, a much more rapid rate ratio of 51 among registrable visually impaired people. Thus, while people aged 75 or over are 15 times more likely than people aged under 16 – 59 to suffer from moderate visual impairment, they are 51 times more likely to suffer from severe visual impairment at registrable levels.

12.3 Multi-handicapped visually impaired people

12.3.1 Hearing impairment

Because vision and hearing are the two senses we use most, we gave additional disabilities resulting from hearing loss special attention in our survey. Pressure on space meant that only four questions were asked, and we were unable to distinguish between degrees of hearing loss.

First of all, we asked if the respondent had a hearing aid, with the results shown in Table 12.3. As with all the questions about hearing, replies were very much age-related and largely independent of residual vision levels. Overall, 22% of respondents said that they had a hearing-aid. The totals for the under-60s, the 60 – 74 year-olds and the 75 + age group were 4, 13 and 28 per cent respectively.

Table 12.3 Visually impaired people with a hearing aid

'Do you have a hearing aid?' (GQ1)

	Age			Total
	16 – 59	60 – 74	75 +	
	%	%	%	%
Yes	4	13	28	22
No	96	87	72	78
Total %	100	100	100	100
Base (population)	77K	180K	500K	757K
(Number interviewed)	(285)	(134)	(176)	(595)

(595 respondents)

Our second question focused on the extent to which impaired hearing hindered normal conversation in everyday settings. As Table 12.4 shows, 22, 34 and 37 per cent in the three age groups said that they found it difficult to hear normal speech.

The hearing impairments encountered were rarely so severe as to prevent the interview being carried out. Deafness was given as the reason for 11 of the 42 proxy interviews that had to be undertaken because the respondent was not able to be interviewed directly, eight of which were with respondents aged 75 or over.

Often the interviews, which were held in the respondent's own home and almost invariably in a quiet room, were only possible if conducted in a very loud voice. As our interviewers were thus able independently to assess whether the respondents had difficulty hearing, we asked them to code their impressions. The results, shown in Table 12.5, are broadly similar to those in Table 12.4. By and large the interviewers' observations confirmed the respondents' self-assessments of their

Table 12.4 Visually impaired people experiencing problems hearing a normal voice

'(When you are wearing your hearing aid) If you are in a quiet room with someone, would you have difficulty hearing them speak to you in a normal voice?' (GQ2)

	Age			Total
	16 – 59	60 – 74	75 +	
	%	%	%	%
Yes	22	34	37	35
No	78	66	63	65
Total %	100	100	100	100
Base (population)	75K	178K	172K	744K
(Number interviewed)	(275)	(131)	(172)	(578)

(578 respondents: no information for 17 cases)

Table 12.5 Interviewers' assessment of respondents' hearing (GRQ12)

Interviewers reported that during the interview respondents had:

	Age			Total
	16 – 59	60 – 74	75 +	
	%	%	%	%
Problems hearing	6	23	45	36
No problems hearing	94	77	55	64
Total %	100	100	100	100
Base (population)	74K	175K	496K	745K
(Number interviewed)	(269)	(130)	(270)	(569)

(569 respondents: no reports on 26 cases)

Table 12.6 Consultations with a doctor about hearing

'Have you ever consulted a doctor about your hearing?' (GQ3)

	Age			Total
	16 – 59	60 – 74	75 +	
	%	%	%	%
Yes	19	32	41	36
No	81	68	59	64
Total %	100	100	100	100
Base (population)	75K	178K	491K	744K
(Number interviewed)	(290)	(121)	(168)	(579)

(Total respondents 579: no information for 16 cases)

hearing difficulties. Overall, 36% of the respondents were reported as having difficulty hearing. Among the 75 + age group, however, the percentage was as high as 45.

As Table 12.6 shows, the proportion of respondents who had consulted a doctor about their hearing is approximately the same as the proportion who admitted to difficulty hearing a normal voice.

Those who had consulted a doctor about their hearing were asked (at GQ4) if they had registered as disabled with their local authority because of their hearing problem. The results provide our best estimate of the numbers of visually impaired people who are also deaf, as opposed to hard of hearing. The 19 of our sample who said that they were registered for hearing loss constituted 3% of those under 75 and 5% of those aged 75 or over.

For people with impaired vision, even a moderate hearing loss has wider consequences than are generally realised. The difficulties the two losses create are much more severe than the difficulties of loss of either vision or hearing alone. While someone who cannot hear the spoken word may be able to manage in social situations by lip-reading and by watching sign language and gestures, a visually impaired person cannot do this. Loss of both senses can prevent people joining in a conversation, isolate them from companionship and prevent them making casual acquaintances. Communication and intense social isolation are the greatest problems for visually impaired people whose hearing is also impaired.

In summary, we find that 22% of visually impaired people under 60 suffer the additional disadvantage of having difficulties hearing normal speech in a quiet room, even if they are wearing a hearing aid. This figure rises to 34% of people aged 60 – 74 and to 37% of people of 75 and over. Interviewers' direct observations of this third age band indicated that 45% had difficulty in hearing during the interview. These figures suggest that people and organisations who work with very old visually impaired people may assume that half are hard of hearing. Communication with such individuals needs to be assessed in the light of this information.

12.3.2 Overall prevalence of additional disabilities among visually impaired people

The data from the OPCS disability survey (Martin et al, 1988a) do not allow precise estimates of how many registrably visually impaired people have a further handicap. Secondary analysis of the OPCS data will be necessary to establish this information (see note 1). However, questions asked in our survey enable us to reach a tentative estimate of other disabilities among visually impaired people, as section 12.3.2.1

shows. This estimate is compared with the results of similar questions asked in the General Household Survey (section 12.3.2.2). In addition, results already published in the OPCS survey allow comparisons with the General Household Survey, and help to set our own findings in perspective.

12.3.2.1 Self-reports of other disabilities by registrable visually impaired people

Among the questions we asked about health and additional disabilities were the following: 'Apart from problems with your eyesight (and hearing), do you have any other permanent illness or disabilities?' (GQ6); and 'Does (illness/disability) make it difficult to do things in the house or get about outside?' (GQ8) The results are set out in Table 12.7.

Table 12.7 Generalised self-reports of other disabilities among registrable visually impaired people (GQ6 and GQ8)

	Age			Total
	16 – 59	60 – 74	75 +	
	%	%	%	%
Reporting of permanent illness/ disability (GQ6)	63	68	68	67
Reporting limiting permanent illness or disability (GQ8)	46	41	46	45
Base (population) = 100%	77K	180K	500K	757K
(Number interviewed)	(299)	(124)	(172)	(595)

(595 respondents)

12.3.2.2 Generalised self-reports of other disabilities by the general population

Every year the government's General Household Survey (GHS) puts the following questions to a national sample of the population living in private households: 'Do you have any long-standing illness, disability or infirmity?'; 'Does this illness or disability limit your activities in any way?'

The GHS results for 1985 (those used in the OPCS report), which vary only slightly from year to year, are shown in Table 12.8. The precise wording of a question can have an impact on the responses received. The GHS estimates include visual and hearing disabilities, but once allowance is made for this the wording of the GHS questions and ours is sufficiently similar for the results to be broadly comparable (see note 2).

158

Table 12.8 Estimates of prevalence of long-standing and limiting disability among the general population, Great Britain 1985

	Age		
	16 – 59	60 – 74	75 +
	%	%	%
Reporting long-standing illness/disability	29	56	63
Reporting limiting long-standing illness/ disability	16	38	48
Base = 100%	15921	2195	1491

Source: GHS data from the OPCS report 1, Table 3.5 (Martin et al, 1988a)

12.3.2.3 Relative frequencies of generalised self-reports of other disabilities among severely visually impaired people

By comparing Tables 12.7 and 12.8 we can compare the prevalence among registrably visually impaired people of disabilities other than vision with the prevalence of these disabilities in the sighted population (see note 3). Although some subsidiary considerations must be taken into account, the comparison reveals, first, that across all age groups the prevalence rate for disabilities other than vision is higher among visually impaired people than among the general population; and, second, that the younger the age group, the more marked the discrepancy. In other words, while the prevalence of all disabilities rises with age, visually impaired people are more likely than sighted people in their age group to suffer from another disability; furthermore, the younger they are, the higher is this probability.

12.3.2.4 Under-estimation in generalised self-reports

The results of the OPCS disability survey demonstrate that the form of the questions on disabilities in the General Household Survey leads to a serious underestimate of prevalence among elderly people; this is likely to be the case with our survey as well. Older people are inclined to discount major disabilities as well as minor ones. This finding has important implications for what should be accepted as the normal

Table 12.9 Prevalence estimates for disabilities in general: GHS and the OPCS surveys compared

	Age		
	16 – 59	60 – 74	75 +
	%	%	%
OPCS survey*	6	27	56
GHS**	16	38	48

*Data computed from Table 3.5 in OPCS report 1, (Martin et al, 1988a)
**See Table 12.8

limitations of ageing, i.e. people are willing to discount very limiting disabilities as a normal consequence of getting old. Table 12.9 sets out the relevant figures.

Two striking points emerge. First, the GHS estimates exceed those produced by OPCS for the two younger age groups, but are lower for the third oldest group. Second, while the OPCS prevalence rate more than doubles between the 60 – 74 and the 75 + age groups, the increase in the GHS rate is relatively modest, about 25%.

Noting the higher prevalence estimate for the under 75s, the OPCS report comments:

> This was to be expected since any limitation in activities is counted for the GHS estimate whereas this survey asked questions about specific activities and only limitations in performing these activities were included in the definition of disability. What is surprising is the lower prevalence estimates for age 75 onwards obtained by the GHS compared with this (OPCS) survey. . . **We suggest that the reason for this is that many elderly people do not think of themselves as having problems or being disabled; they consider limitations in activities a normal consequence of old age.** (RNIB emphasis) On the GHS this probably means that some answer negatively to the first question and thus do not get asked the second, while others who answer 'yes' to the first do not admit to any effect on their activities because they have come to accept their limitations. Both result in lower estimates among the elderly.' (Martin et al, 1988a, page 21)

The same explanation would apply to the questions we asked about the prevalence of other disabilities. As noted above, these questions were similar to the two GHS questions.

These results argue that self-assessments by elderly people themselves provide an insufficient basis for gauging their needs. Elderly people discount the limitations imposed by minor disabilities. OPCS data indicate that the age-related increase in prevalence is even steeper for the more severe disabilities than for the less severe (see note 4).

The conditions elderly people accept as normal and the view they take of their disabilities and of their entitlement to services or social security benefits are both shaped by their expectations. These expectations change over time. Writing in 1978 of the influences that moulded the attitudes and judgements of people then approaching 80, Abrams notes that they matured in the days before the expansion of the welfare state and that many lived most of their lives against a background of abject poverty. 'It would not be surprising if their present criteria of what they need, of what they are entitled to, and of what gives them satisfaction are modest.' (Abrams, 1978, page 7). The next generation of elderly people may not be so accepting of the level of disability regarded as normal for their age. Such changes may already be under way. The 1985 GHS report graphically presents the percentage of respondents reporting a long-standing illness or disability over the previous thirteen years. The graph shows a steady rise over the period. The authors comment: 'As these data were based on people's subjective assessments of their health, any changes over time may reflect changes in people's expectations of good health as well as changes in the incidence or duration of chronic sickness' (OPCS, 1985, page 101).

12.4 The registration of additional disabilities

One indicator of a severe disability is whether a person is registered for it. Local authorities are required to keep registers of people with physical handicaps (called the general classes register) other than vision and hearing disabilities. Respondents who said (at GQ6) that they had disabilities other than vision or hearing were asked (at GQ9) whether they were registered for any of them, with the results shown in Table 12.10.

Table 12.10 Reports of registration for other disabilities[††] (general classes) by visually impaired people

'Can I just check, are you registered for any of these reasons?' (GQ9)

	Age			Total
	16 – 59	60 – 74	75 +	
	%	%	%	%
Reporting:				
Limiting additional illness/ disability*	46	41	46	45
Registered for additional disability	27	15	9	12
No other disabilities	54	59	54	55
Total %	100	100	100	100
Base (population)	77K	180K	500K	757K
(Number interviewed)	(299)	(124)	(172)	(595)

*See table 12.7   [††]Excluding hearing and sight

Table 12.10 shows that visually impaired people aged 75 + compared with younger people with an additional disability are less likely to have their name on the general classes register. Only 20% of those aged 75 + with an additional disability are registered for it, compared with 59 and 39 per cent of the 16 – 59 and 60 – 74 age groups respectively. This is a striking difference. How much reliance can be placed on it?

We noted (in section 2.4.2.1) that checks run with our data showed that most respondents knew whether or not they were registered for visual handicap. However, checks run by Harris in her survey (1971) indicated that less reliance can be placed on respondents' knowledge of registration on the general classes register. Thus, the percentages given in Table 12.10 should accordingly be regarded as only approximate. Even so, they are valid as a rough guide. Using data from actual registers Harris found that, while a higher percentage of the very severely disabled were registered, registration nevertheless declined markedly with age. Among those she categorised as very severely disabled the totals registered in the three age groups 16 – 49, 50 – 64 and 65 + were 47, 39 and 9 per cent respectively. Though we cannot equate levels of severity of disability in her survey and ours, these figures do parallel our own and support the interpretation that the steep fall in registration among the old elderly shown in Table 12.10 is a characteristic of general classes registration.

A very small number of visually impaired people with additional disabilities may be known to, and perhaps receive help from, local authorities by virtue of being on the blind or partially sighted registers rather than the general classes register. Section 3.1 showed that 39, 24 and 19 per cent of registrably visually impaired people in the 16 – 59, 60 – 74 and 75 + age bands respectively are actually registered. If only 1 in 5 of those in the 75 + age group are either registered for their visual impairment or on the general classes register, it follows that the majority (at least 3 in 5) of visually impaired people aged 75 or over are not on either register.

Since local authority registers list people who apply for assistance, part of this under-registration may reflect elderly people's low self-assessment of their own need for help. Anecdotal evidence suggests that the attitudes of statutory workers may make them more sceptical about the necessity of registering older people as disabled.

12.5   Disabilities associated with visual impairment

One third of people under 60 and half those aged 75 + suffer from other disabilities as well as with a serious visual impairment. The most commonly reported problems were arthritis, mobility difficulties, heart conditions and diabetes.

Space did not allow intensive questioning to enable specific medical conditions or other disabilities to be determined with any exactitude. Discussing findings about onset in chapter 5, we noted that about one third of the 16 – 59 age-group said that their eye problems originated at birth. This finding is consistent with the relatively high age-specific rates for further disabilities among the young visually impaired, described in section 12.3.2.1. A distinction is sometimes made between multiple disabilities that are mainly congenital in origin and additional disabilities that are acquired later in life. Most visual impairment in children is congenital and forms part of a syndrome, such as ante-natal rubella infection, linked with other disabilities. The proportion of congenitally disabled people diminishes over successive age groups in relation to the large number of independently acquired visual and other disabilities associated with ageing. Hearing was the only disability about which we asked specifically, the prevalence of which increases markedly with age (section 12.3.1). Any other information we obtained on the nature of disabilities associated with visual impairment rests on the replies to a single question. Those who said that they had an additional permanent illness or disability (apart from problems with vision and hearing, see GQ6), were asked a single, open question: 'What are these illnesses or disabilities?' (GQ7) The answers are shown in Table 12.11. 'Other disability' includes a wide variety of conditions. Particularly mentioned, among many others were: bronchial disorders and emphysema, epilepsy, spinal problems, ulcers, vertigo and Paget's disease.

Table 12.11 Other illnesses and disabilities reported by visually impaired people

	Age			Total
	16 – 59	60 – 74	75 +	
	%	%	%	%
Arthritis	13	21	27	25
Heart condition	14	12	20	18
Legs/mobility	5	17	5	14
Diabetes	7	13	7	9
Bowels/incontinence	#	8	6	6
Hernia	2	4	7	6
Mental handicap	5	#	1	2
Other disability	32	39	22	27
Nothing else mentioned	38	32	32	33
Base (population) = 100 %	77K	180K	500K	757K
(Number interviewed)	(299)	(124)	(172)	(595)

(595 respondents)

To investigate additional disabilities properly would require a series of questions on each disability area (like ours for vision), or at least as many questions as we asked about hearing. The OPCS survey did this for thirteen types of disabilities. Information of the kind given in Table 12.11 as the result of a single open question must be interpreted cautiously, and represents a significant under-estimate among the 75 + group. Furthermore, the exclusion of visually impaired people in residential and hospital accommodation results in an additional underestimate. The respondents themselves are left to define what constitutes a disability, and so the answers themselves tell us nothing about the level of severity that is being measured. These data must be combined with other information in order to obtain prevalence estimates.

In Chapter 15, we asked multi-handicapped visually impaired respondents whether they thought that vision, as distinct from some other disability, is the major factor limiting their ability to perform a variety of tasks.

Notes to Chapter 12

Note 1 (Section 12.3.2)

It is tempting to arrive at an estimate of multi-handicapped visually impaired people from the OPCS published data in the following way. Those with seeing disability scoring 7 – 10 on the severity scale must have at least one further disability. There are 445,000 of these. Inspection of the way OPCS constructed their questionnaire scale for severity of visual impairment suggests that, taking a conservative estimate, those scoring 3 or above should be registrably visually impaired. Of the 1,384,000 with seeing disabilities, 1,022,000 have severity scores between 3 and 10. Assuming that all the latter are registrably visually impaired, this estimate yields a relative frequency of 445/1022 or 44% of the registrably visually impaired with some further disability. The published data also allow this argument to be carried through for separate age bands, yielding percentages of 44, 38 and 46 for those aged 16 – 59, 60 – 74 and 75 + respectively.

The difficulties with this argument are that, first, the correlation between questionnaire answers and sight tests is only approximate, so that the 1,022,000 estimate will include many whose sight loss would not be at registrable levels; and, second, the overall OPCS severity score at any level can be the result of a combination of separate severity scores, taking the three worst areas. Without further analysis there is no way of knowing how the score for visual impairment featured, if at all, in the overall score.

Note 2

In section 12.3.2.2 we made use of comparisons between the GHS and our question on general disabilities. Since both questions were similarly worded, it can be expected that they will share the same biases and that the differences noted between the sighted and the visually impaired populations will be independent of these biases.

Note 3 (Section 12.3.2.3)

Comparing Tables 12.7 and 12.8, and considering first only those aged 75 or over, we note that the entries are about the same. However, Table 12.8 includes replies referring to hearing and eyesight problems which were excluded from Table 12.7 by the form of the question. Comparability therefore requires that we deduct from the percentages in Table 12.8 any replies from respondents who mentioned only hearing or eyesight problems. Although we do not have the data to do this exactly, we know that these problems are very prevalent among those aged 75 or over and that the adjustment, if we could make it, would reduce the percentages in Table 12.8 considerably. The implication of the result for the 75 + age band is therefore that the prevalence rates of other disabilities apart from vision (and also hearing) is considerably greater among visually impaired people than it is among others in this age group.

For younger respondents, comparison of the entries in Tables 12.7 and 12.8 shows directly, even before adjustment, that the latter statement is not only true but applies in increasingly greater measure as we move down the age bands. For those aged 60 – 74 the totals of visually impaired people and of the general population reporting limiting disabilities are 41 and 38 per cent respectively. The corresponding totals for the 16 – 59 age group are 46 and 16 per cent. In this age group about 1 in 2 registrably visually impaired people report a disability other than vision, which is nearly three times the age-specific prevalence rate for all disabilities for this group in the general population.

Note 4 (section 12.3.2.4)

Computations based on Table 4.1 in the OPCS report (Martin et al, 1988a) show that the totals with disabilities in the severity range 7 – 10 are 4, 16 and 44 per cent for the age groups 16 – 59, 60 – 74 and 75 + respectively.

Part D

Mobility and Daily Living

13 Mobility

13.1 Levels achieved

13.1.1 A typical week

Tables 13.1.a. and 13.1.b. classify mobility according to four questions in the survey: whether, in the week preceding the interview, the respondent went out at all (BQ3); whether this was just locally or further afield (BQ4); whether any travelling was done on foot (BQ5); and, if so, whether any travelling on foot was unaccompanied by a sighted person (BQ6).

'Going out' was defined as outside the respondent's house/flat/garden; 'week' as the last seven days. For some respondents, the last week will inevitably have been an exceptional period. Nevertheless, given that fieldwork took place over several weeks in the late autumn and early spring, the results provide a valid general picture of the average

Table 13.1.a. Mobility achieved by residual vision level within two age groups

	Age and residual vision				Total
	16 – 59		60 +		
	B	PS	B	PS	
	%	%	%	%	%
Went out during week? (BQ3):					
No	13	9	34	13	20
Yes	87	91	66	87	80
All going out during week					
Went out locally only? (BQ4):					
Locally only	17	30	31	37	34
Went further	70	62	35	49	46
Went out on foot? (BQ5):					
No	23	23	24	34	30
Yes	64	68	42	52	50
Alone on foot? (BQ6):					
No	13	38	12	6	9
Yes	51	60	30	46	41
Base (population) = 100%	30K	47K	270K	410K	757K
(Number interviewed)	(137)	(162)	(130)	(166)	(595)

Table 13.1.b   Mobility achieved within three age groups

	Age			Total
	16 – 59	60 – 74	75 +	
	%	%	%	%
Went out during week? (BQ3):				
No	10	12	25	20
Yes	90	88	75	80
All going out during week				
Went out locally only? (BQ4):				
Locally only	26	42	32	34
Went further	64	46	43	46
Went out on foot? (BQ5):				
No	23	20	33	30
Yes	67	68	42	50
Alone on foot? (BQ6):				
No	9	9	9	9
Yes	58	59	33	41
Base (population) = 100%	77K	180K	500K	757K
(Number interviewed)	(299)	(124)	(172)	(595)

amount of travelling visually impaired people did in one week. Longer outings are considered in section 13.1.2.

13.1.1.1   All outings during the week

Table 13.1.a. shows that 20% of all visually impaired people did not go out in the last week. In each age group more blind than partially sighted people stayed at home, which confirms vision as a strong determining factor. The biggest difference between blind and partially sighted people is to be found in the 75 + age group; 39% of blind people, but only 15% of partially sighted people, had not gone out in the last week.

It is interesting to note that, of those who did go out, the majority of both the under-60s and the 60 + age group went on trips further afield. However, the 60 + figure masks one interesting variant. Sixty per cent of blind people aged 60 to 74 only travelled locally, while only 40% went further afield.

At 39%, the total of blind people aged 75 and over who had not been out in the last week is significantly higher than their partially sighted counterparts (15%) who had not been out. We shall see later (section 13.1.2.1), it is the independent mobility of visually impaired people as a whole that is restricted.

The data in Tables 13.2.a. and 13.2.b. show that, among those visually impaired people that had been out during the previous week, the frequency of outings is influenced by both age and residual vision.

Table 13.2.a Number of days went out during the week by three age groups

'On how many days did you go out in the last seven days...?' (BQ9)

	Age			Total
	16 – 59	60 – 74	75 +	
	%	%	%	%
1 – 2 days	26	40	50	45
3 – 4 days	14	25	20	21
5 or more days	60	35	30	35
Total %	100	100	100	100
Base (population)	69K	158K	378K	605K
(Number interviewed)	(278)	(108)	(129)	(514)

(514 respondents: 81 had not been out in the previous week)

Table 13.2.b Number of days went out during the week by residual vision within two age groups

'On how many days did you go out in the last seven days...?' (BQ9)

	Age and residual vision				Total
	16 – 59		60 +		
	B	PS	B	PS	
	%	%	%	%	%
1 – 2 days	29	24	39	51	45
3 – 4 days	21	11	22	22	21
5 or more days	51	66	40	27	35
Total %	100	100	100	100	100
Base (population)	26K	43K	180K	356K	605K
(Number interviewed)	(124)	(154)	(95)	(141)	(514)

(514 respondents: 81 had not been out in the previous week)

Overall nearly half (45%) had not been out on more than two days. Older respondents were more restricted in the frequency they go out than younger respondents. We find that 50% of visually impaired people aged 75 + had not gone out on more than two days, compared with 26% of those under 60. Sixty per cent of those under 60 reported going out on five or more days compared with 30% of those aged 75 + .

Looking at both age and residual vision level, a mixed pattern emerges. Sixty-six per cent of partially sighted people under 60 had been out on five or more days compared with 51% of blind people. This pattern is reversed for those aged 60 + where a larger percentage of blind people had been out over the same number of days compared with partially sighted people, 40 and 27 per cent respectively.

This pattern suggests that, while age may have a greater influence on the frequency of going out than residual vision alone, other influences on mobility may also be present, for example the presence or absence of another disability. Furthermore, age, residual vision and another disability have a compound effect on going out.

13.1.1.2 Unguided outings on foot: a measure of independent mobility

In their 1965 survey of the *Mobility and reading habits of the blind* (Gray and Todd, 1968), the authors, having examined a number of possible measures of independent mobility, concluded that the best measure available for survey purposes was whether the respondent had done any unguided travelling on foot during the week preceding the interview. This is our question BQ6, the answers to which appear in Tables 13.1.a and 13.1.b.

Fifty per cent of our respondents said that they went out on foot and 41% on foot alone. There was no difference between the 16 – 59 and 60 – 74 age groups. Extreme old age, the dividing line between the under-75s and those older, is a principal factor that determines whether visually impaired people go out on foot accompanied, and even more so whether they go alone. Sixty-eight per cent of people under 75 and 42% of those aged 75 + went out on foot, while 59 and 33 per cent respectively went out on foot alone. In the younger age band residual vision level made little difference: 51% of blind and 60% of partially sighted respondents went out alone on foot. However, among the 60 + age group sight levels did make a difference. Only 30% of blind people but 46% of partially sighted people went out. Within the latter age band, the corresponding percentages (not shown) were 25 and 39 per cent for those aged 75 and over.

13.1.1.3 Impact of registration

No overall relationship between registration status alone and independent mobility was found. However, a breakdown by age did reveal contrasting relationships. Separate and opposite trends among young and elderly people cancelled each other in the aggregate data. The data appear in Table 13.3.

The greater degree of independent mobility among registered blind and partially sighted people under 60 compared with non-registered people is quite startling. Seventy per cent of the registered group went out alone on foot in the last week, but only 45% of the non-registered. Overall, the registered group suffered from poorer vision than the non-registered, so we must look for other reasons to explain the difference (see Note 1). As successive chapters of this report show, registration is a critical factor determining whether services are received. The impact of services on independent mobility of the younger age group, in particular those offered by mobility officers, is discussed in section 13.4.1.2.

Table 13.3 Relationship between independent mobility, registration status and age

Respondents out on foot during previous week:
'...Was that on your own, or with another person, or both?' (BQ6)

	Age and registration status						Total
	16 – 59		60 +		All ages		
	R	NR	R	NR	R	NR	
	%	%	%	%	%	%	%
Went out on own	70	45	31	39	39	42	41
Went out with help or not out in week	30	55	69	61	61	58	59
Total %	100	100	100	100	100	100	100
Base (population)	29K	48K	140K	540K	170K	587K	757K
(Number interviewed)	(215)	(84)	(137)	(159)	(352)	(243)	(595)

Among the older group, the difference was reversed, although it did not quite reach statistically significant levels. Thirty-one per cent of the registered and 39% of the non-registered went out alone on foot. Why do the services received by registered people of 60 and over fail to have the same impact as on the under 60s? Mobility Officers traditionally spend less time working with individual elderly people than with younger people. Data presented in Table 13.15.a. show how few elderly blind people, even those who are registered, have been given formal mobility training.

13.1.1.4   Comparison with Gray and Todd's 1965 survey results

Gray and Todd surveyed only registered blind people aged 79 and under. We have insufficient data to compare the registered in the older age band, but the results for the roughly comparable younger age bands (16 – 59 in our data, 16 – 64 in Gray and Todd's data) are shown in Table 13.4. There are no significant differences. Despite the twenty-year gap between the two surveys, overall mobility seems scarcely to have altered, at least for young registered blind people. Our results are also consistent with the 1981 survey by the Blind Mobility Research Unit (Clark-Carter et al, 1981, page 21). They too found no significant differences in mobility between registered blind people in their Nottingham sample and those in the 1965 survey, either in the younger or the older age group.

Whatever we make of this comparison over time, it is to be noted that not all registered blind people have had formal instruction in the use of a white cane. Even among those aged 16 – 59, only 55% have had such training (see Table 13.15.b.). When those who have been trained and those who have not are compared, the trained have a clear mobility advantage.

Table 13.4 Mobility of the registered blind – RNIB and Gray and Todd surveys compared

	Registered blind respondents	
	1986 RNIB survey	1965 Gray and Todd survey
	Age group 16 – 59	Age group 16 – 64
	%	%
Did not go out during the week	6	8
Went out but no travelling on foot	11	6
Some travelling on foot but not unguided	17	23
Some travelling on foot, sometimes unguided	66	63
Total %	100	100
Base (population)	17K	24K
(Numbers interviewed)	(74)	(420)

13.1.2   Outings over a year

We asked respondents who had not been out on foot in the previous week if they ever went out on foot (BQ7) and, if so, whether they went on their own (BQ8). We also asked those who said that they had not gone out at all in the previous week (20%) whether they had been out at all in the last 12 months (BQ10); whether any travelling was done on foot (BQ11); and, if so, whether this was done unaccompanied by a sighted person (BQ12). Table 13.5 compares mobility over this longer time span with the results for a typical week, and shows that three-quarters (15% of the 20%) who said that they had not been out in the previous week had been out during the past year. The remaining quarter (5% of the 20%) who said they had not been out of their house during the previous year may fairly be categorised as truly 'housebound'.

Table 13.5 Levels of mobility achieved by visually impaired people during a week and a year

	During a week	Over a year
	%	%
'Housebound'	20	5
Went out with help	39	52
Went out on own	41	43
Total %	100	100
Base (population)	757K	757K
(Number interviewed)	(595)	(595)

The 15% who said that they had been out during the previous year but not the previous week divided 7 to 1 between those who had been out on foot accompanied and those who had been out on their own (39 + 13 = 52 and 41 + 2 = 43). Extending the time period from a week to a year increased the total who had been out accompanied from 39 to 52 per cent and of those who had been out alone by only 2%, from 41 to 43 per cent. The latter marginal difference means that 9 out of 10 people who had not done any unguided travelling during the previous week had also not travelled in this way during the last year. (A point of interest is that the majority of those housebound over the period of a year are aged 75 + .) The result corroborates the view that reference to the previous week provides a very good index of independent mobility.

13.1.2.1   Comparison with the sighted population

The data shown in Table 13.6.a are from Hunt's survey (1978) which covered people aged 65 and over living at home in England in 1976. Hunt's respondents were asked if they could go out on their own or only with help. The closest possible comparison with our survey can be obtained from data for mobility over a year, as shown in Table 13.6.b. While there is no difference in the percentages housebound, the proportion of elderly visually impaired people who can only go out with help vastly exceeds that of the elderly sighted population: 53 and 8 per cent respectively. While the great majority, 87%, of elderly people are able to get out on their own, only 42% of visually impaired people can do so.

Table 13.6.a.   Mobility of the general population aged 65 or over (Hunt survey 1978)

The elderly general population

	Two age bands		All 65 +
	65 – 74	75 +	All 65 +
	%	%	%
'Housebound'	2	10	5
Went out with help	5	13	8
Went out on own	94	77	87
Total %	100	100	100
Population numbers*	4316K	2184K	6500K
(Number interviewed)	(1354)	(1268)	(2622)

*Weighted data (see Hunt, 1978, paras 1.6 and A.3)
Source: Hunt 1978, Table 10.2.1, page 68

Hunt (page 144) suggests that a figure of 6,500,000 people should be used to extrapolate national estimates from her data. On this basis, 8% of elderly people who can only go out with help represent about half a million people. The 53% of visually impaired people who are similarly limited represent about a third of a million people. To give a precise

Table 13.6.b. Mobility of visually impaired people (over a year) aged 60 or over, RNIB survey (1986)

	Two age groups		
	60 – 74	75 +	All 60 +
	%	%	%
'Housebound'	#	7	6
Went out with help	41	57	53
Went out on own	59	36	42
Total %	100	100	100
Base population	180K	500K	680K
(Number interviewed)	(124)	(172)	(296)

(296 respondents: 299 aged 16 – 59 excluded)

comparison, these figures should be adjusted to take account of a number of factors. Nevertheless, they do provide a rough comparison. At the least we can say that visually impaired people represent a very substantial proportion of all elderly people who lack independent mobility. (Data from the OPCS survey are considered in Section 13.1.2.2.)

Since mobility is related to age as well as to visual impairment, comparisons with the general population across broad age bands must take account of the fact that the age profile of visually impaired people is older. However, lack of independent mobility is much more strongly related to visual impairment than to age, and visual impairment itself has a strong impact quite independent of age (see note 2). Evidence for this can be found in the age group relationships in Tables 13.6.a. and 13.6.b. In the 75 + age group, 77% of the general population compared with only 36% of visually impaired people are independently mobile. The corresponding totals in the under-75 age group are 94 and 59 per cent respectively. The age bands for the under-75s are sufficiently similar in Tables 13.6.a. and 13.6.b. for the younger age base of the RNIB data not to negate the differences in mobility between sighted and visually impaired people. It can be shown (see note 2) that the mobility differences persist even when age is completely controlled (i.e. any difference due to age is fully accounted for). (The RNIB data have a wider age range for the younger group, 60 – 74, compared with Hunt's 65 – 74 data. If anything, this means that the comparison understates the discrepancy in mobility needs.)

Elderly people who can only go out accompanied and who live alone are handicapped still more. As section 3.4 shows, the visually impaired population, being much more skewed towards extreme old age, more often live on their own. Hunt found that 30% of her general population sample aged 65 or over living at home were in single person households, while the corresponding total in our sample was 48%.

13.1.2.2 Comparison with people with other disabilities

Report 4 of the OPCS Disability Survey classifies respondents according to whether they are 'housebound', 'usually go out with assistance' or 'usually go out unassisted' (Martin, et al, 1989, pages 22 – 23). Since these categories are approximately the same as those in our survey with reference to mobility over the year, we can compare the overall mobility levels of visually impaired people with those of disabled people in general, as in Table 13.7.

Table 13.7 Levels of mobility of disabled people (OPCS data) compared with visually impaired people

	Visually impaired (RNIB survey)*	General disabled population (OPCS survey)
	%	%
Housebound	5	8
Went out with help	52	14
Went out on own	43	78
Total %	100	100
Population (base)	757K	5780K
(Number interviewed)	(595)	(10479)

OPCS population data from Report 1 (Martin et al, 1988a). OPCS mobility data, Table 3.5, OPCS Report 4 (Martin et al, 1989)
*Mobility in RNIB survey based on that over a year

It is evident that, although registrable visually impaired people are not significantly more housebound than disabled people in general (5 compared with 8 per cent), they enjoy markedly less overall mobility: only 43 compared with 78 per cent are able to go out on their own.

Levels of overall mobility as low as those experienced by visually impaired people occur only among those disabled people who score very high on the OPCS scale that measures severity of disability. Table 13.8 reproduces OPCS data showing the distribution of mobility levels along the severity scale. Without secondary analysis of the OPCS data these severity scores cannot be analysed in terms of registrable visual impairment. However, it is instructive to compare the data as they stand. Some 72% of the disabled population with severity scores as high as 5 – 6 still have independent mobility. Even 50% among those with a score of 7 – 8 are able to go out on their own compared with 43% of registrably visually impaired people (see Table 13.7). Only in cases of the severest disability is overall mobility among disabled people in general (21%) significantly lower than among visually impaired people. However, more disabled people with very high severity scores are housebound than visually impaired people as a whole; 20 and 39 per cent of disabled people with severity scores of 7 – 8 and

9 – 10 are housebound compared with 5% of the visually impaired population. The fact remains that over half (57%) of all registrably visually impaired people are unable to go outside their homes without help. This represents a high level of dependency when coupled with the fact that so many live on their own (Chapter 3), so depending on sighted helpers to arrive before they themselves can venture out.

Table 13.8   Mobility levels of disabled people within the OPCS severity categories

	Severity category					
	1 – 2	3 – 4	5 – 6	7 – 8	9 – 10	1 – 10
	%	%	%	%	%	%
'Housebound'	1	3	10	20	39	8
Went out with help	2	9	18	31	40	14
Went out on own	97	88	72	50	21	78
Total %	100	100	100	100	100	100
Population (base*)	2009	1408	1190	786	387	780

*Estimates in thousands from data in OPCS Report 1 (Martin et al, 1988a)
Source: OPCS 1989, Report 4, (Martin et al, 1989) Table 3.5

13.2   Respondents' perceptions of mobility

13.2.1   Visual impairment as a limiting factor

Respondents were asked (BQ1) to rate the extent to which they considered their sight problem prevented getting about out-of-doors. Table 13.9 shows the relationship between the responses and actual independent mobility (as measured by BQ6 – unguided outings on foot during the previous week). Forty-two per cent of those who reported that they had not gone out on foot alone during the previous week and 17% of those who did go out said that they thought their sight problem 'very much' limited them getting out-of-doors. The corresponding totals of those who said that they thought it was 'not at all' a limiting factor were 28 and 39 per cent. People at the same objective level of mobility differed in the extent to which they thought themselves limited in their mobility by their sight.

Table 13.10 relates self-assessments of mobility limitations (as measured by BQ1) to sight levels in two age groups. The proportions of blind and partially sighted people aged 16 – 59 rating themselves 'very much' limited were 38 and 16 per cent. In the older age band the corresponding proportions were 46 and 24 per cent. Those with better vision considered that their mobility was less limited, as we would expect from the answers given to more objective questioning about the

Table 13.9 Self-assessments of mobility related to actual independent mobility*

'We are interested in the extent to which you get about and the amount of walking you do outside. Would you say that your sight problem limits you getting about out-of-doors?...'(READ OUT) (BQ1)

	Went out alone during the week (BQ6)		Total
	Out alone	Not out alone	
	%	%	%
Very much	17	42	32
To an extent	32	22	26
Very little	13	8	10
Not at all	39	28	32
Total %	100	100	100
Base (population)	311K	447K	757K
(Number interviewed)	(314)	(281)	(595)

*Independent mobility; out alone on foot during the previous week (section 13.1.1.2)

Table 13.10 Self-assessments of visual impairment as a limit to mobility by residual vision within two age groups

'..Would you say your sight limits you getting about out of doors...?' (BQ1)

	Age and residual vision				Total
	16 – 59		60 +		
	B	PS	B	PS	
	%	%	%	%	%
Very much	38	16	46	24	32
To an extent	21	31	19	30	26
Very little	10	12	7	11	10
Not at all	25	41	28	34	32
Total %	100	100	100	100	100
Base (population)	30K	47K	270K	410K	757K
(Number interviewed)	(137)	(162)	(130)	(166)	(595)

extent of independent mobility (BQ6 – see Table 13.1.a.). However, the differences by age group are markedly narrower than those obtained from BQ6. This is likely to be yet another example of the tendency of older disabled people to discount the extent to which they are handicapped by their disability (Chapter 12).

13.2.2 The confidence factor

Table 13.11 compares how much confidence visually impaired people have in their ability to walk alone in (BQ13) and outside (BQ14) the immediate neighbourhood. (These questions were asked only of those who had been outside their homes on foot alone in the previous year.) As might be expected, levels are higher in the immediate neighbourhood. Thus only 1% rated themselves 'not at all' confident in their ability to walk in their immediate neighbourhood, while 26% said that they felt 'not at all' confident outside their immediate neighbourhood. Generally people felt more confident in their immediate neighbourhood than outside it. Thirty-eight per cent were very confident inside their neighbourhood, compared with 23% outside.

Table 13.11   Confidence in ability to walk out-of-doors alone

'How confident do you feel in your ability to walk in...
   —your immediate neighbourhood... (BQ13)
   —outside your immediate neighbourhood... (BQ14)
...on your own?'

	Immediate neighbourhood	Outside neighbourhood
	%	%
Very confident	38	23
Fairly confident	41	25
Not very confident	20	25
Not at all confident	1	26
Total %	100	100
Base (population)	371K	371K
(Number interviewed)	(341)	(341)

341 respondents: all those who had been out on foot alone during the previous year

The answers to the two questions (BQ13 and BQ14) were closely correlated. Knowing a respondent's level of confidence in the immediate neighbourhood enables one to predict their confidence level outside it. For instance, 59% of those who said that they were 'not at all' confident in going further afield came from those who rated themselves 'not very confident' locally. Similarly, 62% of those who said they were 'very confident' locally also said that they were 'very confident' walking alone further afield. When two questions receive such closely correlated responses, they can be taken as equivalent indicators of the same underlying factor, and each can be used to measure that factor, in this case confidence in independent mobility.

Table 13.12 supplies confidence ratings in the ability to walk alone in the immediate neighbourhood by age and residual vision level (BQ13); both variables influence confidence. Among the 16 – 59 year-olds, 65 and 53 per cent of blind and partially sighted people say that they feel 'very confident'. Among the older age group this is lower, 45 and 30 per cent respectively. While the 60 – 74 and 75 + age groups show different levels of confidence in the immediate neighbourhood (BQ13), both these groups of elderly visually impaired people have low levels of confidence further afield (BQ14). In the three age bands 16 – 59, 60 – 74 and 75 + the totals saying that they are very confident in the immediate neighbourhood are 57, 42 and 31 per cent respectively, and outside the immediate neighbourhood 31, 22 and 23 per cent respectively.

Table 13.12   Confidence in ability to walk out-of-doors alone by residual vision within two age groups

'How confident do you feel in your ability to walk in your immediate neighbourhood on your own?' (BQ13)

	Age and residual vision				Total
	16 – 59		60 +		
	B	PS	B	PS	
	%	%	%	%	%
Very confident	65	53	45	30	38
Fairly confident	20	34	30	50	41
Not very confident	14	10	25	20	20
Not at all confident	1	3	0	0	1
Total %	100	100	100	100	100
Base (population)	16K	33K	115K	207K	371K
(Number interviewed)	(151)	(57)	(51)	(82)	(341)

341 respondents: all those who had been out on foot alone during the previous year

13.3   Impact of other disabilities

Section 12.3 noted that half of all visually impaired people also suffer from other limiting disabilities. Table 13.13 breaks down our index of independent mobility (unguided journeys on foot in the previous week, BQ6) by whether or not the respondent has other disabilities. Overall, 41% of visually impaired people make independent outings; however, only 30% of those with additional disabilities do so compared with 52% of those without additional disabilities.

The impact of additional disabilities is most marked among those aged 16 to 59. Eighty per cent of those without additional disabilities went out alone, but only 34% of those with them. Young visually impaired people with additional disabilities do not show vastly differently levels of independent mobility compared with older visually impaired people in general. However, younger visually impaired people without additional disabilities are much more mobile than their older counterparts. If additional disabilities are present the advantages of relative youth

Table 13.13 Impact of other disabilities on independent mobility
(GQ8, BQ6)

	Age and other limiting disabilities						Total
	16 – 59		60 +		All ages		
	Other disabilities		Other disabilities		Other disabilities		
	No	Yes	No	Yes	No	Yes	
	%	%	%	%	%	%	%
Out alone on foot in previous week							
Out alone	80	34	45	36	52	30	41
Not alone/not out	20	66	55	64	48	70	59
Total %	100	100	100	100	100	100	100
Base (population)	38K	39K	341K	340K	379K	379K	757K
(Number interviewed)	(185)	(114)	(140)	(156)	(325)	(270)	(595)

vanish. Young and old visually impaired people with additional disabilities suffer equally from immobility.

Those who said (BQ1) that their sight problem limited their getting about out-of-doors were asked (BQ2) whether their sight problem was the main limitation. Table 13.14 breaks down the answers according to the presence or absence of other limiting disabilities (GQ8). Once again, the impact of such disabilities is marked. The great majority (82% across all age groups – 95% in the 16 – 59 age band) of those without other limiting disabilities said that sight was the main limiting factor, in contrast with half (47%) those with another limiting disability.

Table 13.14 Sight as the main factor limiting mobility by age and other limiting disabilities (BQ2, GQ8)

'Is your sight problem the main reason that it is difficult for you to get about, or is it something else?' (BQ2)

	Age and other limiting disabilities						Total
	16 – 59		60 +		All ages		
	Other disabilities		Other disabilities		Other disabilities		
	No	Yes	No	Yes	No	Yes	
	%	%	%	%	%	%	%
Main reason for mobility problems							
Sight	95	54	80	46	82	47	63
Other reason	5	46	20	54	28	53	37
Total %	100	100	100	100	100	100	100
Base (population)	22K	28K	212K	251K	234K	279K	512K
(Number interviewed)	(115)	(84)	(104)	(117)	(219)	(201)	(420)

420 respondents: 175 respondents who did not consider (at BQ1) that their sight problem limited their mobility were not asked BQ2

Hearing loss was not included in the other disabilities considered, even though it is commonly held that hearing does affect the ability of visually impaired people to move around on their own. Perhaps our data were too unrefined to detect it, but we could find no evidence of any relationship of hearing problems (GQ2) and independent mobility (BQ6).

13.4 Mobility aids and training

We asked the following set of questions under this heading.

'Do you have a white stick or a cane to help you get about outside?' (BQ23)

'Has anyone given you proper lessons in using one (a white cane)? (BQ24)

'Has anyone given you lessons in how to get about outside, or in the home?' (BQ25)

'Have you ever been offered advice on getting about or on the use of a white stick or cane for getting about?' (BQ29)

Tables 13.15.a., 13.15.b. and 13.15.c. break down the results by age, registration status and residual vision levels. Table 13.15.a. also shows the data obtained relating to guide dogs discussed in section 13.4.2.

Table 13.15.a. Mobility advice, lessons and guidance received, by registration status and age

	Age and registration status						Total
	16 – 59		60 +		All ages		
	R	NR	R	NR	R	NR	
	%	%	%	%	%	%	%
Have white stick or cane	62	11	75	7	73	8	22
Received proper lessons in use of white cane*	40	4	13	1	18	1	5
Have guide dog	9	0	1	0	2	0	1
Used to have guide dog	3	0	#	1	1	1	1
Some lessons in getting about	5	4	1	0	2	#	1
No lessons or advice	43	91	82	92	75	92	88
Never go out	0	0	1	7	1	6	5
Base (population) = 100%	29K	48K	140K	540K	170K	587K	757K
(Number interviewed)	(215)	(84)	(137)	(159)	(352)	(243)	(595)

(595 respondents)   *The 4% non-registered aged 16 – 59 here consisted of 2 interviews only, both non-registered partially sighted people. None of the non-registered blind people in the sample had had lessons

183

Table 13.15.b. Mobility advice, lessons and guidance received, by residual vision and age

	Age and residual vision						Total
	16 – 59		60 +		All ages		
	B	PS	B	PS	B	PS	
	%	%	%	%	%	%	%
Have white stick or cane	54	16	32	12	37	12	22
Received proper lessons in use of white cane	33	8	7	1	9	2	5
Some lessons in getting about	6	4	1	0	1	#	1
No lessons or advice	55	84	85	93	82	92	88
Never go out	0	0	6	5	5	5	5
Base (population) = 100%	30K	47K	270K	410K	301K	456K	757K
(Number interviewed)	(137)	(162)	(130)	(166)	(267)	(328)	(595)

(595 respondents)

Table 13.15.c. Mobility advice, lessons and guidance received, by age

	Age		Total
	16 – 59	60 +	
	%	%	%
Have white stick or cane	31	21	22
Proper lessons in use of white cane	18	3	5
Some lessons in getting about	5	#	1
No lessons or advice	72	90	88
Never go out	0	6	5
Base (population) = 100%	77K	680K	757K
(Number interviewed)	(299)	(296)	(595)

(595 respondents)

13.4.1 Use of a white stick or cane

Twenty-two per cent of respondents said (at BQ23) that they used a white stick or cane to get about (population projection 169,000). Usage was heavily concentrated among the registered: 73% (124,000 people) compared with 8% (45,000) of the non-registered were users. Significant age differences occurred only among registered partially sighted people. Eighty-two per cent (89,000) of registered blind people (15,000 under 60, 74,000 60 +); 33% (4,000) of registered partially sighted people under 60; and 63% (31,000) of those aged 60 + said that they used a white stick or cane.

Only 5% (4.6% rounded – population projection of 35,000) of visually impaired people as a whole said that they had received proper mobility lessons in the use of a white stick or cane (BQ24). These consisted of 18% (30,000) of the registered and only 1% of the non-registered. Both age and residual vision had an impact. Fifty-five and 17 per cent respectively of registered blind people aged under 60 and 60 + had received lessons (equivalent to 10,000 and 15,000 people), as had 17 and 6 per cent of registered partially sighted people in the same age bands (2,000 and 3,000 people). Only among registered blind people aged under 60 have a majority (55% – 67% of those with one) received lessons in the use of a white stick or cane as a mobility aid.

If we exclude from the total number of cane users those people who are under 60 and registered blind, 154,000 users remain. From this large group, only 16% (25,000) have had proper lessons in the use of their white cane or stick.

It may be argued that respondents were given more mobility training than they reported, but the fact that such training was not recalled suggests that it was not very significant. Our information on training related to age verifies long-standing assertions about the age bias in the provision of training. (For example, 33% of blind people under 60 have been trained; 18% of those aged 60 to 74 and 5% of those aged 75 + .) It is often said that blind people over 60 are 'too old to get out and about', but this anecdotal opinion should be set against Hunt's evidence (see Table 13.6.a.) that 93% of 65 to 74 year-olds in the elderly population as a whole go out on their own and 77% of the 75 + group. Although more elderly visually impaired people have additional handicaps, there is considerable scope for improving independent mobility.

13.4.1.1   Source and format of mobility lessons

Those who said that they had not received proper lessons (BQ24) were asked, 'Has anyone given you any lessons in how to get about outside, or in the home?' (BQ25). The positive answers to this question resulted in a small increase (population projection 35,000 to 40,000) in the number who had received mobility instruction.

Of the estimated 40,000 people who had received some form of mobility instruction, mobility officers and home teachers were the main source of these lessons, reported (BQ26) by an estimated 13,000 and 9,000 respectively. The remaining mentions were spread across a variety of types of instructor: for instance, doctor/nurse (6,000), RNIB (3,000), social worker or other social services (2,000), rehabilitation officer (1,000), household member (1,000), unspecified other (3,000).

Those who had received lessons were asked (BQ28) 'How long did the training last?' and were given set categories in which to reply: just one or two visits – not proper lessons (34%), 1 – 3 proper lessons (12%),

4 – 10 proper lessons (13%), 11 – 30 proper lessons (18%), more than 30 lessons (8%), residential course (6%). The population projections for BQ26 and BQ28 come from the 114 respondents who had received lessons. The grossed up figures carry sampling errors (Section 21.4), and must accordingly be treated as approximate estimates.

Non-users of a white stick or cane were asked three further questions. First, 'Have you ever been offered advice on getting about or on the use of a white stick or cane for getting about?' (BQ29), to which some 99% said 'no'. They were then asked 'Did you know that people with sight problems can be given training to help them to get about?' (BQ30). Some 25% said that they did know (30% of the registered, 23% of the non registered). Knowledge was related to age, though mainly among the registered. Among registered blind and registered partially sighted people aged under 60 the total saying 'yes' was 73 and 51 per cent respectively, while in other sub-groups the total was 30% or less.

The 1% (rounded) who said (at BQ29) that they had received advice amounts to 10,000 people. However, since this percentage results from interviews with only 31 respondents their replies about sources of advice must be treated with caution. Given the small number of respondents involved, it is more sensible to enumerate exact replies received. Nine, nine, six, three and two respondents mentioned home teacher, mobility officer, social worker, others unspecified from social services and doctor/nurse respectively. The local blind society and RNIB were each mentioned by one respondent.

13.4.1.2   Impact of lessons on mobility

As noted in Section 13.1.1.2, for survey purposes the best measurement of independent mobility was the question whether or not the respondent had done any travelling on foot unguided during the previous week (BQ6). Data on whether the respondent has received proper lessons in using a white stick or cane is provided by BQ24. The answers to BQ6 and BQ24 enable us to compare the independent mobility of those who have received proper lessons with those who have not, as in Table 13.16.

The comparison can only be made for blind people aged 16 – 59, since only this sub-group contains sufficient numbers who have received formal training (see Note 2). The results show that formal training produces a clear advantage: 64% of those who had been trained went out on foot alone in the previous week compared with only 45% of those who had not been trained. However, Table 13.16 includes both registered and non-registered. (All 63 respondents aged 16 – 59 who had received formal mobility training (BQ24) were registered blind; none of the 14 non-registered blind respondents in this age group had received such training.) It should be noted that a similar tabulation

Table 13.16   Independent mobility of blind people aged 16 – 59 who have and have not received lessons in using a white cane

Whether has had proper lessons in use of a white stick or cane (BQ24)

Those who have been out alone in previous week on foot (BQ6)

	Lessons in using a white cane		Total
	Lessons	None	
Went out unguided in last week	%	%	
Went out alone	64	45	51
Went out with guide	36	55	49
Total %	100	100	100
Base (population)	10K	20K	30K
(Number interviewed)	(63)	(74)	(137)

(137 respondents: blind people aged 16 – 59 who have had formal lessons in mobility)

based only on registered blind people aged under 60 (123 interviews, population projection 18,000 of whom 10,000 had received mobility training) did not show that training benefited mobility. While a full explanation of this apparent anomaly will have to await more intensive secondary analysis, we can hypothesise that Table 13.16 provides another demonstration of the registration effect already noted in Table 13.3. That is to say, registration has a trigger effect on the delivery of services in general, and this affects mobility over and above specific mobility training. As noted in section 13.1.1.4, training of this kind has a limited impact on the numbers of visually impaired people who are independently mobile, as the comparison with Gray and Todd's survey shows.

It was noted in section 13.4.1 that only 55% of all registered blind people aged 16 – 59 have received formal mobility training. More extensive formal mobility training would have a considerable impact on mobility levels, even among younger registered blind people. Since none of our non-registered (but registrable) blind respondents had received formal training, there is clear scope for raising the mobility level of this group by extending the service to them. Finally, as noted in section 13.4.1, there is even greater scope for extending the service at least to registered blind people aged 60 and over.

13.4.2   Guide dogs and other mobility aids

We asked 'Do you have a guide dog, or have you ever had one?' (BQ33). Only 21 respondents currently had a guide dog: all were registered blind and only three were over 60 years old (see Table 13.15.a.). This suggests that there are about 4,000 guide dog owners, a figure that is very near the known ownership advised by the Guide Dogs for the Blind Association.

As the last question on mobility, respondents were asked, 'Can you think of any practical help that might make it easier for you to get out more than you do at the moment?' (BQ34). Some 72% could think of nothing. The most frequent suggestions were a human escort and a car (5% each). 'Better health' and 'better sight' were each mentioned by 2%, a 'guide dog', 'a white stick' and 'more wheelchair access' by about 1% each. Some 12% of replies can be classified as 'other', a category that consisted of a large variety of items including (number of mentions in brackets): fewer or no steps leading out of the house/flat (3); mobility allowance (2); bus pass or cheaper bus fares (4); money for taxis (2); wheelchair and someone to push it (1); invalid cars or electric wheelchairs (2); large-print timetables or enlarged route numbers on the front of buses (3); a small telescope to see such (bus) numbers (1); fewer uneven pavements (1); better street lighting (1); painted pavement edges (1); no overhanging branches/hedges (2); no parked cars on pavements (1); no racks of goods or notices outside shops (2); more bleeper crossings (1); more mobility training officers (1); rehabilitation course (1).

13.5   Visits

Questions on visits to and from relatives, friends and neighbours fitted easily into the sequence on mobility, and the answers may be conveniently reported here.

The following questions were asked:

'About how often do you visit relatives?' (BQ17)

'About how often do you visit friends and neighbours?' (BQ18)

'Apart from those living with you do you have any close relatives?' (BQ19)

'About how often do any of your close relatives manage to visit you?' (BQ20)

'Do any friends and neighbours ever come to visit you?' (BQ21)

'How often do your friends and neighbours come to visit you?' (BQ22)

Table 13.17 shows the answers received from all respondents. Since the percentages change little between the various sub-groups, a more detailed breakdown is not required.

No doubt because of their restricted mobility, visually impaired people receive more visits than they make. Weekly visits from relatives or

Table 13.17 Frequency of visits to and from relatives, and friends and neighbours

	Visits to		Visits from	
	Relatives BQ17	Friends BQ18	Relatives BQ20+	Friends BQ22++
	%	%	%	%
At least once a week	23	25	54	47
Less, but at least monthly	15	11	13	14
At least once every 3 months	8	3	4	4
2 – 3 times a year	12	4	9	4
Once a year	5	1	3	1
Less often	6	13	3	1
Never	31	43	14	29
Total %	100	100	100	100
Base (population)	757K	757K	757K	757K
(Number interviewed)	(595)	(595)	(595)	(595)

+ Includes information from BQ19
+ + Includes information from BQ21

friends, at 54 and 47 per cent, considerably exceed those made to relatives or friends, 23 and 25 per cent respectively. Conversely, those who never visit relatives or friends, 31 and 43 per cent, considerably exceed those who never receive visits from relative or friends, 14 and 29 per cent respectively.

The terms 'weekly' and 'friends' are used here, although the actual questions stated 'at least once a week' and 'friends and neighbours'. At least weekly visits do much to help visually impaired people living alone to manage their day-to-day affairs. Although people living alone make and receive slightly more visits, the trend is not so great as to offset their isolation. When the responses of people living alone and with others to BQ17, BQ18, BQ20 and BQ22 were compared, a difference of about 5% emerged. For example, 57% of those living alone received weekly visits from relatives compared with 51% of those living with others. As far as informal contacts are concerned, people living alone who never visit or receive visits are in complete social isolation. (Formal contacts are considered in Chapter 19.) Given our estimate that 346,000 visually impaired people live alone, a significant proportion, 26% (about 90,000 people), say that friends or neighbours never visit them, and 11% (38,000 people) say that they are never visited by a relative. Of respondents living alone, 30, 44, 11 and 26 per cent answered 'never' to questions BQ17, BQ18, BQ20 and BQ22. As far as visits to friends and relatives are concerned, there is no difference from respondents living with others. There was only a marginal difference in visits from friends and relatives; the totals for those living alone and with others were 11 and 17 per cent (relatives) and 26 and 30 per cent (friends).

Breakdowns of the four questions on frequency of visits (BQ17, BQ18, BQ20 and BQ22) were also made by age and residual vision level. The latter produced no significant differences, nor did age have any effect on the frequency with which visits were received. Only one question, on the frequency of visits made to relatives (BQ17), produced any age difference. Some 31% of the younger age group, 16 – 59, visit relatives weekly compared with 23% of those aged 60 or over.

Other findings relevant to the social support network of visually impaired people are reviewed in Chapters 16, 19 and 20.

Notes to Chapter 13

Note 1

The registered in Table 13.3 include both blind and partially sighted people. The correlation between mobility and mobility training among the registered blind sub-group is discussed in Section 13.4.1.2 (Table 13.16).

Note 2

Table 13.16 is restricted to the sub-group of registered blind people aged 16 – 59 for two reasons. Both age and residual vision could affect mobility, and it is necessary to control for both these factors if we wish to assess the true impact of the training variable on its own. If we had sufficient data we would want to make the cross comparison between BQ24 and BQ6 separately within sub-groups controlled for age and residual vision. Blind 16 – 59 year olds constitute one such sub-group. It so happens that this is the only sub-group for which we have sufficient data to analyse with respect to mobility training: of the total sample of 595 respondents, only 100 said at BQ24 that they had had proper lessons and, of these 100, 63 were aged 16 – 59 and registrably blind. In fact, all of them were registered blind.

We have not developed comparisons between the registered and non-registered blind in this age group since (see 21.9) we had only 14 respondents among the sub-group of 16 – 59 year-olds registrably blind people who are not registered. Thus in Table 13.16, whereas all 63 respondents interviewed who had received proper lessons were registered, the 74 who had not received them consisted of 60 registered blind and 14 non-registered blind people. It is to be noted, however, that the percentages for independent mobility are as low as 25% among the non-registered blind compared with 71% of the registered blind in the 16 – 59 age group. The difference is large enough to be statistically significant, but since the 25% results from only 14 interviews, the 95% confidence interval (see 21.4) is about .4 (+ /-); that is, the population value could lie between 65% and zero. It seemed better to leave the statistical statement of the overall effect of registration on mobility to the data in Table 13.3. This shows the dramatic difference of 70 versus 45 per cent, and, since both blind and partially sighted people are included, the numbers interviewed are more substantial. It may be worth noting that, among partially sighted people, 17% (16 respondents) of the registered and 6% (2 respondents) of the non-registered had had lessons (BQ24). The corresponding independent mobility figures for partially sighted people were 75 and 55 per cent (BQ6).

14 Shopping and Transport

14.1 Shopping

14.1.1 Distance to the nearest food shops

At BQ35 we asked 'How long would it take you to walk to your nearest food shop – would it be ...?' The aim of the question was to ascertain information on the average 'walking time' from the respondent's home; the wording was modified for those unable to walk by themselves to 'How long would it take for someone to walk there?' The following alternatives were read out by the interviewer (the percentage of people responding is given in brackets): up to 5 minutes (30%); 6 to 10 minutes (29%); 11 to 15 minutes (15%); 16 to 20 minutes (7%); 21 to 30 minutes (6%); longer (11%). Thus, over half of our respondents live within 10 minutes', and three-quarters within 15 minutes', walk of the nearest food shop.

14.1.2 Shopping and visual impairment

We asked (BQ36) 'Do you do your household shopping on your own most of the time, some of the time, or never?' and received responses of 22, 19 and 59 per cent respectively. Thus, the majority (59%) of visually impaired people rely on others to shop for their basic needs. This applies to all sub-groups except for partially sighted people in the 16 – 59 and 60 – 74 age bands, though even here 49 and 41 per cent respectively never do their own shopping. Thus those who always do their own shopping are in a minority in all sub-groups. In the 16 – 59 age group, 14 and 26 per cent of blind and partially sighted people respectively, and in the 60 + age group 19 and 25 per cent, did their own shopping most of the time. Among those aged 75 and over, only 17% did their own shopping most of the time, and 20% some of the time, with no difference in this age group between residual vision levels.

Visual impairment aside, there are many reasons why people might not do their own household shopping, including the ordinary division of house-keeping roles, immobility because of additional disabilities, distance from the shops, busy road crossings, lack of bleepers (audible signals) at crossings, and the availability of helpers. While more refined analysis might identify some of these reasons, we did ask three more questions (BQ37, BQ38 and BQ39) to help to clarify the picture.

Those who never do their own household shopping were asked (BQ37) 'Is that because you can't manage on your own?' Eighty-three per cent of them responded 'yes', and indicated immobility owing to handicap as the major reason. This finding applies to all sub-groups (though among partially sighted people in the 16 – 59 age group the total fell to 70%).

Those who said (at BQ36) that they do their own shopping most or some of the time were asked (BQ38) 'How difficult do you find the shopping when you do it on your own? Is it very difficult, fairly difficult, or not at all difficult?' Replies to each category were 24, 29 and 47 per cent. In the 'very difficult' category, age rather than residual vision was the major variable; in the 16 – 59, 60 – 74 and 75 + age bands, 10, 11 and 33 per cent respectively gave the 'very difficult' response. We noted above that only 37% of visually impaired people aged 75 or over do their own shopping most or some of the time, and now we find that a third of them find it very difficult. Those who responded 'very difficult' or 'fairly difficult' (at BQ38) were asked (BQ39) 'Is your eyesight the main reason for your difficulty?' Eighty per cent said that it was. The total reached 97% among blind people, and fell to 77% among partially sighted people aged 60 or over.

14.1.3 Local road conditions

Road and traffic conditions encountered on the way are one factor affecting visually impaired people's ability to do their own household shopping. At BQ15 we asked about traffic in the neighbourhood; 40% said that it was very busy, 34% fairly busy and 24% not at all busy. We also asked (BQ16) whether local pedestrian crossings were equipped with audible signals: 12% said that all crossings in their area had them, 23% that some had, 49% that none had, and 17% did not know. Thus the majority of visually impaired people have to negotiate very or fairly busy roads in neighbourhoods where few or none of the pedestrian crossings have audible signals.

14.1.4 Source of help with household shopping

All respondents were asked (BQ40) 'Who usually/sometimes helps you with your household shopping?'. Only 13% overall said 'nobody'. This breaks down to 9% of blind people, 17% of partially sighted, 22% of the under-75s and 8% of those aged 75 or over. The main sources of help mentioned were household member (38%), other relatives (36%), friend (12%) and home help (10%). Age differences were notable: in the age bands 16 – 59, 60 – 74 and 75 + the mentions for household member were, 67, 41 and 32 per cent; for other relative, 15, 29 and 41 per cent; for friend 7, 7 and 14 per cent; and for home help 4, 8 and 12 per cent. A wide variety of other types of helper were mentioned (social worker, voluntary worker, doctor, nurse and unspecified others), but none of these individually scored more than 0.5%.

The older age groups receive more help from people outside the household such as other relatives and less from those relatives in the house and other household members. Although still of minor importance, the amount of help given by friends and home helps also increases with the increase in age of respondents. In short, as spouses die, relatives, friends and neighbours increase their role. This pattern is also seen in Chapter 15.

14.2   Transport

14.2.1   Transport used in a typical week

14.2.1.1   All usage

We noted (section 13.1.1.1, Table 13.1.a.) that some 80% of respondents (about 605,000 visually impaired people) make some sort of outing in a typical week, and that nearly two-thirds (381,000 people, some 63% of those who go out during the week) do so on foot. Thus about one-third of those who make weekly outings rely on some form of transport. In addition, many of those who do go out on foot will also use transport.

The data, shown in Tables 14.1.a. and 14.1.b., were derived from the answers to questions BQ42A and BQ42B:

> 'Now I would like to ask you a few questions about any type of transport you use. Thinking about the last seven days, that is from... up to yesterday, have you used a...?' (BQ42A)
>
> [If yes) 'Was that on your own, or with someone else, or both?' (BQ42B)

Table 14.1.a.   Use of transport by those who had been out during the previous week

'Thinking about the last seven days, have you used a...?' (BQ42A)

	Mode of transport used					
	Car	Bus	Taxi	Train	Coach	Tube
	%	%	%	%	%	%
Used last week	59	33	15	3	3	1
Not used last week	41	67	85	97	97	99
Total %	100	100	100	100	100	100
Base (population)	605K	605K	605K	605K	605K	605K
(Number interviewed)	(514)	(514)	(514)	(514)	(514)	(514)

514 respondents. BQ42A was only asked of respondents who had been out in previous week at BQ3. A few 'no answers' at BQ42A have been counted as not using a vehicle in the week

Table 14.1.b. Independent use of transport during the previous week

'Thinking about the last seven days, have you used a...?' (BQ42A)

IF YES: Was that on your own, or with someone else, or both (BQ42B)

	Mode of transport used					
	Car	Bus	Taxi	Train	Coach	Tube
	%	%	%	%	%	%
Used...						
On own	9	80	61	17	11	22
With someone else	91	20	39	83	89	78
Total %	100	100	100	100	100	100
Base (population)	357K	200K	91K	18K	18K	6K
(Number interviewed)*	(328)	(223)	(86)	(29)	(22)	(14)

*Respondents who had used each mode of transport at BQ42A

The six types of transport mentioned most frequently at BQ42A were: car (59%), bus (33%), taxi (15%), train (3%), coach (3%) and tube (1%). Thus almost as many people (about 357,000) go out by car as go out on foot, about half as many (200,000) use buses, and almost half as many again use taxis (some 90,000 people). Train, coach and tube are relatively little used over the span of a week. (In the London area, the incidence of tube users would of course be greater, but even if the figures were adjusted accordingly the figures for the tube are about the same as those for the relatively little used train and coach.)

An important point to note, not shown in the tables, is that 28% of blind people under 60 took a taxi in the previous week. This will no doubt absorb a considerable proportion of their income, which we have already seen is lower than that of the general population.

14.2.1.2 Independent weekly usage

The extent to which a particular form of transport helps the independent mobility of visually impaired people can be gauged from the percentage of respondents who said (at BQ42B) that they use it on their own rather than accompanied. As Table 14.1.b shows, buses and taxis emerge as the chief means of independent mobility. Eighty and sixty-one per cent of visually impaired people (160,000 and 56,000) who had been out used these two forms of transport. Twenty-two, 17 and 11 per cent using tubes, trains and coaches respectively did so on their own, but as already noted the actual numbers travelling in these ways are very low. Although cars are the dominant means of transport, used by some 357,000 visually impaired people in a week, their use does of course depend on the availability of a sighted companion. (Some 9% of car-users, almost exclusively blind people aged 75 and over, said that they had been out on their own in a car. These respondents either misunderstood the question, or else were travelling with volunteer

drivers whom they hardly knew and so considered that they were going
out 'on their own'.)

14.2.2 Transport over the year

Respondents who had not used a particular mode of transport during
the previous week were asked (at BQ43A) if they had used it during the
previous year. Table 14.2.a. shows the following usage pattern over a
year: car 82% (population projection 285,000 people); bus 34%
(172,000); taxi 31% (187,000); coach 24% (162,000); train 14%
(95,000); and tube 4% (28,000).

Table 14.2.a. Use of transport over a year by those who had
not been out during the previous week

'Now I would like to ask about the different types of transport you use. Have
you used a ...during the last twelve months?' BQ43A

	Mode of transport used					
	Car %	Bus %	Taxi %	Train %	Coach %	Tube %
Used in last 12 months	82	34	31	14	24	4
Not used in last 12 months	18	66	69	86	76	96
Total %	100	100	100	100	100	100
Base (population)	348K	506K	602K	680K	675K	692K
(Number interviewed)+	(243)	(349)	(484)	(543)	(550)	(559)

+Respondents are those who had not used the particular mode of transport
during the previous seven days

Table 14.2.b. Independent use of transport during the
previous 12 months

IF YES to BQ43A: 'Do you go on your own, or with someone else, or both?'
(BQ43B)

	Mode of transport used					
	Car %	Bus %	Taxi %	Train %	Coach %	Tube %
Used...						
On own	1	45	24	43	10	37
With someone else	99	55	76	57	90	63
Total %	100	100	100	100	100	100
Base (population)	287K	177K	188K	92K	164K	27K
(Number interviewed)*	(193)	(149)	(204)	(134)	(187)	(68)

*Respondents are those who have used the mode of transport during the
previous 12 months, but not in the last seven days

These statistics represent occasional travellers in contrast with the
regular travellers previously considered. Comparing Tables 14.1.a. and

14.2.a., in other words those visually impaired people who make weekly outings and those who go out less than once a week, we find that cars, even more than in the latter group, are the dominant means of transport for both groups, but especially for occasional travellers (59 and 82 per cent). Buses are used by much the same proportions, 33 and 34 per cent. Taxis (15 and 31 per cent), trains (3 and 14 per cent) and coaches (3 and 24 per cent), however, are used much more by occasional than by regular travellers. Large numbers of visually impaired people who do not use these forms of transport on a regular weekly basis, nevertheless use them for occasional special journeys during the course of a year.

On the whole, the occasional travellers consist of less mobile visually impaired people, for whom the forms of transport they can use unaccompanied represent a particularly important element of their independence. Table 14.2.b. shows the percentage of occasional travellers who use each form of transport on their own: 45% used buses independently, 43% trains, 24% taxis, 10% coaches and 37% tubes. As might be expected, independent use by occasional travellers is lower than by regular travellers in all categories except the tube and train. Trains in particular are used more often for occasional independent journeys; 43% used a train in the previous year, compared with 17% in the previous week. The pattern varies again for taxis. Occasional travellers resort to a taxi relatively more often than those who go out regularly on a weekly basis (31 and 15 per cent, Tables 14.1.a. and 14.2.a.). However, taxis are used more often by regular travellers as a means of independent travel; 61% of them who use taxis do so on their own, compared with only 24% of occasional travellers (Tables 14.1.b. and 14.2.b.). The tube accounts for only 4% of the journeys made by occasional travellers, but just over one third (37%) are unaccompanied. Coaches are more often used by occasional travellers, but almost always (90%) on an accompanied basis.

15 Daily Living Skills

15.1 The daily living skills assessment tasks

A large part of our survey was devoted to assessing the ability of visually impaired people to look after themselves: or, in welfare jargon, assessing their daily living skills. Respondents were questioned on their ability to carry out a set of everyday tasks, and were also asked to self-assess whether the difficulty in the task was because of their visual impairment or for some other reason.

Fifteen tasks or daily living skills (DLS) were used to assess the ability of respondents to live independently. Six tasks related to personal care; one of these varied according to the sex of the respondents, men being asked about shaving, women about doing their hair. A further six consisted of domestic tasks, and the final three related to dealing with paper work, mail and strangers calling at the house door.

Table 15.1 lists all these tasks for those saying that they found them either 'fairly difficult', 'very difficult' or 'impossible'. When respondents said that they did not carry out a particular task, they were asked how difficult they would find it if they had to do it. Nine out of ten blind and partially sighted people experienced difficulties with one or more of these crucial daily living skills. For three-quarters the difficulty was so great that they had to have help.

15.2 Personal care tasks

Three tasks stand out in this group as causing difficulty. Twenty-six per cent of respondents said that getting about the house caused them difficulty; 32% mentioned washing and bathing, and 81% cutting their toe nails. Toe-nail cutting appears to be a particular problem, with 57% attributing the difficulty mainly to their sight (Table 15.2). A large majority (88%) of those aged 75 or over reported problems with toe-nail cutting, together with 74% of the 60 – 74 year-olds and 54% of those aged under 60.

Table 15.1 Difficulties with daily living skills by residual vision within two age groups

'Can we talk about how you manage in the home. I have here a list of things that some people have difficulty doing at home, and I would like you to tell me how difficult it is for you...' (GQ13) (GQ18) (GQ23)

	Age and residual vision				Total
	16 – 59		60 +		
	B	PS	B	PS	
	%	%	%	%	%
Personal care					
Cutting toe nails	65	47	82	85	81
Washing/bathing	33	21	41	28	32
Getting about the house	34	21	31	22	26
Getting into/out of bed	22	15	20	19	19
Dressing	23	19	24	14	18
Doing hair (women)*	39	20	25	23	24
Shaving (men)*	12	10	20	16	17
All having difficulties with personal care tasks	69	53	84	88	84
Domestic tasks					
Vacuum cleaning	50	36	60	51	53
Making a hot meal	48	21	52	33	39
Tidying up	43	24	48	25	34
Cutting up food	36	22	47	18	30
Wash up and dry dishes	36	17	44	17	24
Making a hot drink	33	13	37	12	22
All having difficulties with domestic tasks	66	43	70	62	64
Mail and other tasks					
Dealing with...					
Paperwork, including bills and letters	86	63	73	55	63
Post through the door	85	45	69	47	56
Strangers calling at door	59	23	52	25	36
All having difficulties with mail tasks	88	64	77	58	66
All having difficulty with one or more task	91	76	89	94	91
No difficulties with any task	9	24	11	6	9
Base (population) = 100%	30K	47K	270K	410K	757K
(Number interviewed)	(215)	(137)	(84)	(159)	(595)

Note: Entries relate to respondents who found the tasks either 'fairly difficult' 'very difficult' or 'impossible'

*Asked of men and women separately

Base population: women: 17K, 27K, 186K, 311K, 542K

               men: 13K, 20K, 84K, 98K, 216K

15.2.1 Sight as the main cause of difficulty

As Table 15.2 shows, sight was an important reason for finding 'getting about the house', 'cutting toe nails', 'doing hair' (women) and 'shaving' (men) difficult. Even if other problems are given as the main cause of difficulty, the additional impact of visual impairment should not be under-estimated. Evidence for this appears in Table 15.1, where for every task but one more blind people than partially sighted people report problems.

Table 15.2 shows that except for 'shaving' a higher percentage of blind respondents than of partially sighted respondents consistently reported sight as the main difficulty. The largest differences was for 'getting about the house' and 'cutting toe nails'.

Table 15.2 Sight as the main cause of difficulty with personal care tasks

'Do you find ... (DLS tasks) difficult mainly because of your sight problem or something else?' (GQ15)

			Sight	Other	Total %	Base (Popltn)	Nos. +
Getting about the house	%	B	54	46	100	91K	(57)
	%	PS	24	76	100	97K	(66)
	%	B & PS	38	62	100	188K	(123)
Getting into/out of bed	%	B	28	72	100	55K	(35)
	%	PS	17	83	100	84K	(53)
	%	B & PS	21	79	100	140K	(88)
Washing/bathing	%	B	32	68	100	120K	(73)
	%	PS	18	82	100	115K	(75)
	%	B & PS	25	75	100	235K	(148)
Cutting toe nails	%	B	69	31	100	238K	(193)
	%	PS	49	51	100	364K	(211)
	%	B & PS	57	43	100	602K	(404)
Dressing	%	B	28	72	100	66K	(51)
	%	PS	10	90	100	67K	(50)
	%	B & PS	19	81	100	133K	(101)
Doing hair (women) + +	%	B	46	53	100	54K	(39)
	%	PS	30	70	100	74K	(38)
	%	B & PS	37	63	100	129K	(77)
Shaving (men) + +	%	B*	57	43	100	14K	(15)
	%	PS*	93	7	100	14K	(19)
	%	B & PS	73	27	100	28K	(34)

+ (Numbers) only asked of respondents who had difficulty with each task

+ + Asked of men and women separately

*Low bases: % differences to be treated with caution (see section 21.4)

15.2.2 Help with personal care tasks

When we asked (at GQ16) who assists with personal care tasks, the helpers most frequently mentioned were someone from the 'health service' and 'someone in the household' (68 and 33 per cent respectively). 'Other relative' (8%) was the only other helper to receive a significant mention. Table 15.3 shows the results in detail.

Table 15.3 Help with personal care tasks by age and residual vision

'You said you need help with some of these things. Who helps with these things?' (GQ16)

	Age			Residual vision		Total
	16 – 59	60 – 74	75 +	B	PS	
	%	%	%	%	%	%
Health service	25	52	77	54	79	68
Someone in the house	78	40	26	46	23	33
Other relative	7	8	9	11	7	8
Friend/neighbour	7	#	5	4	4	4
Home help	10	2	3	4	3	3
Base (population) = 100%	40K	122K	411K	235K	237K	572K
(Number interviewed)	(138)	(89)	(146)	(177)	(196)	(373)

(373 respondents: 222 reported no help needed with personal tasks)

Sources of help vary significantly according to the age group concerned. The patterns for the 16 – 59 and the 75 + groups form almost direct opposites. With increasing age help shifts from within the household to outside sources (in this case the health service). Seventy-eight per cent of respondents aged 16 – 59 were helped by 'someone in the house', but only 40% of those aged 60 – 74 and 26% of the very elderly. The totals for health service helpers were 25, 52 and 77 per cent respectively in the same three age groups. Thus the younger age groups still share the household with relatives able to help with these tasks. The older the visually impaired person, the less likely it is that family carers will be present, a finding supported by the data on single households provided in Chapter 3. And even if family carers are available, they themselves are likely to suffer from poor health. Forty-seven per cent of respondents living with one other person reported that person's health was 'not too good' or 'not at all good' (GQ10).

Table 15.3 also shows that blind people depend far more than partially sighted people on someone in the house (46 and 23 per cent). Dependence on health service support, by contrast, is more prevalent among partially sighted people (79 compared with 54 per cent). A more detailed breakdown by residual vision level within age reveals an interesting inversion among the 75 + group. While 39% of blind people in this age group were helped by someone in the house and 60% relied on health service support, only 17% of partially sighted people had someone living with them and 89% were supported by the health service. These figures suggest that if they are to stay at home, older blind people need someone to live with them; without such support, they are more likely to have to go into care. On the other hand, partially sighted people are more likely to be able to cope on their own but consequently need health service support for personal care arrangements.

A theme can be seen developing. With increasing age the helper shifts from the informal care network, relatives and friends, to the formal care network, someone from the statutory welfare services. The situation is even more difficult when no welfare resources are available. In many cases among older people a family helper is simply not present. Given an ageing population, this situation will not improve. These findings have important implications for community care, especially when the family is expected to take on the role of principal carer; even with the support of welfare services, this may not be possible.

15.3   Domestic tasks

As Table 15.1 shows, the overall level of difficulty with domestic tasks was lower than that for the personal care tasks (64 compared with 84 per cent). Within the two age groups more blind people than partially sighted people consistently reported difficulty with each of the tasks. The overall figures are 66 to 43 per cent and 70 to 62 per cent for young and old visually impaired people respectively.

The average difference between blind and partially sighted people who have difficulty with the tasks is about 20% across both age groups, 'vacuum cleaning' being somewhat lower for older partially sighted people. There was no significant difference in the proportions of younger and older blind people and younger and older partially sighted people who found these individual tasks difficult, which would suggest that the primary difficulty relates to vision.

15.3.1   Sight as the main cause of difficulty

The response to this question (GQ20), shown in Table 15.4, allows us to be fairly confident that performance of domestic tasks depends upon the level of residual vision. These tasks require considerable hand/eye co-ordination, the eye leading the hand to the task in question, in contrast with the personal care tasks which primarily require motor skills to accomplish. It is only to be expected that the tasks which require a far greater degree of visual assessment for their accomplishment are those for which respondents are more likely to state that the difficulty is because of their sight problem.

Table 15.4   Sight as the main cause of difficulty with domestic tasks

'Do you find ... (DLS tasks) difficult *mainly* because of your sight problem, or mainly something else?' (GQ20)

			Sight	Other	Total %	Base (Popltn)	Nos. +
Cutting up food	%	B	74	26	100	132K	(115)
	%	PS	42	58	100	85K	(69)
	%	B & PS	62	38	100	217K	(184)
Making a hot drink	%	B	73	27	100	99K	(72)
	%	PS	55	45	100	55K	(52)
	%	B & PS	67	33	100	154K	(124)
Making a hot meal	%	B	67	33	100	147K	(119)
	%	PS	39	61	100	131K	(91)
	%	B & PS	54	46	100	278K	(210)
Wash up and dry dishes	%	B	66	34	100	978K	(74)
	%	PS	29	71	100	71K	(91)
	%	B & PS	50	50	100	168K	(135)
Vacuum cleaning	%	B	55	45	100	171K	(126)
	%	PS	25	75	100	215K	(128)
	%	B & PS	38	62	100	386K	(254)
Tidying up	%	B	60	40	100	135K	(102)
	%	PS	37	63	100	108K	(82)
	%	B & PS	50	50	100	243K	(184)

+ (Numbers) only asked of respondents who had difficulty with each task

15.3.2   Help with domestic care tasks

Those who said that they needed help with domestic care tasks were asked (at GQ21) who helps. Overall, 'someone in the house' (57%), 'home help' (39%) and 'other relative' (16%) were the most frequent responses, as Table 15.5 shows.

The pattern of assistance with domestic tasks does not alter as dramatically as with personal care tasks, reflecting their rather different nature. However, the trend for increasing help from the welfare services and decreasing reliance on someone in the house with increasing age is still evident. Elderly people, especially those aged 75+, receive a relatively high level of assistance from within the household, together with increased help from the formal care services.

The nature of the tasks alters the outside agency that provides most help. The health service was most frequently mentioned as the agency providing help with personal care tasks. With domestic tasks, home helps provided by social services departments are most frequently mentioned. It is also interesting that the overall level (39%) of outside

Table 15.5 Help with domestic tasks by age and residual vision

'You said you need help with these things...Who helps you?' (GQ21)

	Age			Residual vision		Total
	16 – 59	60 – 74	75 +	B	PS	
	%	%	%	%	%	%
Someone in the house	82	64	52	65	51	57
Home help	21	26	45	28	48	39
Other relative	14	13	17	12	18	16
Volunteer not identified	0	0	4	5	2	3
Friend/neighbour	13	0	1	2	2	2
Health service	3	0	2	1	3	2
Base (popltn) = 100%	32K	88K	290K	180K	230K	410K
(Number interviewed)	(111)	(68)	(105)	(153)	(131)	(284)

(284 respondents: 311 reported no help needed with domestic tasks)

help required for domestic tasks is lower than that for the personal care tasks (68%). This may reflect the fact that not only are domestic tasks generally less urgent but also the lower statutory resources available to fulfil them.

As with the personal care tasks, blind people depend more on someone in the house (65%) than partially sighted people (51%), whereas the latter rely to a greater extent on home helps (48 and 28 per cent). It should be noted that our questions did not distinguish between the various tasks a helper may undertake. A home help may simply vacuum and tidy the house, while a household member will deal with the personal care tasks.

15.4   Mail-related and other tasks

These tasks, which concern dealing with paperwork such as bills and letters, mail and strangers calling at the door cause considerable difficulty. A higher proportion of respondents than for other tasks across all age groups and both sight levels stated that they found these tasks either 'very difficult' or 'impossible'.

Blind people especially find dealing with paperwork and post through the door particularly difficult (86, 85, 73 and 69 per cent of young and old people respectively). That blind people find this particularly difficult is hardly surprising since most official communications and unsolicited mail is in print form.

Strangers calling cause twice as many blind people difficulty compared with partially sighted people (53 and 25 per cent).

15.4.1 Sight as the main cause of difficulty

As Table 15.6 shows, sight is the overwhelming cause of difficulty with mail-related tasks; almost equal proportions of blind and partially sighted people reported difficulty, over 80% for both paperwork and post. This obviously has implications for direct postal communication with visually impaired people, even though a large proportion of visually impaired people can read some print (Chapter 7), while those who cannot have someone who reads to them (Chapter 9).

Twice as many blind compared with partially sighted people found dealing with strangers calling difficult. While 84% of blind people said that sight was their main difficulty, a still overwhelming majority (65%) of the latter did so.

Table 15.6   Sight as the main cause of difficulty with mail-related tasks

'Do you find ... (DLS task) difficult *mainly* because of your sight problem or *mainly* something else?' (GQ25)

			Sight	Other	Total %	Base (Popltn)	Nos. +
Paperwork including	%	B	87	13	100	222K	(228)
bills and letters	%	PS	80	20	100	246K	(201)
	%	B & PS	83	17	100	468K	(429)
Post through the door	%	B	90	10	100	213K	(221)
	%	PS	83	17	100	200K	(163)
	%	B & PS	87	13	100	413K	(384)
Strangers calling at the	%	B	84	16	100	150K	(137)
door	%	PS	65	35	100	107K	(92)
	%	B & PS	76	24	100	257K	(229)

+ (Numbers) only asked of respondents who had difficulty with each task

15.4.2 Help with mail-related tasks

Overall, as Table 15.7 indicates, the most frequently mentioned helpers with these tasks were 'someone in the house' (53%), 'other relatives' (35%), and 'friend/neighbour' (11%). The main source of help for these tasks is the informal care network, a stark contrast with personal care and domestic tasks where the formal care network is a significant source of help. These communication tasks represent a far more extensive problem, and fewer respondents stated that they had 'no problem' or 'did not need any help' with them. This may reflect their visual nature—there is no alternative method of coping with printed material that comes through the door.

Table 15.7   Help with communication tasks by age and residual vision

'You said you need help dealing with paperwork or post and things that come through the door. Who helps you with these things?' (GQ26)

	Age			Residual vision		Total
	16 – 59	60 – 74	75 +	B	PS	
	%	%	%	%	%	%
Someone in the house	88	57	46	58	47	53
Other relative	7	18	45	32	37	35
Friend/neighbour	7	12	12	10	12	11
Home help	2	8	10	7	10	9
Base (popltn) = 100%	44K	105K	299K	226K	222K	448K
(Number interviewed)	(187)	(86)	(126)	(229)	(170)	(399)

(399 respondents: 106 reported no help needed with mail and strangers calling at the door)

In all age groups, the statutory welfare services received negligible mentions for these tasks. It is interesting to speculate whether this is because of the nature of the tasks or because welfare services are not allocated to do these jobs. With callers, this is only to be expected, since a helper would have to be present all the time.

Many people prefer family and friends to deal with mail, perhaps for reasons of privacy. This is in contrast with many aspects of intimate personal care, where someone from the health service is a major helper. Furthermore, an appreciable number of respondents lived alone and were visited only infrequently by family, friends and neighbours.

As with the other tasks, help from someone in the house decreases with increasing age, while assistance from outside the household increases. It is noticeable that 'other relative' (relatives outside the household) is more frequently mentioned than 'friend/neighbour', reflecting the private nature of the tasks; these mentions probably related to the first two tasks rather than to strangers calling at the door. Respondents are likely to wait for a relative to visit to read mail rather than ask a neighbour. For instance, one respondent interviewed at the pilot stage waited for his daughter's weekly visit when she read his mail.

Respondents were given the opportunity to say which other household tasks they found difficult. The ones most frequently mentioned, though not by many people, were: household activities (14%); food preparation (14%); cleaning (11%); electrical (4%); decorating (3%).

15.5   Overall difficulty with daily living tasks

Counting the number of tasks respondents find difficult gives us an overall view of the restrictions that visually impaired people experience in these tasks essential to daily life. Table 15.8 provides this information.

Table 15.8 Overall difficulty with daily living tasks, by residual vision within three age groups

Number of tasks found difficult (BQ13, BQ18, BQ25)	16 – 59		60 – 74		75 +		All 16 +		Total
	B	PS	B	PS	B	PS	B	PS	
	%	%	%	%	%	%	%	%	%
None	9	24	10	18	11	1	11	8	9
1 – 3	25	37	22	33	20	46	21	42	34
4 – 7	23	20	34	30	23	30	25	28	28
8 – 10	18	11	19	14	21	11	20	11	15
11 or more	25	9	15	5	25	12	23	10	15
Total %	100	100	100	100	100	100	100	100	100
Base (population)	30K	47K	65K	115K	205K	295K	300K	457K	757K
(Number interviewed)	(137)	(162)	(55)	(69)	(75)	(97)	(267)	(328)	(595)

Various points are worth emphasising. First, blind people of all ages have significantly more difficulties than partially sighted people; the only marginal exception is cutting toe nails among those aged 60 and over (Table 15.1). For example, 66% of blind people aged 16 – 59 have problems with four or more tasks, in contrast with only 40% of partially sighted people; this approximate ratio applies to both the 60 – 74 and 75 + age groups. Second, increasing difficulties correlate with increasing age, although to a lesser extent than in other areas our survey investigated, since younger people too experience considerable difficulties with these daily tasks. (For reasons not immediately apparent, more people under than over 60 had difficulty with communications tasks; see Table 15.1.) Third, those tasks that caused more difficulty generally also produced a larger differentiation between blind and partially sighted people.

15.6 Household devices and gadgets

15.6.1 Awareness of household devices and gadgets for visually impaired people

Respondents were asked (at GQ31) whether they had heard of some of the more popular devices and gadgets for use in the home. As Tables 15.9.a. and 15.9.b. show, awareness varied with both age and residual vision. More blind respondents had heard of the devices. Both younger people and blind people are more often registered and thus more likely to be in contact with the agencies that carry relevant information.

Residual vision level affects awareness in two ways. First, it may determine the actual or perceived need for these devices, and so

Table 15.9.a Awareness of popular devices and gadgets by residual vision within three age groups

'There are various devices and gadgets which are available for people with sight problems, to help them do things that otherwise they couldn't do very well. Can I check whether you have heard of such devices?' (GQ31)

	Age and residual vision						Total
	16 – 59		60 – 74		75 +		
	B	PS	B	PS	B	PS	
	%	%	%	%	%	%	%
Special timers	75	55	62	25	37	27	36
Special marker for cooker	65	32	47	29	29	15	27
Writing template/guide	54	31	39	15	31	7	21
Liquid level indicator	53	31	33	9	8	10	15
Other devices	23	19	15	8	10	2	8
Unaware of any devices	26	42	30	59	44	65	53
Base (population) = 100%	30K	47K	65K	115K	205K	294K	756K
(Number interviewed)	(137)	(162)	(55)	(69)	(75)	(97)	(594)

(594 respondents: no information for 1 respondent)

Table 15.9.b Awareness of popular devices and gadgets by residual vision

	Residual vision		Total
	B	PS	
	%	%	%
Special timers	46	29	36
Special marker for cooker	36	20	27
Writing template/guide	35	12	21
Liquid level indicator	18	12	15
Other devices	8	12	5
Unaware of any devices	53	52	61
Base (population) = 100%	300K	456K	756K
(Number interviewed)	(267)	(327)	(594)

(594 respondents: no information for 1 respondent)

influence whether the individual concerned seeks information about them. Second, and more important, it may also influence whether service-providers inform the individual concerned about the existence of the devices.

Age also plays a complex role. As an individual's sight deteriorates with increasing age, he or she may develop coping techniques or else, more drastically, avoid doing difficult tasks. From the perspective of the welfare services, they thus become a coping individual who does not 'need' sight aids. This process is compounded by the fact that elderly people are likely to suffer disabilities or long-standing illnesses that may limit their activities. Even though their sight may be very restricted, the presence of other disabilities deflects attention from the benefits sight aids may offer. Hence, while awareness of these typical technical aids is quite high among younger blind people, it is worryingly low among blind people aged 75 or over.

15.6.2   Possession of popular devices and gadgets

Respondents who were aware of the named devices were asked (at GQ32) if they possessed the item. Respondents were able spontaneously to report whether they used the item, (although this is reported in the text it is not shown in the table). Table 15.10 shows the results to questioning at GQ32. Special timers (which include watches) were the most popular devices and also the ones most likely to be used. Both age and residual vision level determine possession and usage. Those aged 75 and over are less likely to possess these aids, and if they do possess them are also less likely to make use of them.

Table 15.10   Possession of devices and gadgets by residual vision and age

'Do you actually have a ...?' (GQ32)

	Age and residual vision						Total
	16 – 59		60 – 74		75 +		
	B	PS	B	PS	B	PS	
	%	%	%	%	%	%	%
Writing template/guide	24	6	21	9	18	1	10
Special timers	43	8	23	4	9	4	9
Special marker for cooker	19	4	19	7	2	2	5
Liquid level indicator	22	3	15	1	3	2	4
Other devices	23	19	15	8	10	2	8
Have no gadgets	50	75	63	88	69	92	80
Base (population)	30K	47K	65K	115K	205K	295K	757K
(Number interviewed)	(137)	(162)	(55)	(69)	(75)	(97)	(595)

(595 respondents)

The data in Table 15.10 suggest a problem relating to elderly visually impaired people. They are least likely to possess devices and gadgets. When they do possess them they do not appear to use them. Even with popular devices such as special timers, those aged 75 + spontaneously express a high non-user rate. This trend may reinforce the perception among welfare agencies that it is not worthwhile providing elderly people with aids of this kind. Reasons linked to other disabilities, such as lack of manual dexterity, may explain why elderly people do not use these devices and gadgets.

Table 15.10 shows that writing templates or guides (10%) and special timers (9%) are the items most frequently possessed. Special timers were possessed by 43, 23 and 9 per cent of blind people in increasing age order, compared with 8, 4 and 4 per cent of partially sighted respondents. Only 18% of those who have timers report not using them. Writing templates and guides were possessed by 24, 21 and 18 per cent of blind respondents. Among partially sighted respondents, the possession rate was much lower, 6, 9 and 1 per cent, increasing in age order. Non-use of templates was spontaneously reported by 42% of those who possessed them.

It is clear from Table 15.10 that at all ages very few partially sighted respondents possessed the aids listed. Tables 15.9.a. and 15.9.b. indicate that fewer have heard of them. None of this, however, should cause much surprise.

15.6.3 Registration status and devices and gadgets

If awareness of devices and gadgets is examined according to registration status (Table 15.11), it is clear that registered respondents are more aware than non-registered respondents. The differences resulting from residual vision level and age remain. In other words, registered and younger respondents are more likely to be aware of the devices and gadgets available. This adds to the developing theme of this report that while welfare agencies claim to offer help to all individuals with a visual impairment, in reality they provide most assistance to younger visually impaired people, particularly those who are registered.

Table 15.11 Awareness of popular devices and gadgets among the registered and non-registered, within two age groups (GQ31)

	Age and registration				Registration status		Total
	16 – 59		60 +				
	R	NR	R	NR	R	NR	
	%	%	%	%	%	%	%
Special timers	84	48	57	27	62	29	36
Special marker for cooker	70	29	48	19	52	19	27
Writing template/guide	67	23	47	12	50	12	21
Liquid level indicator	71	20	32	7	38	8	15
Other devices	32	13	15	5	18	5	8
Unaware of any devices	14	50	24	62	22	61	53
Base (population) = 100%	29K	48K	139K	540K	169K	587K	756K
(Number interviewed)	(215)	(84)	(136)	(159)	(351)	(243)	(594)

(594 respondents: no information for 1 respondent)

Table 15.12 shows that registration is a clear influence on possession of devices and gadgets. This is to be expected, since the registered are also most aware of them.

Table 15.12 Possession of popular devices and gadgets among the registered and non-registered

'Do you actually have a ...?' (GQ32)

	Registration status		Total
	R	NR	
	%	%	%
Writing template/guide	32	3	10
Special timers	31	2	9
Special marker for cooker	16	2	5
Liquid level indicator	15	1	4
Other devices	18	5	8
Have no devices	44	90	80
Base (population) = 100%	170K	587K	756K
(Number interviewed)	(351)	(243)	(594)

(594 respondents: no information for 1 respondent)

16 Leisure

16.1 Radio and television

16.1.1 Radio ownership

Some 19% of visually impaired people either do not own a radio (9%) or own one but do not listen to it (10%). This total of those not owning a radio – or owning one but never listening – increases with age: 7, 12 and 22 per cent respectively in the age bands 16 – 59, 60 – 74 and 75 +.

16.1.2 Stations most listened to

Respondents owning a radio were asked (at BQ45) which of the following radio stations they listened to most: BBC Radios 1, 2, 3 and 4, local radio for the blind, local radio (BBC and commercial), or other radio station. As Table 16.1 shows, local radio proved the most popular choice, 34% of respondents selecting it overall: 48% of those aged 16 – 59; 44%, 60 – 74; 28%, 75 +. (Note that our survey was

Table 16.1 Radio stations most listened to

'Which radio station do you listen to most?' (BQ45)*

	Age			Total
	16 – 59	60 – 74	75 +	
	%	%	%	%
Radio 1	11	#	3	4
Radio 2	14	32	22	23
Radio 3	3	2	#	1
Radio 4	19	13	24	21
Local radio for the blind	#	0	#	#
Local radio	48	44	28	34
Other radio station	#	2	#	1
Never listen to radio	3	7	11	10
Do not own a radio (BQ44)	4	5	11	9
Base (population) = 100%	77K	180K	500K	757K
(Number interviewed)	(299)	(124)	(172)	(595)

*Respondents were allowed to mention two stations if they were unable to decide between them; in the event most chose a single station

undertaken before BBC Radio 5 came into existence.) Twenty-three and 21 per cent respectively overall listened to Radios 2 and 4.

The preferences were broadly the same across all the age groups. Radio 1 was listened to almost exclusively by the 16 – 59 age group (11%); Radio 2 was more preferred by people aged 60 and over than by younger listeners (25 and 14 per cent). Local radio was a clear leader among people aged under 75, 45% of whom preferred it, against 28% of those aged 75 or over.

16.1.3 Other stations listened to

That a station is not listened to most often does not of course mean that it is never listened to. We asked (at BQ46) to which other stations respondents listened. Table 16.2 combines the results of BQ45 and BQ46 to show the total percentage listening to each station. Radios 1 and 3 were each mentioned by 15% overall; Radio 1's largest audience was among the under-60s (37%). Half of all visually impaired people (well over one third of a million in all) listen to a local radio station, although the numbers decline with age: 71, 56, and 34 per cent respectively of the three age bands. Hardly anyone (2% overall), even among our blind respondents, mentioned local radio for the blind, and only slightly more (5% overall) said that they listened to other radio stations.

Table 16.2   All radio stations that are listened to

'Which radio station do you listen to most?' (BQ45)

'Do you listen to any of these other radio stations at all?' (BQ46)

	Age			Total
	16 – 59	60 – 74	75 +	
	%	%	%	%
Radio 1	37	9	12	15
Radio 2	46	47	41	43
Radio 3	18	13	14	15
Radio 4	36	34	37	36
Local radio for the blind	3	1	3	2
Local radio	71	56	34	50
Other radio station	8	6	3	5
Never listen to radio	3	7	11	10
Do not own a radio (BQ44)	4	5	11	9
Base (population) = 100%	77K	180K	500K	757K
(Number interviewed)	(299)	(124)	(172)	(595)

About one-fifth of all blind and partially sighted people listen regularly or occasionally to Radio 4's *In Touch* programme, which is specifically aimed at people with a visual impairment. Overall, only 28% of blind and partially sighted people know about the programme. Awareness was highest among blind people under 60 (53%). Thirty-eight per cent of young elderly blind people, and 31% of those aged 75 or over, were aware of it.

Of those who do know about *In Touch*, over three-quarters listen either regularly (20%) or occasionally (56%). These overall figures hide some interesting variations. An extremely high percentage of blind and partially sighted people aged 75 or over, 90 and 82 per cent respectively, listen either regularly or occasionally, the majority occasionally. The equivalent totals for blind and partially sighted people aged 16 – 59 are 65 and 45 per cent.

These figures suggest that the programme should be more vigorously promoted among its potential audience, since it is clear that once people are aware of it a significant majority do tune in. For both the voluntary and statutory services the programme is a very useful vehicle for reaching their client groups.

16.1.4 Changing radio stations

Sixty-six per cent of visually impaired people who listen to the radio said (at BQ47) that they change stations on their radio by themselves; the total was 77% of those aged under 60, falling to 62% of those aged 75 + . Differences in residual vision level have a marked impact with increasing age. The percentage (77%) of those who change stations themselves hardly changes with sight level in the younger age group. Sixty-three per cent of blind people aged 60 – 74, and 77% of partially sighted people, change stations by themselves; among those aged 75 + the numbers are 51 and 71 per cent respectively.

The fact that nearly one half of blind people aged 75 and over cannot switch radio stations on their own only serves to emphasise the importance of producing easy-to-operate equipment.

16.1.5 Television

While it might be expected that visually impaired people would have much less use for television than sighted people, our survey does not bear this out. We asked respondents (at BQ50) if they had a television set and, if so, whether they watched or listened (BQ51). Some 94% said that they did have one, the percentage hardly varying between blind and partially sighted respondents.

It is the extent, rather than the mere fact, of television viewing or listening among blind and partially sighted people that is surprising. That 90% watch or listen makes it a vital communication medium for the statutory and voluntary services. Organisations representing visually impaired people should therefore urge programme makers to avoid 'vision only' representation of information on programmes that consist primarily of 'talking'; one example is the use of sub-titles alone to translate foreign-language interviews shown on news programmes.

16.2 Hobbies

16.2.1 Spontaneous versus prompted replies

BQ52 in the leisure section asked 'Still thinking about your spare time; we've already talked about radio and television, and the different ways of reading. Apart from these things, do you have any hobbies or interests?' This was an open, unprompted question and respondents gave spontaneous replies. It is likely that the things people mention spontaneously are more important than those named only after prompting. However, we also named a number of activities – gardening, knitting or needlework, listening to music, outdoor sports and indoor games – and asked respondents (at BQ53) if they did any of these things. The prompt list partly consisted of activities which, as the pilot suggested, many people did but failed to mention. We also wanted to collect more detail about the types of indoor games played.

Table 16.3 shows both spontaneous (BQ52) and prompted replies (BQ53), bringing together the data obtained on any item for which both spontaneous and prompted replies were obtained. The text analyses the information in three sub-sections on the most popular activities; substantial minority interests; and miscellaneous minority interests.

16.2.2 The most popular activities

Before we examine the most popular hobbies, it is worth recalling the popularity of television, radio and tapes. Ninety per cent of visually impaired people listen to or watch television, 81% listen to radio and 46% to tapes. Even individual services score relatively high, with 12% listening to RNIB Talking Books and 8% to talking newspapers.

Television, radio and tapes aside, the five most popular activities are: gardening, knitting or needlework, outdoor sports, indoor games and listening to music.

16.2.2.1 Gardening

Gardening was mentioned spontaneously by 15% of respondents overall, and is the activity *par excellence* favoured by elderly visually impaired people, and particularly by blind people. Nineteen per cent of blind, and 14% of partially sighted, people aged 60 + mentioned

Table 16.3 Hobbies of visually impaired people as revealed by spontaneous and prompted replies (BQ52 and BQ53)

	Age and residual vision						Total
	16 – 59		60 – 74		75 +		
	B	PS	B	PS	B	PS	
	%	%	%	%	%	%	%
Gardening:							
spontaneous	7	9	20	24	19	10	15
prompted	33	38	26	42	29	33	32
Knitting/needlework:							
spontaneous	12	29	19	35	25	22	25
prompted	16	37	18	44	8	34	26
Listening to music:							
spontaneous	6	4	4	2	0	0	1
prompted	95	83	92	88	81	67	77
Playing music:							
spontaneous	6	2	3	0	1	#	2
Outdoor sports:							
spontaneous –							
swimming	14	2	1	#	0	0	1
walking	12	9	0	#	0	0	1
other	11	3	0	#	0	0	1
Outdoor sports:							
prompted	18	10	0	3	0	#	2
Indoor games:							
spontaneous –							
snooker	3	4	2	2	0	2	2
other	1	1	2	3	3	2	3
Indoor games:							
prompted –							
card games	11	7	10	21	4	8	9
dominoes	9	3	11	4	2	2	3
Scrabble	6	5	3	7	0	3	3
snooker	5	4	0	0	0	0	1
other	10	9	1	8	0	7	5
Substantial minority interests:							
spontaneous –							
handicrafts	6	6	6	6	2	2	4
dancing	1	5	0	6	#	2	2
pubs	8	2	#	1	2	2	2
church	2	4	6	3	1	#	2
committees/meetings	2	4	6	3	1	#	2
voluntary work	3	9	0	0	1	0	1
other	34	37	24	19	8	16	14
Base (popltn) = 100%	30K	47K	65K	115K	205K	295K	757K
(Number interviewed)	(137)	(162)	(55)	(69)	(75)	(97)	(595)

gardening spontaneously, compared with only 8% of those aged 16 – 59. After prompting, the mention of gardening rose to 32%.

Gardening is almost as popular among blind people as among partially sighted people. Nor is it particularly age-related. It is just as popular among the older generation as among younger visually impaired people, with 29 and 33 per cent of blind and partially sighted people aged 75 or over mentioning it as a hobby, in comparison with 32% for the whole blind and partially sighted population.

Though both sexes engage in gardening, it is more popular among men. Roughly twice as many men as women mentioned gardening spontaneously, the same proportion that Hunt's (1978) survey of sighted elderly people found. This survey also revealed that gardening is one of the most popular hobbies of sighted elderly people. Twenty-six per cent of respondents aged 65 or over mentioned gardening spontaneously compared with 15% in our roughly similar age group. While it can be expected that more sighted people would mention gardening, nevertheless a remarkable number of both blind and partially sighted people do not let their handicap prevent them pursuing what would appear to be a hobby requiring visual skills.

Our results reveal that blind and partially sighted people of all ages do engage in gardening. That more could probably do so is suggested by the lower participation levels in comparison with sighted people of the same age. These findings suggest that organisations representing visually impaired people should explore ways of providing additional support and encouragement, e.g. through additional technical aids, gardening hints and support services.

16.2.2.2   Knitting and needlework

The word 'knitting' is used as a shorthand for replies such as knitting, sewing, crocheting, and using a knitting- or sewing-machine. Twenty-five per cent of respondents mentioned knitting spontaneously. Knitting is almost exclusively a woman's activity, 34% overall engaging in it. In the three age bands, 16 – 59, 60 – 74 and 75 +, the totals were 36, 47 and 29 per cent.

Prompting produced only a very small increase in mentions of knitting, which suggests that this is a very definite preoccupation, and important to those who do it. They do not have to be prompted to remember it.

Hunt found that 34% of sighted women aged 65 or over (40, 26 and 23 per cent respectively in the age groups 65 – 74, 75 – 84 and 85 +) mentioned knitting spontaneously, much the same level as we found. However Hunt put 'needlework' in a separate category which was mentioned by 20, 22 and 20 per cent of sighted women in these three age groups. Although we are not told how much double counting there was (women who gave replies in both categories), it is safe to assume that fewer visually impaired than sighted women engage in knitting and related activities. Again, the remarkable fact is the number of women who do follow this activity despite their sight loss. 'I knit by touch' was a common comment. The popularity of knitting is a tribute both to the knitters' ingenuity and also to those organisations that supply special patterns and technical aids.

16.2.2.3   Outdoor sports

Outdoor sports are a very popular activity only among the 16 – 59 age band. Because of the extreme bias in the age distribution of visually impaired people, it is easy to lose sight of the importance of this group of activities. Across all age groups, only 3% of respondents spontaneously mentioned an outdoor sport, and among those aged 60 and over less than 1% did so. Of the 16 – 59 age group, however, 25% mentioned outdoor sports. No other activity so dramatically separates young and old visually impaired adults.

Swimming and walking were the two main activities, mentioned by 14 and 2 per cent and 12 and 9 per cent of blind and partially sighted respondents respectively. The difference for swimming is statistically significant. No other major sporting activity emerged, but 11% of blind people, and 3% of partially sighted people, aged under 60 mentioned a wide variety of different activities that are categorised in Table 16.3 as 'other' outdoor sports (the difference is statistically significant). These included sailing, skiing, riding, fishing and archery, none of which was pursued by more than 1 or 2 per cent of the age group. Prompting did not result in an increase in the numbers who said that they participate in outdoor sports, and a breakdown by sex showed no significant differences.

Our results demonstrate that younger blind rather than young partially sighted people take most interest in outdoor sports in general, and in swimming in particular. Although the popularity of sports among younger blind people may surprise many sighted readers, it is at least partly explained by the active sports programmes in schools for blind people and the activities of the many specialist sports organisations of blind people. Sports activity among younger blind people is a success story and as such particularly worthy of support.

16.2.2.4   Indoor games

Very few respondents mentioned indoor games spontaneously, perhaps because they did not perceive these as a hobby or interest. Only 'snooker' was mentioned sufficiently to be singled out. When prompted, however, many respondents said that they did play them and named a variety.

Dominoes is a great favourite, especially among blind people aged under 75, 10% of whom mentioned dominoes against 4% of partially sighted people of the same age. (The difference is not statistically significant.) Only 2% of those aged 75 and over play dominoes.

Card games were fairly popular among the under-60s, with little difference between partially sighted and blind respondents (7 and 11 per cent). Among the two older groups, however, cards were much more popular among partially sighted people. Twenty-one per cent of partially sighted and 10% of blind respondents aged 60 – 74 mentioned card games, 8 and 4 per cent of those aged 75 + . Overall, 9% mentioned card games after prompting, a total exceeding any other indoor game.

Scrabble was mentioned by 6% of the under-60s and 5% of those aged 60 – 74, with no significant differences between partially sighted and blind respondents. Among those aged 75 and over, 3% of partially sighted respondents mentioned Scrabble, but none of the blind respondents.

Snooker is used to cover a number of related activities, including billiards and other ball games. This pastime mainly interested the under-60s, 4% of whom mentioned it. Only one respondent from the older age groups claimed any interest.

The term 'other' indoor games covers a range of activities, including Ludo and Monopoly, although no single example counted for more than 2%. Ten per cent of blind people under 60, but less than 1% of the older age groups, together with about 7% of partially sighted respondents across all age bands, gave replies in this category.

16.2.2.5   Music

Two per cent of respondents overall mentioned spontaneously that they played a musical instrument or sang; 6, 2, 3, 0, 1 and under 1 per cent of blind and partially sighted people respectively in the three age bands. Only 1% mentioned spontaneously that they listened to music as a pastime. This may have been because of the way the question was framed. Over 80% across all residual vision groups said that they listened to music when specifically prompted, except among partially sighted people aged 75 + where the total was 67%. The total reached 95% among young blind people.

16.2.3   Substantial minority interests

This group of hobbies and interests, while not individually as popular as those described above, still had a sufficient following to warrant being percentaged in Table 16.3. They consisted of spontaneously-given replies under the following headings: handicrafts, dancing, pubs, church, committees and voluntary work.

Replies mentioning pottery/woodcarving/basket work/other handicrafts/ making things were coded as 'handicrafts'. This is the most popular of all the substantial minority interests, and its classification was a borderline decision. Six per cent of respondents aged under 75, and 2% of those aged 75 +, with no differences according to level of residual vision, mentioned handicrafts.

While mentions of handicrafts totalled 4%, the remaining activities reached only 2% overall and were mainly confined to respondents aged under 75, at about the 5% level, though there were minor (non-significant statistically) variations with sight and age level. 'Pubs', which also covered social centres and clubs, were mentioned most often by younger blind people (8%). 'Church' and 'committees' covered mentions of membership either of a committee or, more generally, of an association. (See section 16.3 for more detailed information.) 'Voluntary work', which included replies relating to 'helping people', was mainly mentioned by respondents in the 16 – 59 age group.

16.2.4   Miscellaneous minority interests

These minority interests are represented by the substantial 'other' category in Table 16.3, which accounts for 14% overall and is particularly extensive among the under-60s. Mentions were made by 34, 37, 24, 19, 8 and 16 per cent of blind and partially sighted people respectively in the three age bands. The category consists of a large number of diverse activities, all mentioned spontaneously, but none by more than 2% in any of the age groups. These activities included computing, typing, keeping pets or animals, visiting friends, bingo, going to the cinema/theatre/concert/opera. The percentages in Hunt's similar 'other' category were approximately the same as those reported here.

16.2.5   Visually impaired people without hobbies

In evaluating our data on visually impaired people without hobbies, it is important to bear in mind the wording of the relevant question (BQ52), which asked respondents to disregard reading, radio and television.

As Table 16.4 shows, a substantial proportion of respondents (46%) failed to mention spontaneously any hobbies or interests. The proportion varied more according to age than to residual vision, from 34% of the under-75s to 52% of those aged 75 and over. Overall, 54% of visually impaired people account for the 78% of hobbies mentioned spontaneously, or an average of 1.4 hobbies each.

Table 16.4   Visually impaired people without hobbies

'Still thinking about your spare time; we've already talked about radio and television, and the different ways of reading. Apart from these things, do you have any hobbies or interests?' BQ52

	Age and residual vision						Total
	16 – 59		60 – 74		75 +		
	B	PS	B	PS	B	PS	
	%	%	%	%	%	%	%
Has no hobby	39	32	38	32	51	53	46
Has hobby	61	68	62	68	49	47	54
Total %	100	100	100	100	100	100	100
Base (population)	30K	47K	65K	115K	205K	295K	757K
(Number interviewed)	(137)	(162)	(55)	(69)	(75)	(97)	(595)

Sections 16.1.2 and 16.1.5 on radio and television listening show that some 80% of visually impaired people listen to radio and television, with radio listening well distributed over all stations. The analysis of reading habits in Chapters 7, 8 and 11 demonstrates the large numbers of visually impaired people who use some form of reading medium. As a result, excluding radio, television and reading substantially inflates the number of people without hobbies. These are indisputably leisure activities, and if they were included the total of 46% without hobbies would fall substantially. The reduction would be greatest among elderly people, since the data show that reading and radio listening are more common among people aged 60 and over.

Hunt's survey provides broadly comparable data about sighted elderly people. In reply to an open, unprompted question, which was similar to ours but did not exclude reading and radio listening, about 17% of those aged 65 – 74 and 30% of those aged 75 + were unable to name a hobby or interest. Our comparable figures are 34 and 52 per cent. In Hunt's data, spontaneous mentions of reading and radio/TV were high, about 25% in each category. If this 25% is added, Hunt's figures reach 42 and 55 per cent of respondents without hobbies in the 65 – 74 and 75 + age groups, discounting reading and radio/TV.

These are only rough and approximate comparisons. But we can at least be confident that in relative terms the proportion of visually impaired people without hobbies or interests is no greater than among the general population.

16.2.6   Diversity of hobbies and interests

In so far as hobbies and interests contribute to the quality of life, visually impaired people compare quite positively with the general population, pursuing a wide variety of interests. Among older people, who can be compared with Hunt's survey of sighted people, we find the same catalogue of activities. Even activities one might expect loss of vision to preclude have a substantial following among visually impaired people.

16.3 Clubs and social centres

Respondents were asked (at BQ58) 'Do you ever go to ...'

'A social club or day centre just for people with sight problems?'

'A day centre or social centre *not* just for people with sight problems?'

'A club or society for the elderly?' (if over retirement age)

'A sports club or sports centre?'

'A church or a church group?'

'Any other kind of club or society which has regular meetings or activities?'

For brevity, the first five options are referred to as blind club, ordinary club, elderly club, sports club and church group. Although not included in this list, respondents spontaneously mentioned working men's clubs sufficiently to warrant the creation of a separate sixth category in Table 16.5. These spontaneous mentions suggest that these clubs are probably more important, in comparison with the prompted list of clubs, to the individuals concerned than the percentages in the table reflect.

16.3.1 Attendance at clubs and social centres

Table 16.5 shows attendance rates. Overall, 45% of respondents attended one or more social clubs. The most frequently mentioned types were: church group (22%), elderly club (15%), ordinary club (10%), working men's club (7%), blind club (3%), sports club (2%). Six per cent of replies were categorised as 'other club'. Church groups were the most frequently named 'social centre'. However, this term embraces both services and church-organised social activities.

Many respondents mentioned more than one type: the total of clubs mentioned was 65% suggesting attendance at an average of 1.4 clubs by each visually impaired person who goes to a club or social centre. Although the overlap has not been analysed, since church groups predominate in the sub-groups, it seems likely that church groups are the club most frequently attended plus one other. This is most readily seen among the partially sighted 16 – 59 group, where 42% mentioned that they went to one or more clubs, and a total of 61% of clubs were mentioned, with 30% alone mentioning church groups; none of the other clubs exceeded 9%.

Attendance at elderly clubs reached a peak of 28% among partially sighted respondents aged 75 + , but was only about 8% in the other sub-groups aged 60 and over. Attendance at ordinary clubs is about twice as high (16%) among those aged 60 – 74 as among the other age groups.

Working men's club's were attended overall by 7% of visually impaired people. They were mentioned most by young blind people compared with older blind people (17 and 2 per cent respectively). More women than men mentioned working men's clubs, but here residual vision levels and sex brought pronounced differences among older people, with partially sighted women aged 60 – 74 and especially 75 + attending most often, and blind women rarely.

Blind clubs (those catering solely for people with sight problems) are discussed in greater detail in section 16.4. Here it is worth noting that these clubs are attended exclusively by people who are registered, and mainly but not entirely by those registered blind rather than partially sighted. Twenty-seven per cent of the registered attended a blind club. No non-registered respondents mentioned attending a blind club.

However, it should be noted that overall attendance at clubs was not influenced by registration status. Similar percentages (45 and 44 per cent) of both registered and non-registered people attended one or more clubs.

Table 16.5 Attendance at social clubs

'I would now like to ask you about groups, clubs and social centres you go to. Do you ever go to...(read out descriptions)?' (BQ58)

	Age and residual vision						Total
	16 – 59		60 – 74		75 +		
	B	PS	B	PS	B	PS	
	%	%	%	%	%	%	%
Church groups	23	30	20	18	16	27	22
Elderly club	–	–	8	6	9	28	15
Ordinary club	13	6	14	19	8	8	10
Working men's club	17	9	3	12	2	8	7
Blind club	10	2	9	1	4	#	3
Sports club	17	9	1	7	0	0	2
Other club	10	5	5	15	3	4	6
Total % of clubs mentioned	90	61	60	78	42	75	65
Go to one or more club	63	42	35	50	29	53	45
Don't go to any club	37	58	65	50	71	47	55
Base (popltn) = 100%	30K	47K	65K	115K	205K	295K	757K
(Numbers interviewed)	(137)	(162)	(55)	(69)	(75)	(97)	(595)

Attendance at sports clubs is concentrated among the 16 – 59 age band (17% of blind people, 9% of partially sighted people) as would be expected from their hobbies. The impact of registration on attendance is important. Of people under 60 who attend a club or social centre, 36% of the registered blind, but only 6% of the non-registered blind, attend a sports club. The corresponding totals for registered and non-registered partially sighted people are 31 and 43 per cent.

Although 'other club' reached 6% overall, no individual club was mentioned by more than 1% of respondents. Bingo, luncheon and social clubs, rotary/masonic clubs and Services clubs were most frequently mentioned by blind people aged 16 – 59 (7%). The following received very few mentions (under 0.5%) overall and without bunching within the sub-groups: dancing clubs, music clubs and Women's Institutes.

16.3.2 Frequency of attendance

We also asked (at BQ59) how often respondents went to the clubs they mentioned: once a week or more; once a fortnight; once a month; or less than once a month. For people going to church groups the percentages attending at the above rates were 65, 16, 7 and 13; for elderly clubs 51, 12, 23 and 14; for ordinary clubs 90, 5, 3 and 2; for working men's clubs 35, 7, 56 and 2; for blind clubs 24, 36, 38 and 2; and for sports clubs, 60, 2, 10 and 28, respectively.

With the exception of working men's clubs and blind clubs, over half visually impaired people attend their clubs at least once a week, which suggests a high level of commitment to the club and its corresponding importance in their life. A notable point is that fewer than a quarter attend a blind club weekly.

16.3.3 Non-attendance at clubs or social centres

16.3.3.1 Relationship with living alone

As Table 16.6 shows, more people living alone than living with others go to social clubs (51 and 38 per cent). This finding establishes the important role social clubs have for visually impaired people who live on their own. Perhaps those who live alone make more efforts to get out for that very reason, while those living with others receive the social support they need from the people they live with. Analysis by age does not reveal any strong consistent differences.

Another striking fact revealed by the data is the larger proportion of blind people living alone who go to social clubs compared with blind people living with others. Among partially sighted people there is no statistically significant difference (section 21.4) between those living

224

alone and those living with others (52 and 49 per cent respectively). Forty-seven per cent of blind people living alone go to social clubs compared with only 27% of those who live with others. We can only speculate why such a high total (73%) percentage of blind people who live with others do not go to social clubs. Are they being more protected? Or do they simply get their support from home?

Table 16.6 Attendance at social clubs, by living alone/with others within residual vision levels

	Residual vision and living alone						Total
	B		PS		B & PS		
	Live alone	Not alone	Live alone	Not alone	Live alone	Not alone	
	%	%	%	%	%	%	%
Don't go to any club	53	73	48	51	49	62	55
Go to one or more club	47	27	52	49	51	38	45
Total %	100	100	100	100	100	100	100
Base (population)	102K	199K	244K	213K	346K	412K	757K
(Numbers interviewed)	(65)	(202)	(126)	(202)	(191)	(404)	(595)

16.3.3.2 Reasons for non-attendance

All respondents who said (at BQ58) that they did not attend any clubs were asked (BQ60), 'Why don't you go to any clubs or social centres? Is it that you're not interested, or you would have difficulty getting there, or some other reason?'

Most replies fell into the two prompted categories, 56% saying that they were not interested and 25% that they would have difficulty getting there. 'Other reasons' covered a variety of categories, each of which obtained only a few mentions: like to do other things (7%), health problems (6%), nobody to go with (5%), don't like clubs or being organised (4%), can't leave dependents – children, sick spouse or aged parents (3%), never thought of it (3%), financial reasons (1%).

That over half (55%) of visually impaired people, many living alone, do not go out to any social clubs or centres is a major cause of concern. People have the right to choose privacy. However, a quarter reported difficulties reaching a club, and the answer of those who said that they were 'not interested' are also open to interpretation. If one feels unable, for whatever reason, to participate in an external activity, self-respect and self-defence can easily lead to a 'not interested' answer.

The very high level of non-attendance (over 60% among elderly blind people) offers major opportunity to club and centre organisers, social workers and volunteers to introduce or re-introduce elderly visually impaired people to these social activities.

16.4   Clubs and day centres for visually impaired people

16.4.1   Impact of registration on attendance

As has already been noted (section 16.3.2), although overall only 3% attend blind clubs, 60% of those attending doing so at least once a fortnight. Since our answers came from only 47 respondents, caution is necessary in drawing conclusions based on such small numbers. The population projection for those involved is 21,000 (subject to sampling error, section 21.4)

The chief characteristic of those who attend blind clubs is that they are registered. No respondent who was not registered said that they attend, while 27% of the registered do so. People registered blind rather than partially sighted are the main attenders, with a slight relative predominance of the elderly. Twenty-four and 9 per cent of blind and partially sighted respondents aged 16 – 59 attended, and 39 and 10 per cent of those aged 60 + .

Section 16.3.1 shows that similar proportions of registered and non-registered attend a club or day centre. However, the attendance of so many registered at blind clubs has an impact on their membership of clubs for the elderly. Of people aged 60 + who attend a club or day centre, only 17% of those registered blind compared with 37% of the non-registered went to an elderly club. The corresponding figures for the registered and non-registered partially sighted are 31 and 43 per cent.

Thus once again registration is a key predictor and catalyst of access to service. In this case, registration does not have a wholly benign impact in that attendance correlates with lower rates of attendance at other forms of clubs and social activities. Service-givers must try to present attendance at clubs and centres for visually impaired people as an additional activity, rather than as a substitute for attendance at gatherings where visually impaired and sighted people mingle.

16.4.2   Principal activities at blind clubs

Respondents were asked about activities at their blind club in both unprompted (BQ62) and prompted (BQ63) questions, as follows:

Unprompted:

'What sorts of things do you do at your social club or day centre?' (BQ62)

Prompted:

> 'Can I just check, do you do, or take part in any of the following
> things there?
> Indoor games
> Handicrafts
> Lunch clubs
> Listen to talks on how to cope with loss of vision?'

Table 16.7 sets out the answers to both questions. Despite the low actual numbers on which the percentages are based (only 47 respondents attended a blind club), a clear pattern emerges from the spontaneously mentioned activities. A group of six popular items – music/singing/recitals (mentioned by 45%), meeting friends/chatting (44%), talks (of an entertainment rather than instructional kind) (38%), having lunch (28%), indoor games (23%), and handicrafts (23%) – was mentioned significantly more often than a group of seven less popular activities: trips/outings (11%), typing class (8%), parties (4%), bring and buy sales (4%), raffles (4%), and talks on sight problems (2%).

The numbers saying that they take part in indoor games and handicrafts hardly changed when these items were specifically prompted. Only 10% said that they took part in luncheon clubs (as distinct from just having lunch) when this item was prompted. Fourteen per cent said they participated in talks on sight problems when this item was prompted.

Following these questions on club activities, those who attended a blind club were asked (at BQ64): 'Is there anything your social club or day centre could be doing that would be helpful or interesting for you personally?' This question yielded very thin information. Sixty-two per cent could not think of anything. The remaining replies were mainly of a general, unspecific nature: more/different activities, activities should be available more often, more or better entertainment. The only specific items mentioned were 'simple manual tasks, screwing nuts and bolts together', 'cooking lessons', 'involving families of the blind in the centre', 'a sound chip for the computer at the centre', 'talks from British Telecom about telephones'.

One thing stands out from the information obtained about activities at blind clubs, and that is the lack of social rehabilitation activities. Clearly, people do not wish to be battered remorselessly with rehabilitation and training. However, the unique feature of these clubs and centres is that they are attended by visually impaired people alone, unlike other clubs and centres. There is considerable scope for using these separate settings as an opportunity for low-key rehabilitation and training activities.

Table 16.7 Activities at social clubs for visually impaired people

'What sorts of things do you do at your social club or day centre?' (BQ62)

'Can I just check, do you do, or take part in any of the following things there?' (BQ63)

	BQ62 Unprompted %	BQ63 Prompted %
Music/singing/recitals	45	–
Meet friends/chat	44	–
Entertainment talks	38	–
Have lunch/lunch clubs	28	10
Indoor games	23	24
Handicrafts	23	24
Trips/outings	11	–
Typing class	8	–
Tea	8	–
Parties	4	–
Bring and buy sales	4	–
Raffles	4	–
Talks to do with vision	2	14
Other	3	–
Base (population) = 100%	21K	21K
(Number interviewed)	(47)	(47)

(47 respondents: those who say they attend blind clubs)

16.4.3   Reasons for non-attendance

Those who said (at BQ58) that they did not attend a blind club were asked: 'Why don't you go to a club/day centre for people with sight problems? Is it that you don't know of one round here, or that you have no-one to go with, or because you would have difficulty getting there, or some other reason?' (BQ60)

The most frequent reason given was 'don't know of one' (44%). This was also the only reason that varied between the registered and non-registered respondents, being mentioned by 35% of the former and 47% of the latter. Nineteen per cent said that they had 'difficulty getting there', and 17% said that they preferred to go to clubs that were 'not just for those with sight problems'. This answer was given as frequently by blind as by partially sighted people aged under 75. Among those aged 75 or over, 8% of blind and 19% of partially sighted people mentioned it.

The answer 'my sight problem is not serious enough' produced the main difference between blind and partially sighted respondents. Twelve per cent of the latter but none of the former gave this reason.

A variety of other reasons was also given, none of which individually amounted to more than 2%. These included 'no time', 'health prevents', 'too old', 'never thought of it', 'don't like clubs'. Some 15% simply said 'not interested'.

16.5 Pubs, bingo, theatres, concerts

Pubs, bingo, theatres and concerts are all recreational situations in which visually impaired people can participate with the general sighted and non-disabled public. We asked (at BQ65) whether respondents ever participated. Table 16.8 classifies the results by age, the main factor producing a variation in response. Overall, 62% of respondents said that they never took part, while 38% went to at least one. In the age bands 16 – 59, 60 – 74 and 75 + , the totals saying that they did not participate showed a steep rise from 31 and 51 to 69 per cent; conversely, the totals attending at least one fell from 69 and 49 to 31 per cent respectively.

Table 16.8 Attendance at pubs, bingo, theatre, concerts

'Do you ever go to...?' (BQ65)

	Age			Total
	16 – 59	60 – 74	75 +	
	%	%	%	%
Goes to:				
pubs	56	23	10	18
concerts	27	24	13	17
theatres	27	19	12	15
bingo	7	8	8	7
Go to at least one of these	69	49	31	38
Go to none of these	31	51	69	62
Base (population) = 100%	77K	180K	500K	757K
(Number interviewed)	(299)	(124)	(172)	(595)

Across all age groups the totals saying that they went to pubs, concerts, theatres and bingo, were 18, 17, 15 and 7 per cent. The age gradient just noted is almost entirely explained by the decline with increasing age in pub-visiting, from 56% in the 16 – 59 age group to 23 and 10 per cent in the 60 – 74 and 75 + age bands respectively. Theatre-going also declined across the three age bands, though less precipitously – 27, 19 and 12 per cent respectively; concert-going showing a similar decline – 27, 24 and 13 per cent. Bingo-going proved relatively stable across the three age bands, although it was the only one of these four activities much affected by residual vision level. Only 3% of blind people went to bingo compared with 11% of partially sighted people.

16.6 Holidays

16.6.1 During the last five years

The inability to take a holiday can be used as an indicator of poverty. For this report a holiday was defined as a week or more away from home. Question BQ66 enquired about holidays in the last five years, with the results shown in Table 16.9. Thirty-eight per cent of visually impaired people had not taken a holiday in the previous five years. Across the three age bands 16 – 59, 60 – 74 and 75 + the totals were 26, 30 and 44 per cent. Residual vision level produced no difference among those aged under 75. But of those aged 75 + 55% of blind and 35% of partially sighted people had not taken a holiday over the previous five years. Seventeen, 20 and 25 per cent of respondents had taken one holiday, two to four holidays or five or more holidays respectively.

The data reveal that only about a quarter of visually impaired people take a regular holiday. The remainder fall into two groups of just over a third each who either never go on holiday (38%) or who do go on holiday but not regularly (37%).

Table 16.9   Holidays in the previous five years, by residual vision within three age groups

'How many holidays have you had in the last 5 years? By holiday, I mean spending a week or more away from home, or staying with friends or relatives for a week or more.' (BQ66)

	Age and residual vision						Total
	16 – 59		60 – 74		75 +		
	B	PS	B	PS	B	PS	
	%	%	%	%	%	%	%
None	25	24	28	30	55	35	38
One holiday	16	22	19	16	11	20	17
2 – 4 holidays	25	22	29	18	13	25	20
5 or more	34	32	24	36	21	20	25
Total %	100	100	100	100	100	100	100
Base (population)	30K	47K	65K	115K	205K	295K	757K
(Number interviewed)	(137)	(162)	(55)	(69)	(75)	(97)	(595)

16.6.2 During the last twelve months

Table 16.10 provides detailed data on the 62% of visually impaired people who had not taken a holiday during the previous twelve months. Comparative data for the general population shows that 40% of adults in Great Britain had not taken a holiday in 1988, (Central Statistical Office, 1990, page 160).

230

Table 16.10 compares the different sub-groups with respect to those who have not had a holiday for either 5 years or 12 months.

Table 16.10 Holidays in the previous twelve months and five years, by residual vision within three age groups

'How many holidays have you had in the last 5 years?...' (BQ66)

'Have you spent a week or more away from home in the last 12 months?' (BQ67)

	Age and residual vision						Total
	16 – 59		60 – 74		75 +		
	B	PS	B	PS	B	PS	
	%	%	%	%	%	%	%
No holiday in last 5 years	25	24	28	30	55	35	38
No holiday in last 12 months	43	51	61	44	68	68	62
Base (popltn) = 100%	30K	47K	65K	115K	205K	295K	757K
(Numbers interviewed)	(137)	(162)	(55)	(69)	(75)	(97)	(595)

16.6.3 Holidays and elderly blind people

Most visually impaired people have taken at least one holiday over the previous five years, with the major exception of blind people aged 75 or over. Fifty-five per cent of this group had not had a holiday in the previous five years, and 68% had also not had a holiday in the previous twelve months. We estimate that this group amounts to 205,000 people, nearly three-quarters of them women (Chapter 3). The population projection for the 55% is thus 113,000. Chapter 13 showed that a considerable number of this same group live alone, and that many had not been outside their home during the previous year.

16.6.4 Registration and holidays

Among people experiencing the severest visual loss (that is, registrably blind people), more of those who are registered have taken a holiday, and have taken five or more holidays, over the previous five years. The details are shown in Table 16.11. As happens with other services, registration (as blind) shows a significantly increased likelihood of having a particular service, in this case a holiday. Eighty per cent of registered blind people under 60 have taken a holiday. Among blind people aged 60 or over, 66% of the registered have had a holiday compared with 46% of the non-registered. However, registration seems to have little effect on the number of holidays taken by partially sighted people.

Table 16.11 Holidays during previous five years, by registration status and residual vision within two age groups

'How many holidays have you had in the last 5 years?...' (BQ66)

	\multicolumn{8}{c}{Age, residual vision and registration}	Total
	\multicolumn{4}{c}{16 – 59}	\multicolumn{4}{c}{60 +}	
	\multicolumn{2}{c}{B}	\multicolumn{2}{c}{PS}	\multicolumn{2}{c}{B}	\multicolumn{2}{c}{PS}	
	R	NR*	R	NR	R	NR	R	NR	
	%	%	%	%	%	%	%	%	%
None	20	36	24	27	34	54	45	33	38
One holiday	12	22	9	26	16	10	12	20	17
2 – 4 holidays	29	19	29	18	17	15	15	23	20
5 or more	41	22	39	30	33	18	26	24	24
Total %	100	100	100	100	100	100	100	100	100
Base (population)	18K	12K	12K	35K	91K	179K	49K	361K	757K
(Number interviewed)	(123)	(14)	(92)	(70)	(74)	(56)	(63)	(103)	(595)

*Low unweighted base, caution with percentages

As Table 16.12 shows, our data indicate that registration has a similar impact on holiday-taking over a 12-month period. Overall, younger registered people were more likely to have had a holiday in the last 12 months than their older counterparts; similarly for the non-registered. Within the residual vision sub-groups registered blind people are more likely to have taken a holiday during this time than non-registered blind people. This difference is especially evident among blind people aged 60 and over where the largest difference occurs. Forty-seven per cent of registered blind people over 60 took a holiday in the last 12 months compared with only 26% of the non-registered.

Thus registration helps to ameliorate the very poor holiday prospects noted above for elderly blind people. However, at these severe sight loss levels the non-registered are more than twice as numerous as the

Table 16.12 Holidays during the last twelve months, by registration status, residual vision and two age groups

'Have you spent a week or more away from home in the last 12 months?' (BQ67)

	\multicolumn{8}{c}{Age, residual vision and registration}	Total
	\multicolumn{4}{c}{16 – 59}	\multicolumn{4}{c}{60 +}	
	\multicolumn{2}{c}{B}	\multicolumn{2}{c}{PS}	\multicolumn{2}{c}{B}	\multicolumn{2}{c}{PS}	
	R	NR*	R	NR	R	NR	R	NR	
	%	%	%	%	%	%	%	%	%
Yes	62	49	57	47	47	26	30	40	38
No	38	51	43	53	53	74	70	60	62
Total %	100	100	100	100	100	100	100	100	100
Base (population)	18K	12K	12K	35K	91K	179K	49K	361K	757K
(Number interviewed)	(123)	(14)	(92)	(70)	(74)	(56)	(63)	(103)	(595)

registered (section 3.1), and only a minority of the non-registered, about one in three, enjoy a holiday in the course of a year.

16.6.5 Special holidays for visually impaired people

As we have seen, 38% of visually impaired people (population projection 288,000) had spent a week or more away from home during the previous twelve months. They were then asked (BQ68): 'Thinking now of your *most recent* holiday, was this one specially arranged for people with sight problems?'

Only 4% replied 'yes' to this question, giving a population projection of 12,000. All of them were registered. The population projection for the registered who had been away in the last 12 months was 76,000. So among the registered who had been away in the last 12 months, 16% had been on a holiday for people with sight problems.

Out of the 12,000 special holidays, some 9,000 were taken up by registered blind people age 60 and over. Twenty-one per cent of registered blind people age 60 and over who had been away in the last twelve months had been on a special holiday, compared with 12% of registered blind people under 60 (around 1,000). (We saw in the last section that some 47% of the registered blind aged 60 or over, giving a population projection of 43,000, took a holiday in the last 12 months.) The registered blind aged 60 and over are the sub-group with the greatest concentration of specially arranged holidays.

Among the registered partially sighted, even among those aged 60 and over, such holidays are relatively uncommon. Around 9% (approximately 1,000), who had been away in the last twelve months took such holidays. (These percentages, subject to sampling error, section 21.4, apply only to those taking a holiday in the last 12 months.)

16.6.6 Demand for specialised hotels for visually impaired people

Only 13% of visually impaired people express a preference for staying in a hotel for people with sight problems, and a further 12% could not say either way. Table 16.13 breaks down the responses by age, residual vision and registration status. Registered blind people aged 60 and over express the highest preference for staying in a special hotel (37%), with another 23% uncertain. Registered partially sighted people express the next highest preference (23%). This explains, and to a large extent justifies, the specialised concentration of hotel provision on elderly people, especially blind people.

However, a not-insignificant minority of both non-registered blind and partially sighted people aged 60 and over also express a preference for holidays in specialised hotels (14 and 5 per cent respectively). While

Table 16.13 Preferences for specialised hotels by registration, residual vision and age

'If you were going to stay at an hotel for a holiday, would you prefer to stay in one solely for people with sight problems?' (BQ70)

	Age, residual vision and registration								Total
	16 – 59				60 +				
	B		PS		B		PS		
	R	NR*	R	NR	R	NR	R	NR	
	%	%	%	%	%	%	%	%	%
Yes	11	6	11	7	37	14	23	5	13
No	82	79	85	91	40	76	61	84	75
Don't know	7	15	4	2	23	10	16	11	12
Total %	100	100	100	100	100	100	100	100	100
Base (population)	18K	12K	12K	35K	91K	179K	49K	361K	757K
(Number interviewed)	(123)	(14)	(92)	(70)	(74)	(56)	(63)	(103)	(595)

*Low unweighted base, caution with percentages

these percentages are small, they are on relatively large bases and reflect a substantial, largely unmet demand for holidays in specialised hotels. In numerical terms, the equivalent population projections are 25,000 and 19,000. It also is worth noting that approximately the same number of elderly people answered 'don't know', in other words expressed no objection to holidaying in a specialised hotel.

17 Employment

17.1 Paid employment

Table 17.1 shows that not being in paid employment is normal for visually impaired people of working age. (It should be noted that, in contrast with other sections of this report, the analysis is based on the conventional working ages of men, 16 – 64, and women, 16 – 59.) The OPCS disability survey states that 31% of all disabled people under pension age are in work (Martin et al, 1989). Our findings are that 25% of visually impaired people are in work, 17 and 31 per cent of blind and partially sighted people respectively.

While it is the case that only 4% of all visually impaired people are in work, this is a misleading statistic because of the disproportionate number of retirement age. Of those of working age, 25% were in work at the time of our survey, approximately 22,000 people. The total number in work increases to about 30,000 since about 8,000 people over normal retirement age said that they were still in work. Perhaps not surprisingly, almost all of these were women, since, because of their chequered work pattern, the retirement pension often does not provide sufficient income; as a result, a large number of women have to continue working beyond retirement age. Practically all those over retirement age and working were doing so part-time rather than full-time.

The lower part of Table 17.1 provides a brief work history of visually impaired people in general. Overall, most visually impaired people have worked at some time in their lives. However, sight level does have an impact. Overall 13% of blind, but only 4% of partially sighted, respondents reported that they had never worked, a ratio of 3 to 1. There is also some indication that women are more likely never to have done any paid work.

The data show that, while only 17% of blind people of working age are in work, nearly three-quarters have worked at some time; only 11% have never worked at all. This suggests that, even though some blind people may not have worked since acquiring their visual handicap, many did so beforehand. The conclusion to be drawn is that large numbers of blind people are unemployed not because they are unable to work but simply because employers will not offer them jobs.

Table 17.1   Paid employment and past employment by two age groups and residual vision

'Now I would like to move on to talk about jobs and employment. Can I just check. First of all are you in paid employment at the moment?' (PQ1)

'Have you ever done any paid work?' (PQ2)

	Age and residual vision						Total
	16 – 59/64 +			60/65 plus*			
	B	PS	B & PS	B	PS	B & PS	
	%	%	%	%	%	%	%
Yes, in paid employment	17	31	25	#	1	1	4
No, not in paid employment	83	69	75	99	99	99	96
Working pattern of those not in work							
Worked in the past	72	64	68	86	95	91	88
Never worked at all	11	5	8	14	4	8	8
Total %	100	100	100	100	100	100	100
Base (population)	41K	50K	91K	260K	406K	666K	757K
(Number interviewed)	(147)	(170)	(317)	(120)	(158)	(278)	(595)

+women 16 – 59; men 16 – 64
*women 60 + ; men 65 +

This chapter shows that the first few years after onset of sight loss are a crucial period in which resources should be concentrated on working with blind and partially sighted people and their employers. Job retention rather than retraining and job-finding seems to be the key to improving the employment prospects of blind and partially sighted people. Once people lose their jobs they enter a period of long-term unemployment. While current practice tends to provide help when a visually impaired person has lost his or her job, our data suggest that by then it is often too late. To be most effective, the emphasis should be on early intervention.

17.2   Reasons for not working

17.2.1   People who have never worked

As we have seen, only 11% of blind people of working age, and 5% of partially sighted people, have never held any paid employment. A brief enquiry was made (at PQ3) about the reason why these people had never worked; no table is shown because of the low number of respondents. Reasons given were fairly evenly divided among 'sight problems', 'other disabilities', 'studying' and 'other reasons'.

17.2.2   Reasons for leaving last job

Table 17.2 shows the reasons given by people of working age for leaving their last job. Nearly half (46%) blind people of working age left their last job because of deteriorating vision, and a further third (35%) left because of injury at work. Chapter 5 shows that very few people lose their sight due to accident, and so it is likely that a significant number of these injuries at work did not cause the visual impairment. Conversely, however, a pre-existing sight problem may have contributed to the injury. (Data are available for people of retirement age group, but the majority of their responses are misleading, since they acquired their visual impairment after retirement age.)

Table 17.2 Reasons given by people of working age + not in paid work for leaving their last job, by residual vision and sex

'What was the main reason why you left your last job?' (PQ6)

	Residual vision		Sex		All not working
	B	PS	Men	Women	
	%	%	%	%	%
Made redundant	3	15	12	6	9
Business closed	1	2	2	1	2
Temporary/seasonal work	1	3	3	1	2
Retired/retired early	1	8	3	7	5
Dismissed because of visual handicap	2	2	2	1	2
Left due to visual handicap	46	14	44	11	29
Left due to injury at work	35	41	31	47	38
Left for family reasons	10	10	2	20	10
Other reasons	3	5	2	6	4
Total %	100	100	100	100	100
Base (population)	29K	32K	34K	27K	62K
(Number interviewed)	(88)	(106)	(98)	(96)	(194)

(194 respondents: working-age respondents not in work who have worked in the past)   +Women 16 – 59; men 16 – 64

The pattern for partially sighted people is similar, except for one important respect which has an impact on all the other reasons. Whereas 46% of blind people left their last job because of visual handicap, only 14% of partially sighted people did so. However, many more partially sighted people were made redundant (15% in comparison with 3%) or retired/retired early (8% in comparison with 1%). It is possible to conjecture that these figures reveal a form of surrogate dismissal because of visual handicap by which employers use redundancy and early retirement to ease out partially sighted employees.

Table 17.2 also separates the reasons men and women gave for leaving their last job. Overall 10% left for family reasons, but with a significantly larger percentage of women (20%) compared with men (2%), almost certainly to have children and raise a family. This means that many of the women concerned will have left work long before the onset of their visual impairment. This may explain the lower numbers of women leaving due to visual handicap (11% compared with 44%). One difference difficult to explain is the greater total of women (47% compared with 31%) leaving due to injury at work.

Overall, more than two-thirds (69%) of respondents reported leaving work because of disability or injury. This covers those who were 'dismissed because of visual handicap', who 'left due to visual handicap' and who 'left due to injury at work'.

17.2.3   People of retirement age

People of retirement age produced a very different pattern of reasons for leaving their last job (no table shown). Well over a third said that they had 'retired'; about a quarter that they had left for 'family reasons'; about a sixth left due to 'injury at work' or because of their visual handicap. The difference between blind and partially sighted people was insignificant, which reflects the fact that their working life was complete before the onset of their handicap (see also section 17.8.3).

As with people of working age, there is a major sex difference among people of retirement age, 73% of men compared with 31% of women saying that they have 'retired'. Thus a large proportion of men have worked until retirement. Expressed another way, just under 3 in 10 of men stopped work prematurely, compared with nearly 7 in 10 of women, with all the implications for post-retirement income and benefits. For example, many women will not have worked enough years to provide sufficient National Insurance contributions for a full pension in their own right (see also section 17.5.2). 'Family reasons' were given for stopping work by 32% of women compared with 1% of men. Having to stop work because of disability shows no real difference for those of retirement age.

17.3   Last paid work undertaken

Table 17.3 shows the number of years since respondents of working age last worked, calculated from their current age and the age at which they reported having last worked. The data reflect the difference between the working patterns of men and women. Women reported a longer time since they last worked, a large percentage having stopped work for family reasons.

In 1987, of the general sighted population, 43% of unemployed people had been out of work for more than a year, 47 and 30 per cent for men and women respectively (Central Statistical Office, 1988). According to our survey, 88% of unemployed visually impaired people had not worked for over a year. Thus, once visually impaired people lose their jobs they are much more likely than sighted people to remain unemployed for a long period of time.

Table 17.3 Number of years since unemployed people of working age+ last did paid work, by sex

'How old were you when you last did any paid work?' (PQ4)

	Men %	Women %	Men and Women %
1 year or less ago	13	12	12
2 – 5 years ago	45	19	33
6 – 10 years ago	28	22	25
11 or more years ago	14	47	30
Total %	100	100	100
Base (population)	34K	26K	60K
(Number interviewed)	(95)	(94)	(189)

(189 respondents; no information for 5; working age respondents not in work)
+Women 16 – 59; men 16 – 64

17.3.1 Onset of visual impairment and ceasing work

In an attempt to establish whether any relationship exists between the onset of visual impairment and not working, Table 17.4 shows the period between onset and when the respondent 'last did paid work' for those of working age. The differing pattern of men and women is again evident. About half (51%) of women left their last job before the onset of visual impairment, in most cases presumably to start a family. Similar departures from the job market were very small for men (6%). Approximately one-third of men (34%) lost their last job within two years of the onset of visual impairment. While the comparable figure for women (18%) appears lower, the differing work pattern of women needs to be taken into consideration. If the 51% of women stopping work before onset are excluded from the base, the number of women stopping work within two years of onset now becomes equal to that for men (35%).

Lower job mobility among visually impaired people is likely to mean that many of the 40% (of men) who worked for over five years after onset are likely to have remained with the same employer. In other words, if a visually impaired employee and his or her employer can stay in partnership for the first two or three years after onset the chances of long-term employment are very good.

The high rate of job loss in the first two years after onset supports much anecdotal evidence, now quantified here, of a lack of contact with statutory and voluntary support agencies until employment has either ceased or seems likely to stop. Employers are unaware of the

Table 17.4 Relationship between onset of visual impairment and stopping work, by residual vision and sex

'How old were you when you first realised your sight problem was affecting everyday things...?' (YQ16)

'How old were you when you last did any paid work?' (PQ4)

| | Residual vision | | Sex | | All not working |
| | B | PS | Men | Women | Total |
	%	%	%	%	%
Onset 19 or under	14	25	16	23	19
10 or more years after*	11	11	16	5	11
5 – 9 years after	15	18	24	7	16
3 – 4 years after	2	8	5	5	5
Onset to 2 years after	38	16	34	18	27
1 – 5 years before*	16	11	6	23	13
6 or more years before	4	11	#	28	8
Total %	100	100	100	100	100
Base (population)	29K	32K	33K	26K	59K
(Number interviewed)	(84)	(98)	(91)	(91)	(182)

(182 respondents: question asked of those of working age, not working; no information on onset for 7, no information for 5 on age last worked)
Working age; women 16 – 59, men 16 – 64
*After/before onset of sight problem

rehabilitation and retraining services available (for which they currently have to pay); nor are they aware of the wide range of technical aids and the personal reader service (which are provided free). The same applies to employees with a recent visual impairment, who may well 'hide' the extent of their disability from their employer. Statutory and voluntary agencies should undertake much more significant public education campaigns aimed at employers, trade unions and employees.

Sixty-eight per cent of respondents of retirement age had stopped work before onset or within two years after onset. A further 10% experienced onset before the age of 20.

The conclusions drawn in Section 17.3 on employment retention are strengthened. We have seen that many years of unemployment are likely to face the one-third who lose their job shortly after onset. While most help with employment for visually impaired people is currently provided after job loss, our evidence supports the case for early intervention with employers at the stage of onset to encourage and support employment retention.

17.4 Desire to work

Those currently in work were asked (PQ7) whether they would like to work, if they could find the right job. The question was deliberately phrased in this way so as to elicit an initial response based on the desire to work. This was followed by a question concerning registration as unemployed with the local job centre as a more objective measure of the desire to work.

Table 17.5   Desire to work among those of working age + if the right job was available, by residual vision and sex

'Would you say you would like to work now, if you could find the right job ...?' (PQ7)

	Residual vision		Sex		Total
	B	PS	Men	Women	
	%	%	%	%	%
Would like to work	46	57	62	38	52
Would not like to work	47	39	30	60	43
Don't know	7	6	8	3	5
Total %	100	100	100	100	100
Base (population)	33K	29K	33K	29K	62K
(Number interviewed)	(102)	(109)	(102)	(109)	(211)

(211 respondents: question asked of those of working age not working)
+Women 16 – 59; men 16 – 64

As Table 17.5 shows, more men than women (62% compared with 38%) express this simple desire to work. Based on respondents of normal working age, there is no statistically significant difference in the desire to work between blind and partially sighted people. However, when the age range is reduced to 16 – 59 for both men and women, 59% of partially sighted people compared with 39% of blind people express a desire to work. This difference is most likely accounted for by excluding from the analysis men approaching retirement who have no real desire to return to work.

Only 10% of those not working were 'registered as unemployed or looking for work' with their local job centre (PQ8). One interpretation of the difference between the expressed desire for work and action taken, in terms of registration for work, is that visually impaired people are highly realistic about their chances of gaining work! Based on an assessment of both the large percentage not working and those out of work for a year or more, the chances of finding work are very slim indeed.

17.5   Occupational structure of the visually impaired population

17.5.1   Occupational structure of those not in work

Those not currently working were asked (PQ5) what their last job was, and their answers were graded on the professional/manual scale (Table

17.6). More women than men held 'clerical/other non-manual' and 'unskilled manual' jobs. By contrast, men were more likely to be found in 'skilled manual' and 'senior professional' jobs than women. This pattern replicates that found in the general population.

Table 17.6 Occupational structure of visually impaired people of working age not in paid work, by sex

'Thinking about your last job, what was your job title, and what did the job involve?' (PQ5)

	Working age 16 – 59/64 +		
	Men	Women	Total
	%	%	%
Senior professional	13	7	10
Junior professional	4	14	9
Professional	17	21	19
Clerical/other non-manual	7	22	14
Skilled manual	35	2	20
Unskilled manual	41	54	47
Not stated	0	#	#
Total %	100	100	100
Base (population)	34K	27K	61K
(Number interviewed)	(98)	(96)	(194)

(194 respondents: those who have worked in the past not now working; no information for 4)   + Women 16 – 59; men 16 – 64

17.5.2   Occupational structure of those in work

Table 17.7.a. shows the occupational structure of visually impaired people in work. Since the categories do not match exactly, the occupational structure of jobs can only be compared on a limited basis with the data from the general disabled population in the OPCS disability survey (Martin et al, 1989) Table 17.7.b. shows that the job profile of visually impaired people has some similarities with that of the disabled population as a whole. The main difference is in the 'professional' category, where 14% of visually impaired people, 25% of disabled people in general and 34% of the general population are found. By contrast, visually impaired and disabled people in general make up a larger proportion of the 'semi-skilled' and 'unskilled' categories (36 and 31 per cent, compared with 23% of the general population).

Visually impaired people are less likely to be employed than both the general sighted population and the disabled population in general. When employed, they suffer additional economic disadvantage in that fewer are employed in professional and skilled occupations.

Table 17.7.a. Occupational structure of visually impaired people currently in paid employment

	All in paid employment +
	%
Senior professional	10
Junior professional	4
Professional (total of above)	14
Clerical/other	18
Skilled manual	28
Unskilled manual	36
Not stated	4
Total %	100
Base (population)	22K
(Number interviewed)	(93)

(93 respondents: working age respondents in work)

+Women 16 – 59; men 16 – 64

Table 17.7.b. Occupational structure of the general population (GHS), disabled people (OPCS) and visually impaired people (RNIB) of working age +

	GHS* 1985	OPCS* 1985	RNIB 1986
	%	%	%
Professional	5	2	} 10
Employer or managerial	15	11	} –
Intermediate non-manual	14	12	4
Professional (total of above)	34	25	14
Junior non-manual	19	18	18
Skilled manual and own account non-professional	25	26	28
Semi-skilled manual and personal services	18	22	} –
Unskilled	5	9	} 36
Not stated	–	–	4
Total %	100	100	100
Base	10326	1138	22K
Number interviewed in RNIB survey			(93)

(93 respondents: working age respondents in work)

+ Women 16 – 59; men 16 – 64

Source: OPCS, report 4, Table 7.20 (Martin et al, 1989). GHS data also from OPCS report

*The OPCS and GHS data both refer to 1985, the OPCS fieldwork date

17.5.3 Protected or open employment environments for visually impaired people

Table 17.9 shows that a large majority (80%) of working visually impaired people are employees in open employment. Thirteen per cent are self-employed, slightly more than the 10% of the general population in 1985 (Central Statistical Office, 1988). Five and three per cent respectively work in sheltered schemes or as homeworkers.

Table 17.9   Employment status of working visually impaired people

'Do you work in a sheltered employment scheme, or work as a homeworker, or work for an employer somewhere else?' (PQ10)

	All in paid employment +
	%
Working for 'normal' employer	80
Self-employed	13
Sheltered employment scheme	5
Homeworker	3
Total %	100
Base (population)	21K
(Number interviewed)	(91)

(91 respondents: no information for 2: working age respondents in work) +Women 16 – 59; men 16 – 64

17.6   Specialist employment officers

Those working or who had worked in the past were asked (at PQ12) about registration as disabled for employment purposes, often termed as having a 'green card'. (Registration was with the then Manpower Services Commission (MSC).) As Table 17.10 shows, overall 26% said that they were registered disabled for employment purposes. Only 18% had spoken to a specialist employment officer responsible for helping handicapped people to find jobs. Of those not working, 10% were registered with their local job centre.

Registration for employment purposes was greater among blind than partially sighted people (37 and 18 per cent); among those registered with their local social services than those not registered (36 and 15 per cent); and among those working than not working (35 and 23 per cent). In addition, more men than women (36 and 15 per cent) were registered.

Only 18% of respondents overall (26% of blind people, 11% of partially sighted people) had discussed work prospects with one of the variety of

Table 17.10 Visually impaired people of working age + and specialist employment help, by residual vision, registration status, and working status

'The Manpower Services Commission keeps a register of people who are disabled or have a handicap. Are you on this register – it's sometimes called the "green card"?' (PQ12)

'There are specialist employment officers who help handicapped people find jobs. If someone already has a job, they offer advice on how to manage the job more easily. Have you ever talked to someone who offers specialist help and advice like this?' (PQ13)

'People with a disability which affects their work can sometimes get retraining to continue with the job they are already in, or be trained in new skills for a job or other work. Have you ever been offered any retraining or help like this?' (PQ17)

	Residual vision		Registration status		Work status		Total
					In work	Not in work	
	B	PS	R	NR			
	%	%	%	%	%	%	%
PQ12, on MSC register	37	18	36	15	35	23	26
PQ13, spoken to employment officer	26	11	37	6	23	16	18
PQ17, offered training or retraining	9	8	18	3	10	8	9
PQ8, registered with job centre	5	9	13	4	na	10	7
Base (popltn) = 100%	37K	47K	31K	53K	22K	62K	84K
(Number interviewed)	(131)	(158)	(204)	(85)	(95)	(194)	(289)

(289 respondents: working age respondents in work or worked in the past)
+ 16 – 59 for women, 16 – 64 for men

specialist employment officers, such as a Disabled Resettlement Officer or Blind Persons' Resettlement Officer. Given the high level and long duration of unemployment among visually impaired people, such limited contact with specialist advice suggests a major defect in the system as currently operated by the Department of Employment. Registration with the local social services department as blind or partially sighted does, however, increase the likelihood of such contact: further evidence that registration triggers service provision (section 3.10.1).

17.6.1   Services and advice offered

As Table 17.11 shows, a range of services offered by specialist employment officers was described. Just under two-thirds (62%) of respondents said that they were satisfied, and 38% that they were dissatisfied, with the help that they had received. Among a wide variety of reasons for dissatisfaction, the two most frequently mentioned were that the officer 'took no action' on the respondent's behalf or that the respondent was assumed to be 'too handicapped' to be helped.

Table 17.11   Help offered by specialist employment officers

'I'd like to check about the things that this officer did for you – I'll read out a number of things and you can tell me whether you were helped that way. So first, did they...?' (PQ14)

	%
Suggest types of jobs for you to consider	56
Tell you about special equipment or aids for work	41
Suggests any training course to prepare you for work	38
Find jobs you could apply for	37
Suggest that you went to a centre to prepare you for work you could do	37
Give you advice on how to apply for jobs	21
Offer to accompany you to interviews	21
Give you help in a job you were already doing	14
Help you when you started a job	13
Help you to retrain in a job you were already doing	7
Base (population) = 100%	16K
(Number interviewed)	(96)

(96 respondents: only asked of those of working age who had seen employment officer)

When respondents of working age were asked (PQ17, see Table 17.10) if they had been offered any training or retraining, either to help in the job they were doing or for a new job, only 9% said that they had been offered such assistance, and slightly over half (59%) said that they had accepted it. It should be remembered that only 26% of respondents of working age were registered with the employment services through which such help is generally offered, that even fewer (18%) had spoken to an employment officer, and that only half of those had been offered any training or retraining (9%).

All this said, given the relatively small numbers of people who experience 'early onset', the majority of this age group experience it while in work. They may therefore either have left their job due to the sight problem (see table 17.2) or have learnt to cope on their own in the job they were doing. The outcome is that relatively few people actually see a specialist employment officer.

Several issues emerge concerning registrable blind people, who are the most disadvantaged visually impaired workers and potential workers.

Tables 17.1 and 17.4 show that about 4 in 5 blind people of working age are unemployed, and that two-thirds left work after the onset of their visual impairment. The first two years after onset, when just over one-third of unemployed blind people became unemployed, are particularly critical. The findings shown in Table 17.10 explain the reasons, although they do not justify them. First, only a quarter of blind people of working age even speak to a specialist employment officer. Of this quarter, only 14% were given 'help in a job (they) were already doing' (Table 17.11). Overall, probably as few as 4% (3.5% rounded) of blind people have ever received help and advice in the job they were doing, despite the fact that well over three-quarters of them subsequently lost that job.

The high level of dissatisfaction expressed with the help from specialist employment officers gives a bleak picture of the help offered to blind and partially sighted people wanting to work.

17.7 Use of special equipment or services in work

As Table 17.12 shows, overall only 14% of respondents of working age had used either specially adapted equipment and aids or special clerical services to help them to overcome their disability at work. However this figure conceals wide variations between blind and partially sighted people. For example, 45% of blind but only 13% of partially sighted people currently in work use special equipment, and 23% of blind, compared with 13% of partially sighted, people use special clerical or other services.

Table 17.12   Use of special equipment or aids, or clerical or other services at work, among those working and not working, by residual vision

'Do you use any aids or equipment specially designed or adapted to help you overcome your disability at work?' (PQ27)*

'Do you use any special clerical or other services, to help you over come your disability at work?' (PQ28)*

	Residual vision and work status						Total
	In work			Not in work			
	B	PS	B & PS	B	PS	B & PS	
	%	%	%	%	%	%	%
Use/used aids and equipment	45	13	23	12	2	6	11
Use/used special services	23	13	16	4	2	3	7
All using aids or services	48	24	31	13	4	8	14
No aids or services used	50	66	62	69	82	77	73
No response	2	10	7	3	6	4	5
No sight problem in last job	na	na	na	15	8	11	8
Total %	100	100	100	100	100	100	100
Base (population)	7K	15K	22K	30K	32K	62K	84K
(Number interviewed)	(43)	(52)	(95)	(88)	(106)	(194)	(289)

(289 respondents: working age respondents in work or worked in the past)
*Those not working were asked about such use in their last job at PQ29 and PQ30

Perhaps the most dramatic conclusion to be drawn from Table 17.12 concerns the reason why some blind and partially sighted people are still working and others are not. In a nutshell, it is that blind and partially sighted people still working are far more likely to be using special equipment and additional clerical services than unemployed blind and partially sighted people were in their last job. Among blind people, for example, the totals for special equipment are 45 and 12 per cent, and the pattern is similar for additional clerical services and overall among partially sighted people. Common sense suggests that greater use of appropriate additional help would increase the chances of holding down a job, and Table 17.12 provides the necessary quantitative evidence.

The apparent success of the technical aids and additional clerical services (primarily the personal reader service), funded by the Department of Employment and supported by RNIB, is an overwhelming argument for increased effort in this area. The penetration-rate for special equipment of 45 and 13 per cent among blind and partially sighted workers respectively still leaves room for expansion. Even more potential exists in the area of clerical services or other services where the penetration-rate among blind and partially sighted workers is only 23 and 13 per cent respectively. Take-up of these services needs to be dramatically improved.

17.8 Employment status and onset of sight problems

Table 17.13 shows the relationship between respondents' employment status and their onset of visual impairment. Overall, 54% of those who were working or had worked said that they had a job when they first experienced sight difficulties (PQ19). This figure rises to 64% if people who experienced onset at under 20 years old are excluded (Table 17.14). This latter figure, 64%, is one of the most significant indications of the extent of unemployment among blind and partially sighted people.

Table 17.13 also shows that, of people currently in work, 43% were working at the time of onset, 21% have changed their job since onset, and 9% said that their job change was because of their sight problem.

Fifty-eight per cent of those not in work when the survey was carried out were working at the time of onset. Eleven per cent had stopped work at some time because of their visual handicap. Just under a third (31%) said that they had left their last job because of sight difficulties. This statistic more than any other indicates yet again the crucial importance of concentrating resources and service activity into this period, at or just after onset, of a visually impaired person's working life. Visually impaired people might be better served if resources and support were focused on keeping them with their current employer.

There is a simple explanation for the apparent paradox that only 43% of those currently working were in work at the time of onset, compared with 58% of those not currently working. As Table 17.13 shows, the base on which the 43% is calculated contains a larger proportion (62%) of people whose age of onset was 19 and under, compared with 20% for those not in work.

Table 17.13 Employment status, time of onset and work history of those working and not working, by residual vision

'When you first had a sight problem, did you have a job at the time?' (PQ19)

'Were you doing the job you already described or a different one?' (PQ20)

'Did you change job because of your sight problem, because of some other disability or illness, or for some other reason?' (PQ22)

'Was there ever a time when you had to stop doing your job because of your sight problem?' (PQ25)

	Residual vision and work status						Total
	In work			Not in work			
	B	PS	B & PS	B	PS	B & PS	
	%	%	%	%	%	%	%
PQ19							
Yes, in work at time of onset	35	46	43	67	49	58	54
Not in work at time of onset	65	54	57	33	51	42	46
PQ22 & PQ25							
Sight direct reason stopped working	20	3	9	18	5	11	11
PQ6*							
Sight reason left last job	na	na	na	47	15	31	22
PQ20							
Change of job since onset	26	19	21	10	12	11	14
Onset aged 19 or under	71	57	62	14	25	20	31
Base (popltn) = 100%	7K	15K	22K	30K	32K	62K	84K
(Number interviewed)	(43)	(52)	(95)	(88)	(106)	(194)	(289)

(289 respondents: working age respondents working or worked in the past)
*From Table 17.2

Table 17.13 shows that, for 58% of those not in work, the last job they held was the one in which onset started. This suggests that their sight problem may have been a contributory factor in their job loss. This suggestion is supported by the fact that 31% clearly state that their sight problem was the reason that they left their last job. It is further strengthened by the fact that residual vision produces a clear difference, with 47% of blind people giving sight as the reason for leaving their last job compared with 15% of partially sighted people.

249

Table 17.14 Employment status and work history of visually impaired people of working age+ with onset at age 20 or over

	Work status		Total
	In work	Not in work	
	%	%	%
PQ19			
Yes, in work at time of onset	74	62	64
Not in work at time of onset	26	38	36
PQ22 & PQ25			
Sight direct reason stopped working	13	13	13
PQ6			
Sight reason left last job	na	34	29
PQ20			
Change of job since onset	29	12	15
Base (population) = 100%	9K	48K	57K
(Number interviewed)	(33)	(126)	(159)

(159 respondents: only working age respondents with onset age 20 or over considered)   +Women 16 – 59; men 16 – 64
Note: The base for those working is too small to allow any firm judgements about differences between those working and not working

Table 17.14 repeats the data in Table 17.13 but excludes respondents whose onset occurred at age 19 or under. It provides further evidence of the contribution of the sight difficulty to the loss of the last job for those not in work. Sixty-two per cent were in work at the time of onset, 12% had changed job since onset; excluding the 12% from the 62% produces 50% where there is some familiarity with the job and the employer before onset; 34% that said the reason they left their last job was because of their sight problem. Conservatively this allows one to say that 68% of those who were not in work left their job because of their visual impairment, which will also be a barrier to future employment.

17.8.1   Employment continuity

Table 17.15.a. shows that overall only a quarter (26%) of those who had a job at onset had changed job since then. Half of those currently in work had changed jobs since onset, while, for 80% of those not in work, the job they had at onset was the last one they held.

Those who had a job at onset were asked (PQ25) if they had ever stopped work because of their visual impairment. As Table 17.15.b. shows, just over half (55%) said that they had stopped. A quarter had to stop immediately, the rest some time after onset.

Table 17.15.a. Employment continuity among those of working age+ employed at onset, by working status

'Were you doing the job you have already described, or a different one?' (PQ20)

	Work status		Total
	In work	Not in work	
	%	%	%
Same job as at onset	50	80	74
Different job from that at onset	50	19	26
Total %	100	100	100
Base (population)	10K	35K	45K
(Number interviewed)	(40)	(104)	(144)

(144 respondents: working age respondents, in work at the time of onset)
+Women 16 – 59; men 16 – 64

Table 17.15.b. Employment stoppage among those of working age+

'Was there ever a time when you had to stop doing your job because of your sight problem?' (PQ25)

	Work status		Total
	In work	Not in work	
	%	%	%
Yes	39	60	55
No	61	36	42
Don't know	0	4	3
Total %	100	100	100
Base (population)	10K	35K	45K
(Number interviewed)	(40)	(104)	(144)

(144 respondents: working age respondents in work at the time of onset)
+Women 16 – 59; men 16 – 64

The data also suggest a difference between those currently in and out of work. Those not in work are more likely to have stopped work because of their sight problem (60 and 39 per cent). We have seen in section 17.8 that, for approximately two-thirds of those not currently in work, the last job they held was the one they had when their sight problems started. This shows the importance of retaining the job held at onset, or at least staying with the same employer.

17.8.2   Changes in job status resulting from onset

Those respondents who had changed jobs since the onset of their sight difficulties were asked about the nature of the change. Comparing the broad economic status of the job held at onset and the last or current job could reveal a shift in job status. Since only fifty-one respondents fell into this category, the evidence set out in Table 17.16 must be treated cautiously.

Few respondents had made a positive job move. Since most individuals were in the non-professional job categories, any move would have been to a similar category, even though to a different employer. The only broad conclusion possible is that onset, far from causing people to 'change' jobs is more likely to 'force' them out of the job market altogether. However, the situation is not entirely bleak. Contrary to the perhaps natural expectation of a clear 'downward' shift, less than half the moves (43%) were into lower-status jobs. A quarter of the moves involved promotion and 32% were moves to jobs of the same status.

Table 17.16   Changes in job status

'What was the job title of the job you were doing when your sight problems first started? What did the work involve?' (PQ21)

'What was the title of the job you changed to? (PQ24)

	All who have changed job since onset
	%
Same status job	32
Lower status	43
Higher status	25
Total %	100
Base (population)	12K
(Number interviewed)	(51)

(51 respondents: working age respondents currently working and not working who had changed jobs since onset)

17.8.3   Employment history of visually impaired people of retirement age

Well over half (60%) of visually impaired people of retirement age had retired or stopped work before onset. Retired blind people were slightly less likely to have retired before onset than partially sighted people (52 and 64 per cent respectively).

Since more visually impaired people of retirement age are women and women generally stop work earlier than men, the combination of these two factors results in the relatively large percentage of people of retirement age who stopped working before the onset of their visual impairment.

Part E

Support Services

18 Allowances and Benefits

18.1 Visually impaired people receiving state allowances and benefits

Our questioning on welfare allowances and benefits sought only basic information. This was in line with our objective of complementing, rather than replicating, the information obtained in the OPCS disability survey (Martin, et al, 1988b), which contained substantial sections on these topics.

While there are a variety of benefits available to disabled people to compensate them for their handicap, for visually impaired people only blind registration status brings any entitlement; registration as partially sighted confers no statutory rights.

Table 18.1 shows that overall 86% of respondents receive a retirement pension, reflecting the age structure of the visually impaired population; 46% receive housing benefit (rent and rates rebate); and 25% receive supplementary benefits (replaced since our survey was carried out by income support).

18.2 Allowances and benefits received by visually impaired people of retirement age

The pattern of benefit receipt based purely on age is not unexpected. Receipt of retirement pension is almost entirely age-dependent, 97% of visually impaired people of retirement age saying that they draw a pension. More interesting is the fact that a substantial proportion of people of retirement age also receive additional benefits because of their low income. Nearly half (48%) receive some form of housing benefit, and just over a quarter (27%) draw supplementary benefit.

Few people of retirement age draw any other benefits. Nine per cent receive attendance allowance, just over a third (38%) at the higher rate. Only 2% receive the mobility allowance, and 4% receive either invalidity or sickness benefit. (Though these are two separate benefits no distinction is made between them in this report; they both cover inability to work because of illness or disability, invalidity benefit being

Table 18.1   Allowances and benefits received by visually impaired people of working and retirement age by registration status

'Can I just check whether you yourself receive any of these allowances or benefits? Do you get...?' (PQ41)

	Registration status within working and retirement age						Total
	Working age +			Retirement age			
	R	NR	Total	R	NR	Total	
	%	%	%	%	%	%	%
Retirement pension	1	10	6	94	98	97	86
Housing benefit	31	36	34	45	48	48	46
Supplementary benefit	21	10	14	34	25	27	25
Attendance allowance							
all rates	8	17	13	17	7	9	10
higher rate	3	9	7	7	2	3	4
lower rate	4	6	5	8	3	4	4
don't know rate	#	2	1	1	2	2	2
Invalidity or sickness benefit	35	46	42	5	3	4	8
Mobility allowance	15	31	25	4	1	2	5
Severe disablement allowance	21	11	15	4	4	1	3
Invalid care allowance	0	0	0	8	0	0	2
Child benefit	18	10	13	0	0	0	2
Unemployment benefit	5	2	3	0	0	0	#
Family income supplement	#	0	#	0	0	0	#
Receive no allowances or benefits	27	19	22	1	0	#	3
Base (population) = 100%	35K	56K	91K	135K	531K	666K	757K
(Number interviewed)	(228)	(89)	(317)	(124)	(154)	(278)	(595)

+ 16 – 59 for women, 16 – 64 for men

paid after the first six months in which sickness benefit is paid.) This latter figure reflects the generally late onset of visual impairment and of any other disability that may prevent work (Chapter 17). Practically all the recipients of this last benefit are men (13% compared with under 1% of women of retirement age), which reflects the fact that many women have stopped work before making sufficient National Insurance contributions to be entitled to this benefit.

The invalid care allowance is paid to carers of people who require some form of care at home because they are unable to look after themselves. Although our question concerned benefits received, 2% of respondents of retirement age said that they received this benefit. While this may reflect either a misunderstanding of the question or the fact that they do care for someone else themselves, it also suggests that these respondents may be in need of 'care' in their own home and the carer is receiving the allowance to look after the visually impaired person.

This latter hypothesis is strengthened by the fact that most of those who said that they received this allowance were aged 75 or over, reflecting the increased need for help in daily living that increasingly severe disabilities among older people bring (Chapter 15).

18.3 Allowances and benefits received by visually impaired people of working age

As Table 18.1 shows, only 22% of respondents of working age said that they did not receive any benefits. This statistic demonstrates that a large majority of visually impaired people depend on some form of income from the state welfare system. Put another way, four out of every five visually impaired people of working age and living in private households depend on some form of social security benefit or allowance.

Invalidity or sickness benefit is received by 42% of people of working age, housing benefit by 34% and mobility allowance by 25%. Other benefits received are severe disablement allowance (15%), supplementary benefit (14%) and attendance allowance (13%).

18.3.1 Registration status

As Table 18.2 demonstrates, registration as blind is not a major determinant of receipt of benefits (the percentage differences in the receipt of the individual benefits between registered and non-registered respondents were not statistically significant, see section 21.4). Receipt of benefits is one of the most often stated reasons for registration. The blind person's tax allowance (BPTA) is practically the only benefit that a visually impaired person is entitled to receive when registered blind, to compensate for the additional cost of the visual handicap. (However, the disability premium on income support may also be available to those registered blind.) So, while registration may be a pathway into the welfare support system, it does not seem to have a large bearing on the welfare benefit system.

18.3.2 Working status

When receipt of benefits is analysed by working status (Table 18.2), a pronounced difference emerges between those in and those not in work. A third of those in work receive some form of discretionary benefit or allowance, chiefly housing benefit (10%) and mobility allowance (9%). Excluding housing benefit and retirement pension, only 1% of those respondents in work reported receiving any form of income maintenance benefit. Nine per cent of those in work reported receiving one of the disablement allowances (attendance allowance or mobility allowance), compared with 33% of those not in work.

The benefits received by people not in work make rather more revealing reading. Over half (56%) receive either invalidity or sickness benefit, and over two-thirds (68%) receive one of these benefits or the severe disablement allowance. It is worth comparing the 56% receiving invalidity or sickness benefit with the tiny 4% receiving unemployment benefit. These statistics indicate that the majority are not working because of a long-term illness or disability, but have worked during a long period in the past, since in order to qualify for invalidity benefit it is

Table 18.2 Allowances and benefits received by visually impaired people of working age+ by work status and registration status (PQ41)

	Work status		Registration status			Total
	In work	Not in work	Registered			
			B	PS	NR	
	%	%	%	%	%	%
Child benefit	11	14	19	15	10	13
Supplementary benefit	1	18	18	27	10	14
Family income supplement	0	#	0	1	0	#
Retirement pension	1	8	1	1	10	6
Unemployment benefit	0	4	2	9	2	3
Invalid care allowance	0	0	0	0	0	0
General income maintenance excluding HB, including pensions	**2**	**28**	**18**	**28**	**22**	**22**
Housing benefit (HB)	10	42	31	29	36	34
All maintenance benefits including HB and excluding pensions	**11**	**50**	**38**	**43**	**40**	**40**
Maintenance benefits excluding HB and excluding pensions	**1**	**20**	**18**	**28**	**12**	**16**
Invalidity or sickness benefit	1	56	37	32	46	42
Severe disablement allowance	0	20	24	16	11	15
Disablement benefits paid	**1**	**68**	**54**	**42**	**53**	**52**
Mobility allowance	9	30	15	13	31	25
Attendance allowance	0	17	10	4	16	13
Disablement allowances paid	**9**	**33**	**21**	**15**	**32**	**27**
All disablement allowances and benefits paid	**10**	**71**	**57**	**44**	**59**	**56**
Not in receipt of any disablement allowances	90	29	43	56	41	44
Base (population) = 100%	22K	69K	22K	13K	56K	91K
(Number interviewed)	(95)	(222)	(130)	(98)	(89)	(317)

+16 – 59 for women, 16 – 64 for men

necessary to build up substantial national insurance contributions. As Chapter 17 shows, a large proportion of those not working have not worked for well over two years.

One-third (33%) of those not working were receiving one of the disablement allowances compared with 21% of those registered blind. Not working seemed to be a greater determinant of receipt of the mobility allowance than registration as blind (30 and 15 per cent). This suggests that receipt of this allowance is determined not by the sight problem *per se* but by some other disability affecting mobility. Seventy-one per cent of those not in work reported receiving one of the disablement allowances and benefits, compared with 57% of those registered blind.

The data in Table 18.2 suggest that being registered blind confers no additional entitlement to benefits; 57 and 59 per cent of those registered blind and the non-registered respectively were receiving benefits. Either visually impaired people are failing to claim benefits or the welfare benefit system is failing to recognise the degree of handicap that a visual impairment causes.

18.3.3   The blind person's tax allowance

Overall only 5% of visually impaired people receive this tax allowance. This figure is low for two main reasons. First, the allowance is only available to registered blind people; and, second, the income of many visually impaired people is too low to attract taxation. Table 18.3 shows that 42% of registered blind people of working age said that they receive this allowance. A similarly large proportion said that they did not

Table 18.3   Registered blind people of working age+ receiving the blind person's tax allowance by work status

'Do you get the blind person's tax allowance?' (PQ43)

	Work status		Total
	In work	Not in work	
	%	%	%
Yes	91	18	42
No, don't pay tax	3	63	44
Don't know what BPTA is	0	9	6
Don't know if get it	2	9	7
No response	3	0	1
Total %	100	100	100
Base (population)	7K	15K	22K
(Number interviewed)	(42)	(87)	(129)

(129 respondents: only respondents registered blind of working age)

+Women 16 – 59, men 16 – 64

259

pay tax (44%). Of those in work 91% said that they receive it; of those working full time 96% said that they receive the allowance. Rather surprisingly 18% of those not in work said that they receive the allowance, indicating that they have sufficient income to pay tax.

18.4 Advice on entitlement to benefits and allowances

Table 18.4 shows that overall 21% of respondents had been advised about benefits to which they might be entitled. The OPCS survey obtained a similar figure of 19% (Martin et al, 1988b). Differences occurred between respondents of working age and retirement age (35 and 19 per cent); men and women (27 and 19 per cent); and the registered and non-registered (29 and 19 per cent). The interaction among these factors should be noted. There are more women than men in the older age group, older visually impaired people are less likely to be registered, and most of the registered are of working age.

Table 18.4   Advice received on benefit entitlement, by age, sex and registration status

'Have you ever spoken to anyone to get advice on what benefits you may be entitled to?' (PQ44)

	Working and retirement age		Sex		Registration status		Total
	WA	RA	M	F	R	NR	
	%	%	%	%	%	%	%
Yes	35	19	27	19	29	19	21
No	65	81	73	81	71	81	79
Total %	100	100	100	100	100	100	100
Base (population)	91K	666K	215K	542K	170K	587K	757K
(Number interviewed)	(317)	(278)	(245)	(350)	(352)	(243)	(595)

WA = working age, women 16 – 59, men 16 – 64; RA = retirement age, 60 and 65 plus

The largest gap between those who have and have not sought advice is among people of working and retirement age. It can be surmised that people of retirement age consider their retirement pension to be their main benefit and may make little effort to seek other benefits. (Indeed, most other benefits are only available to people of working age.) It is well known that elderly people in general are reluctant to claim social security benefits and allowances.

That 65 and 81 per cent of visually impaired people of working and retirement age respectively have not received any advice on benefit entitlements should be a spur to action for statutory and voluntary organisations serving blind and partially sighted people. It is all the more urgent that action should be taken to increase the take-up of benefits since, at the time the survey was undertaken, registered blind and partially sighted people received few benefits as of right. An

260

additional barrier to access to information on benefits is that such information is most often provided in print which is not readily accessible to visually impaired people.

18.4.1 Source of advice on benefits and allowances

Respondents who had sought advice on benefits and allowances were asked to whom they had spoken. As Table 18.5 shows, social/welfare workers (31%) were most frequently mentioned followed by local DHSS offices (23%) and the Citizens Advice Bureau (CAB) (10%). Further mentions of social services included unidentified personnel (5%) and social workers for the blind (4%).

Table 18.5 Sources of advice on benefit entitlement by age and registration status

'Who did you speak to?' (PQ45)	Working and retirement age		Registration status		Total
	WA	RA	R	NR	
	%	%	%	%	%
Social/welfare worker	28	31	38	27	31
Local DHSS office	26	22	27	21	23
Citizens Advice Bureau	30	5	14	8	10
Others from social services	4	5	4	5	5
Health service	4	5	1	6	5
Relative	0	6	2	5	5
Social worker for blind	8	3	11	1	4
Friend/colleague	1	3	5	1	2
Someone in the house	1	1	3	0	1
RNIB	4	0	1	1	1
All mentions of social services	37	34	48	28	35
Don't know	0	7	0	8	6
No information recorded	3	16	5	18	14
Base (population) = 100%	32K	128K	50K	110K	160K
(Number interviewed)	(110)	(65)	(119)	(56)	(175)

WA = working age, women 16 – 59, men 16 – 64; RA = retirement age, 60 and 65 plus

The OPCS report (Martin et al, 1988b) found that the two main sources of information for the disabled population in general were the DHSS office (68%) and social services/social worker (20%), the same as in this survey; the third source they reported, doctor (9%), differed from our own.

That visually impaired people refer more often to social workers for advice than disabled people as a whole (35 and 20 per cent) indicates the problems that visually impaired people experience gaining advice. Though better informed than the lay person, social workers in general do not claim to be experts on the benefit system and are unlikely to be well informed about particular benefits for visually impaired people.

Although registration itself has little influence on the receipt of benefit, it does provide a way into the system (section 3.9.1). Twenty-nine per cent of registered respondents had received advice on benefits, but only 18% of those not registered. Table 18.5 also indicates that the registered are more likely to have spoken to one of the sources who may at least have some 'knowledge' of welfare benefits; 48% compared with 28%, had spoken to someone from the social or welfare services.

18.5 Benefits received by visually impaired people and by disabled people in general

Table 18.6 shows that for the most part a similar proportion of visually impaired people and disabled people in general receive the various benefits available. Such dissimilarities as exist reflect the differing age structures of the two populations. Although the extent of disability increases with age, the visually impaired population contains a greater proportion of people of retirement age; the ratio is 7:1 compared with 1.6:1 in the general disabled population. Thus percentages based on the total sample for the visually impaired population become heavily skewed towards the percentage found in the retirement age group.

An example of this is the total percentages in receipt of the retirement pension shown in Table 18.5. While the percentages for the working and retirement age groups are similar within the two samples (about 6 and 96 per cent respectively), when based on the total sample they become markedly different (86 and 62 per cent for the visually impaired and disabled populations respectively).

Table 18.6 shows that 89% of our respondents, but only 74% of OPCS respondents, received general income maintenance benefits including pensions but excluding housing benefit. This is because there is a greater proportion of people of retirement age in the visually impaired population.

The two disability-based benefits – invalidity and severe disablement – also reveal some major differences. (Note that our questionnaires, unlike those of OPCS, combined the invalidity benefit and sickness benefit. However, since only 3% of the OPCS working age respondents received these benefits, this has little impact on the results.) While 42% of our working age respondents received invalidity or sickness benefit, the equivalent OPCS figure was 30%. Severe disablement allowance was received by 15 and 5 per cent respectively. The attendance and

Table 18.6 Benefits received by visually impaired people and by disabled people in general, of working and retirement age*

	RNIB			OPCS		
	WA	RA	Total	WA	RA	Total
	%	%	%	%	%	%
Child benefit	13	0	2	25	0	10
Family income supplement	#	0	#	1	0	#
Supplementary benefit	14	27	25	23	23	23
Retirement pension	6	97	86	8	96	62
Unemployment benefit	3	0	#	3	0	1
Sickness benefit	+	+	+	3	0	1
Invalid care allowance	0	2	2	0	0	0
General income maintenance excluding HB, including pensions	**23**	**99**	**89**	**36**	**97**	**74**
Housing benefit (HB)	35	50	48	41	55	56
All maintenance benefits including HB and excluding pensions	**40**	**55**	**53**	+	+	+
Maintenance benefits excluding HB and excluding pensions	**16**	**28**	**27**	+	+	+
Invalidity or sickness benefits	42	4	8	27	2	12
Severe disablement allowance	15	1	3	5	0	2
Disablement benefits paid	**52**	**5**	**11**	**35**	**6**	**17**
Attendance allowance	13	9	10	7	9	8
Mobility allowance	25	2	5	13	3	7
Disablement allowances paid	27	10	12	15	11	13
All disablement allowances and benefits paid	**56**	**14**	**19**	+	+	+
Not in receipt of any disablement allowances or benefits	44	86	81	+	+	+
Base (population) = 100%	91K	666K	757K	3808	6174	9982
(Number interviewed)	(317)	(278)	(595)			

+ Not applicable to this survey
WA = working age, women 16 – 59, men 16 – 64; RA = retirement age, 60 and 65 plus
*OPCS refer to the two age groups as pensioner and non-pensioner respectively. Their report also takes the household as the unit
Source: OPCS survey of disability in Great Britain, Report 2; Table 3.4, page 20 (Martin et al, 1988b)

mobility allowances show a similar pattern, with a larger proportion of visually impaired people receiving them (27 and 15 per cent respectively of working age respondents).

It is difficult to suggest reasons why a larger percentage of the visually impaired population than of the disabled population in general meets the criteria for receipt of state disability benefits and allowances.

Table 18.6 shows that, since 25% of visually impaired people of working age receive the mobility allowance compared with 13% of disabled people in general, sight problems themselves are not the major factor. The data in Table 18.2 raise the same point, showing that twice as many non-registered as registered people receive it. Given that the registered have a lower level of residual vision than their non-registered counterparts (section 3.9.4), if sight were the determining factor then the percentages of registered and non-registered would at the very least be equal. It is more likely that the presence of other disabilities combines with the visual impairment to produce the higher proportion receiving the mobility allowance.

The consequence of later onset is that visually impaired people are initially eligible for the contribution-based benefits. Fourteen per cent of visually impaired people of working age receive supplementary benefit (a non-contribution benefit) compared with 23% of the disabled population; after retirement the totals are similar, 27 and 23 per cent respectively. Invalidity or sickness benefit (contribution-based benefits) is received by a greater number of visually impaired people of working age, 42 and 27 per cent. Receipt of disablement allowances also evens out in a similar fashion.

18.5.1   Housing benefit

As Table 18.6 shows, 48% of visually impaired people receive housing benefits, compared with 56% of disabled people in general. Fewer working-age than retirement-age people received them (35 and 50 per cent respectively), a difference replicated among disabled people in general (41 and 55 per cent respectively).

Table 18.7 provides a more detailed breakdown by tenure and working-/retirement-age households. Owner-occupiers are less likely to receive housing benefits than the main tenant groups (local authority and housing association). The proportions receiving housing benefit are 24 and 50 per cent among working-age households, 21 and 73 per cent among retirement-age households.

Table 18.7 also shows that among owner-occupiers, similar proportions of working- and retirement-age households receive housing benefits (24 and 21 per cent). Among tenants, however, the totals are 50 and 73 per cent respectively, which may reflect the generally lower incomes of pensioners.

The summary total in Table 18.6 supports this assertion. Excluding housing benefits and pensions, 16% of working age respondents compared with 28% of retirement-age respondents receive some form of income maintenance benefit or allowance.

Table 18.7 Visually impaired people receiving housing benefits by form of tenure and working and retirement age (percentaged across rows)

		Get HB	No HB	Total %	Base Popl	Number interviewed
Working age households						
Owner occupiers	%	24	76	100	41K	(153)
Rents; LA and HA	%	50	50	100	40K	(128)
Other tenants	%	13	87	100	8K	(17)
Total non-pensioners	%	**35**	**65**	**100**	**89K**	**(298)**
Retirement age households						
Owner occupiers	%	21	79	100	263K	(102)
Rents; LA and HA	%	73	37	100	309K	(140)
Other tenants	%	69	31	100	48K	(17)
Total pensioners	%	**50**	**50**	**100**	**620K**	**(259)**
All households						
Owner occupiers	%	21	79	100	304K	(255)
Rents; LA and HA	%	65	35	100	348K	(268)
Other tenants	%	61	39	100	56K	(34)
All households	%	**48**	**52**	**100**	**709K**	**(557)**

(557 respondents; 36 live with others; no information for 2)

LA = Local authority; HA = Housing association

19 Local Authority Social Services

19.1 Introduction

None of the questions asked so far in this survey has explicitly mentioned local authority social services departments (SSDs for short) or their field workers. This was the result of a deliberate policy decision designed to overcome problems associated with obtaining a fair assessment of the role of SSDs, even though much information had already been gathered about the extent of SSD provision. Enquiries about rehabilitation services were also left to this late point in the interview.

The mandatory services local authorities are required to provide for visually impaired people are limited. There is uncertainty about the precise obligations laid down by legislation (note 1), and the standards of provision vary enormously. Moreover, some local authorities have delegated their duties (or certain aspects of them) to appropriately registered voluntary societies, who act as their agents.

The terms social services and welfare services are used to cover the broad range of provision for visually impaired people, whether delivered by local authority SSDs, their agents or the local society or association for the blind. In some cases the services may actually be provided through the health service, but in this section we are primarily concerned with local SSDs and/or their agents.

As far as our respondents, the service-receivers, were concerned, it seemed important to concentrate on obtaining information about the actual services received, not on knowledge of who provided the service. The study by the Research Institute for Consumer Affairs (Epstein, 1980) and our own pilot survey showed that elderly people in particular are often confused about which agency provides which service. In addition, we wished to ascertain the extent of existing knowledge of service-providers and therefore used 'open' questions that allowed respondents to answer in their own words. Interviewers were given a list of possible service-providers and recorded the answers accordingly. Prompting the names would have resulted in greatly exaggerated knowledge in the extent of respondents' awareness of service-providers (note 2).

This chapter, however, is concerned with more specific questioning about SSD services. Knowledge of the local SSD and its field workers is tested by means of prompts from an itemised check list (section 19.2). In practice, the boundaries between support services provided by SSDs to all elderly and disabled people, specialised services for visually impaired people, and full-scale rehabilitation work are blurred. The frequency of SSD visits, and their relation to registration, varies greatly (note 3). Although some SSDs do offer specialist services to all visually impaired people regardless of registration, this is very unusual, as our data confirm (Table 19.11.b.). It was chiefly our earlier lengthy questioning about the specific services provided to meet particular needs that enabled respondents to make sense of our 'over-arching' questions (note 4) about the overall range of services supplied by the local SSD. Our pilot work suggested that respondents did not necessarily have any clear concept of this, and it would therefore not make sense to ask, for example, how satisfied respondents were with their SSD as a service-provider unless they had some idea of what those services consisted.

Similar considerations surrounded the use of the term 'rehabilitation', which is a matter of debate even among professionals. Many non-registered respondents, and even some registered, were unfamiliar with the expression. We could hardly ask them about the rehabilitation services they had been offered without spelling out what we meant. It was easiest to do this (section 19.5) at a late stage, following lengthy questioning about specific need areas.

Our questioning sequence also helped to overcome problems associated with memory and recall. Shore's study of local authority rehabilitation services was based on respondents who had been registered blind during the previous three years (Shore, 1985). Ours, by contrast, also included the registered partially sighted and the non-registered, a large proportion of whom sustained their sight loss up to fifteen years before the survey. The recall factor alone would therefore have limited the detail with which many of our respondents could be expected to remember the relevant facts. However, our pilot work showed that placing the questions on SSD services towards the end of the interview, following lengthy questioning about specific services that the respondent might have received in the past, helped to aid recollection of any initial SSD help received.

These are the considerations that determined the placing and structure of the questions reviewed in this chapter. The questions attempt to distinguish initial assessments and offers of services and aid (section 19.4) from more extensive visits ranging up to fully-fledged rehabilitation courses (19.5, 19.6); early support from continuing specialised support (19.7, 19.8); and to distinguish both from non-specialised SSD support services such as meals on wheels and home helps (19.11, 19.12).

19.2 General awareness of social services

19.2.1 Awareness as a whole

Table 19.1 shows the level of awareness of eight types of prompted items relating to social and welfare services. The list prompts for both specific field workers and the broader 'social services'. Although most respondents had heard of 'the social services or the welfare services' as such, no less than 16%, mainly the non-registered aged 75 or over, said that they had not. A similar pattern of replies was received for the second inclusive general item, 'social workers or welfare workers'. Overall, 57% said that they had heard of 'voluntary services or voluntary workers'. Awareness was again lowest among the non-registered aged 75 or over (about 50%), reaching 70% in other sub-groups.

Table 19.1 Knowledge of social services

'I'd like to ask you a few questions now about any assistance you have had to help with your sight problems. Can I just check first of all whether you have *heard of* various things. Have you heard of ...?' (CQ1)

	Age and registration status				Total
	Registered		Non-registered		
	16 – 59	60 +	16 – 59	60 +	
	%	%	%	%	%
The social services or the welfare services	96	94	92	80	84
Social workers or welfare workers	97	91	91	78	82
Voluntary services or voluntary workers	71	70	77	51	57
Social workers for the blind or home teachers	76	52	37	27	34
Mobility officers	71	27	34	20	24
Rehabilitation officers	72	33	45	16	23
Technical officers	37	12	6	4	8
Visual handicap adjustment officers	18	13	6	4	6
Not heard of any	2	4	5	14	11
Base (population) = 100%	30K	140K	47K	540K	757K
(Number interviewed)	(215)	(137)	(84)	(159)	(595)

19.2.2 Knowledge of job titles of SSD specialist workers

Awareness of the other items in Table 19.1 fell sharply. Only 34% overall said that they had heard of 'social workers for the blind or home teachers'. Registration was the key factor here. Among the registered aged 16 – 59 and 60 or over, the totals were 76 and 52 per cent respectively, while among the non-registered the totals were 37 and 27 per cent.

Twenty-three per cent overall were aware of 'mobility officers'. Awareness of these workers was an interaction between age and registration. Seventy-one and 27 per cent of the registered aged 16 – 59 and 60 or over respectively had heard of 'mobility officers', compared with 34 and 20 per cent of the non-registered.

The percentages were similar for 'rehabilitation officers' except that some 45% of the non-registered in the 16 – 59 age band said they had heard of them.

Very few respondents, only 8% overall, said that they had heard of technical officers, and these were concentrated among the registered aged 16 – 59 (37%).

We created the title 'visual handicap adjustment officers' to test for 'false positives' in responses. Overall, 6% said that they had heard of these fictional officers. Among the registered aged 16 – 59 and 60 or over, the figures were 18 and 13 per cent respectively. These results enable us to draw the general conclusion that most of the generalised officer/service titles encouraged a degree of false positive response. In other words, awareness among respondents was appreciably lower than our results show.

Registered blind people showed greater awareness of all these items than the registered partially sighted. However, the differences between these two sub-groups were marginal compared with the differences relating to age and registration status noted above.

19.2.3 Awareness of entitlement to specialised help

Rather than prompt item by item for awareness of the specialised services available to visually impaired people, we followed our first question (CQ1) with a statement reviewing the services followed by a further general question (CQ2) about awareness of the availability of these services. Table 19.2 shows the results.

Some correlation between awareness of specialised workers for visually impaired people (CQ1) and awareness of the kind of specialised help available (CQ2) is to be expected. Overall, the 39% who say that they are aware of entitlement to specialised services (Table 19.2) is roughly equivalent to the 34% who had heard of 'social workers for the blind or home teachers', the best known of the specialised workers. The totals aware of specialised services varied from 65% of the registered to 33% of the non-registered.

Table 19.2   Knowledge of specialised help

'(As you may know) these are people who work for the local social or welfare services. In many areas these workers visit people who have sight problems to give them advice on how to cope in the home. They may also offer aids such as braille, a talking book, and a white stick, and give advice on how to get about in the street, local social or day centres, and any benefits you can get and so on.

Did you know that someone with sight problems may be entitled to this kind of help from their local social or welfare services?' (CQ2)

	Age and registration status				Total
	Registered		Non-registered		
	16 – 59	60 +	16 – 59	60 +	
	%	%	%	%	%
Yes	69	63	38	33	39
No/uncertain	31	37	62	67	61
Total %	100	100	100	100	100
Base (population)	30K	140K	47K	540K	757K
(Number interviewed)	(215)	(137)	(84)	(159)	(595)

Awareness of entitlement to specialised services depends mostly on registration status and owes little to age. This contrasts with awareness of social services generally (Table 19.1), where age is a significant factor. While elderly visually impaired people are less knowledgeable than young visually impaired people about the official titles used by blind welfare professionals, they are not equally unaware of the availability of specialised help.

Question CQ2 was deliberately worded in a practical way so as to emphasise the basic social welfare services with which visually impaired people could be expected to be familiar. Thus, the fact that one-third of registered and two-thirds of non-registered blind and partially sighted people are not aware of these services is extremely alarming. This finding has important implications. First, planners and service providers must actively attempt to increase awareness of the available services among these vulnerable groups. Second, as more and more visually impaired people become aware of the services to which they are entitled, voluntary and statutory agencies will be faced with significant resource implications.

19.3   Attitudes to and awareness of services among the non-registered

19.3.1   Awareness of registration

At an earlier point in the interview, following the enquiry into registration status, we asked respondents who said that they were not registered if they had heard about registration (YQ21). Forty-nine per cent said that they had not. There was no difference by age, but blind respondents (62%) were more aware of registration than partially sighted respondents (44%).

We then asked (YQ22) those among the non-registered who were aware of registration if an eye specialist had ever examined them to determine whether they should be registered. Only 8% had undergone such an examination, with no significant difference by residual vision level. When asked (at YQ23) what happened after the examination, most said that their sight loss was not found to be severe enough to qualify for registration.

19.3.2   Awareness of benefits of registration

The data given in section 19.3.1 suggest that one simple reason for not being registered is unawareness of the possibility of registration. However, those who are aware could still be uninformed about the possible benefits resulting from registration. Following the general enquiry (at CQ2) into awareness of entitlement to specialised social services help, we asked all the non-registered: 'Did you know that being registered as blind or partially sighted can help a person to get this kind of help?' (CQ3) Some 71% of the non-registered said that they did not know this, slightly more than those who said that they were unaware of the possibility of specialised help (CQ2), and some 20% more than those who said that they were unaware of registration (YQ21). There was little difference by either age or residual vision level.

19.3.3   Reasons for not being registered

We also asked all the non-registered: 'What would you say was the main reason for not being registered? Was it that you have...?' (CQ4) Three possible reasons (derived from the pilot work) were then suggested. 'Heard of it, but didn't think your eye problem was serious enough' was chosen by 53%; 'never heard of registration' by 19%; 'heard of it, but didn't think there was much advantage for you' by 9%; a further 5, 8 and 6 per cent 'did not want to register', 'didn't know' or gave a variety of 'other' answers respectively.

The finding that so many of the unregistered do not consider their eyesight problem serious enough to warrant registration has considerable implications. Among those giving this reason there was little difference between age groups and, most important, there was no significant difference between respondents at registrably blind and partially sighted levels. This reflects not so much an objective appraisal of their sight problems as a shared underlying attitude towards registration. The answers to CQ3 show that there is little awareness of the potential benefits of registration among the non-registered. Combined with the present results, the conclusion is that the non-registered perceive registration mainly in terms of stigmatisation rather than as a source of help. Registration would represent an official, public categorisation of themselves as having a serious impairment. Since they are unaware of any compensating advantages, it is understandable that they should avoid it rather than positively seek it.

There is an accepted wisdom that registration brings few advantages, and may not be 'worth it'. This is true in that registration brings automatic entitlement to only a handful of services. However, our research shows very clearly something that has never been fully understood until now: namely, the high correlation between registration and take-up of a wide variety of discretionary services for which registration is not technically a qualifier. Conversely, there is a high correlation between failure to register and failure to receive services.

In short, policy planners and service providers have a choice between delivering services to non-registered people as widely as they do to the registered or actively campaigning to increase registration. Probably both are required. Such decisions will no doubt be taken with the resource restraints uppermost in the policy-makers' minds.

19.4   Initial visits from the social services

19.4.1   Visits at the time of onset

Professional help obtained at the time when loss of vision first seriously impinges on daily living activities can be crucial for the subsequent adjustment of the individual. Social services are the main source of this help. For children and young people of school age, intervention and support are primarily an educational responsibility with social services support.

Respondents had already been asked about when they experienced onset of sight loss (Chapter 5). We now asked those who had lost their sight at age 16 or over the following question: 'Thinking back to the time when you first had your eyesight problems, did someone from the social or welfare services visit you at that time?'(CQ5)

The results are shown in Table 19.3. Only 17% overall answered 'yes' to this question, but with a sharp division between the registered and non-registered. Fifty-three per cent of the registered compared with only 6% of the non-registered answered 'yes'. Neither age nor type of registration (blind or partially sighted) made any significant difference.

Ideally, after being examined by a consultant ophthalmologist and found eligible for registration, a visually impaired person should be visited by a social worker, who explains the significance of registration. He or she should provide details of benefits and services available, and make provision for social and emotional rehabilitation and adjustment to disability, including assistance in overcoming mobility or communication limitations. Our data show that this ideal was achieved for only 53% of registered people; nearly half of those who register do not have the advantage of this visit from a social worker. The data confirm on a national basis the results established by an earlier RNIB study on a more restricted sample (Shore, 1985).

Table 19.3 Visits from SSDs at onset of sight loss

'Thinking back to the time when you first had your eyesight problems, did someone from the social or welfare services visit you at that time?' (CQ5)

	Age and registration status				Total
	Registered		Non-registered		
	16 – 59	60 +	16 – 59	60 +	
	%	%	%	%	%
Yes	52	53	2	8	17
No	41	44	98	90	82
Don't know	8	4	0	1	2
Total %	100	100	100	100	100
Base (population)	13K	114K	32K	502K	661K
(Number interviewed)	(91)	(109)	(57)	(149)	(406)

(406 respondents: 144 early onset not asked CQ5; no response to CQ5 for 45)

In overall percentage terms, the likelihood that any registrably visually impaired person was visited by a social worker or other blind welfare worker at the time they first had eyesight problems is very small. In numerical terms, the age profile of visually impaired people means that among the 17% of respondents who received such visits (population projection 109,000 people) are a great many elderly non-registered people. Table 19.3 shows that 8% of the non-registered aged 60 and over were visited. This translates into an estimated 42,000 people, compared with 60,000 (53%) of the registered in the same age group who were visited.

It is nevertheless clear that the great majority of visually impaired people are not receiving support from SSDs when it would be most valuable, at the time of the onset of serious visual loss. The lack of a visit (or its insignificance, in that it could not be recalled) for people newly certified blind must be traumatic. Even among the registered, only one in two of those who lose their sight at age 16 or older are visited by their SSD at the time of loss. Among the non-registered the chances of receiving such a visit are minute, scarcely more than 1 in 20.

19.4.2 Timing of the first visit after registration

We asked all those registered, including those with early onset, the following question: 'You mentioned earlier that you are registered as blind/partially sighted. Thinking back to the time when you had your eyes examined for registration, about how long after that was it that someone from the social or welfare services came to see you?' (CQ6). The answers were as follows: 'less than 6 weeks', 32%; '6 weeks to 3 months', 13%; '3 to 6 months', 5%; 'over 6 months to 12 months', 3%; 'more than a year', 5%. Of the remaining 42%, 30% said that they did not know and 12% they had never been visited. There were no differences by age or type of registration.

Among those who do register for sight loss, and who did receive a visit from their SSD, 45% were visited within three months of registration. However, the crucial area of concern is for the 47% of the registered who have to wait over a year for a visit or do not receive one.

19.4.3   Satisfaction with the first visit

We asked two questions bearing on satisfaction of those (population projection 109,000) who said (at CQ5) that they had been visited by someone from the social or welfare services at the time they first experienced eyesight problems. The first question was: 'Did you feel that they understood the sort of help you needed to cope with your loss of sight?' (CQ7) Seventy-two per cent answered 'yes'. There were no statistically significant differences by age, while insufficient non-registered respondents had received a visit to make a comparison of registered and non-registered possible.

The second question was a straightforward satisfaction rating. We asked: 'How satisfied were you with the help you got to cope with your loss of sight *at that time*. Would you say you were very satisfied, quite satisfied, a bit dissatisfied or very dissatisfied with the help they gave you then?' (CQ8) The responses were 'very satisfied', 18%; 'quite satisfied', 48%; 'a bit dissatisfied', 18%'; and 'very dissatisfied', 16%. There were no statistically significant differences according to age or registration status.

Subjective satisfaction ratings require cautious interpretation (note 5) and should be examined alongside objective evidence of the conditions rated. Generally, people rate themselves as 'very satisfied' in most situations, and even small departures from this represent relative dissatisfaction. It is rare to find substantial numbers of respondents opting for ratings that express degrees of dissatisfaction, as happened in response to our question. Our statistics indicate that those who did receive an initial visit from the social or welfare services at this crucial point did not feel very satisfied with the help they were offered to cope with their sight loss.

Objectively, these ratings support our evidence (sections 19.5 and 19.8) that few respondents, even among the registered, were offered home instruction, counselling, or more systematic rehabilitation and/or advice on aids, either during the initial visit or later.

19.5 Rehabilitation

19.5.1 Offers

We enquired about offers of rehabilitation made to respondents. We did not try to distinguish between the depth of coverage of rehabilitation in the three locations mentioned in our question: 'We talked earlier about difficulties you may have with doing things in the home because of your eyesight problems. In some areas people with sight problems are offered courses of practical training or rehabilitation to help them overcome the effects of sight loss. This training can either be done in your own home, or in a local day centre, or at a residential centre in another area. Have you ever been *offered* a course like this?' (CQ9)

The detailed replies, shown by age and registration status in Table 19.4, reveal that offers of rehabilitation are made almost exclusively to the registered, and primarily to those aged 16 – 59. Thirty-five per cent of the registered in this age group said that they had been offered rehabilitation, compared with 11% of the older registered and 1% of the non-registered. Among the younger registered, 45% of those registered blind had been offered training, compared with 25% of those registered partially sighted. Among the registered aged 60 or over, the type of registration made no difference.

Table 19.4 Offers of rehabilitation

'We talked earlier about difficulties you may have with doing things in the home because of your eyesight problems. In some areas people with sight problems are offered courses of practical training or rehabilitation to help them overcome the effects of sight loss. This training can either be done in your own home, or in a local day centre, or at a residential centre in another area. Have you ever been *offered* a course like this?' (CQ9)*

	Age and registration status						Total
	Registered		Non-registered		Registration		
	16 – 59	60 +	16 – 59	60 +	R	NR	
	%	%	%	%	%	%	%
Yes – at home	3	1	0	0	2	0	#
Yes – at day centre/special centre	7	6	0	1	6	1	2
Yes – at residential centre	29	4	2	0	9	#	2
Total offered training	35	11	2	1	16	1	4
No training offered	65	89	98	99	83	98	95
Base (popltn) = 100%	30K	140K	47K	540K	170K	587K	757K
(Number interviewed)	(215)	(137)	(84)	(159)	(352)	(243)	(595)

*Though the question allowed for more than one response, few respondents gave more than one answer

Because many more people fall into the older age groups, even small percentages correspond to relatively large numbers of people in absolute terms. The population projection for all those who have been offered training is 30,000, of whom: 12,000 are aged 16 – 59; 8,000, 60 – 74; 10,000, 75 or over; 26,000 are registered and 4,000 non-registered.

19.5.2 Location

As Table 19.4 shows, based on the location of the rehabilitation, the 39% of offers for the registered aged 16 – 59 divided 3, 7 and 29 per cent between locations at home, at a day or special centre and at a residential centre. The population projection of the 35% for the registered aged 16 – 59 is 11,000.

Among the 11% of the registered aged 60 or over (population projection 15,000) the split was 1, 6 and 4 per cent. The data suggest that younger people are being offered fuller rehabilitation. It should be noted that a larger part of residential rehabilitation focuses not on daily living or independence skills but on employment rehabilitation.

19.5.3 Take-up

Respondents who had been offered rehabilitation were asked: 'Did you accept the training you were offered?' (CQ10) Sixty-one per cent of respondents (population projection 18,000) had accepted the rehabilitation course offered to them. The small number of interviews (70) does not permit a reliable breakdown by sub-groups.

19.5.4 Unsatisfied demand

Respondents who had not been offered rehabilitation and those who had been offered but not accepted were asked: 'If it were possible, would you like to have a course of practical training or rehabilitation?' (CQ11) Some 10% responded positively (population projection 67,000 – nearly four times the number who had accepted training). In relative terms, unsatisfied demand was greatest among younger respondents: 23% of the registered and 32% of the non-registered aged 16 – 59 (population projections 5,000 and 13,000) but only 8% of those aged 60 or over (population projection 10,000 registered and 39,000 non-registered).

19.6 Home instruction visits

19.6.1 Those who have received home instruction

Some SSDs offer practical instruction by social workers on how to cope at home. These visits supplement the initial visit (if offered) at onset, but fall short of full-scale rehabilitation as described in question CQ9. We asked all those (population projection 755,000) who had not received a full-scale home-based rehabilitation course this question: 'Has anyone from the social or welfare services ever come to your home to give you *practical advice* and instructions on how to overcome these day-to-day problems caused by your eyesight?' (CQ12) Only 4% overall said 'yes' to this question. Table 19.5 combines the response to question CQ12 with those who said that they had accepted rehabilitation offered to them at home at question CQ9. Eleven per cent of the registered compared with 2% of the non-registered had had a home visit.

Table 19.5 Home instruction visits by registration status

'Has anyone from the social or welfare services ever come to your home to give you *practical advice* and instructions on how to overcome these day-to-day problems caused by your eyesight?' (CQ12)

	Registration status		Total
	R	NR	
	%	%	%
Yes – have had home rehabilitation*	11	2	4
No	89	98	96
Total %	100	100	100
Base (population)	170K	587K	757K
(Number interviewed)	(352)	(243)	(595)

*Also includes those who accepted rehabilitation offered at home from CQ9

The population projection for visually impaired people who have received a home visit is 31,000; these divided 19 and 9 per cent of those registered aged 16 – 59 and 60 and over (population projections 6,000 and 13,000), and 3 and 2 per cent of the non-registered (population projections 1,500 and 10,500). Among the under-60s, the registered blind were twice as likely (25%, population projection 5,000) as the registered partially sighted (10%, population projection 1,000) to have received home instruction. Among those registered blind or partially sighted aged 60 or over the equivalent totals were 10 and 8 per cent (population projections 9,000 and 4,000).

19.6.2 Source of home instruction

We asked (CQ13) those who had home instruction (at CQ10 or 'yes' at CQ12) about who had provided it. The answers indicate that the main providers are 'social workers/welfare workers', 47%; 'social workers for the blind/home teachers', 39%; 'mobility officers', 5%. 'Technical officers' and 'local blind association' were mentioned by 2%, and other unidentified individuals mainly from the social and welfare services by 16%. 'Occupational therapist' and 'physiotherapist at the health centre' were other sources mentioned. For the reasons given in the discussion of false positives in section 19.2.2, these figures should be regarded with caution. In particular, at the time of our survey at least as many technical as mobility officers were working in SSDs. The low number of mentions of the former probably results from unfamiliarity with the job title; responses referring to this group of workers are likely to have been given as social worker for the blind.

The difference in the responses of blind and partially sighted people is worth noting. In general, blind respondents were more likely to mention having been visited by a 'social worker for the blind', while with partially sighted respondents an ordinary social worker was more likely to have been mentioned. Over half the blind people in all three age groups were instructed by a social worker for the blind. The figure for partially sighted people aged 16 – 59 was 35%, 10% for those aged 60 – 74, and under 1% for those aged 75 or over.

19.6.3   Timing

We asked: 'How old were you when this person first came?' (CQ14) The answers were analysed in relation to those at question YQ16, which asked how old the respondents were when they first realised that their sight problem was affecting their everyday lives (section 5.2.3). This enabled us to estimate the time interval between the onset of sight loss and the first practical instruction visit in the home. As Table 19.6 shows, the timing of home instruction, for those who receive it, is largely unrelated to the onset of sight loss. Only 12% received this instruction within one year of onset; 9% after 1 to 2 years, and 18% after 3 to 5 years. For 42% there was a gap of at least 10 years between onset and introduction.

Table 19.6   Time interval between onset of sight loss and any practical rehabilitation instruction in the home

	All who have had rehabilitation instruction at home %
Less than one year	12
1 to 2 years	9
3 to 5 years	18
6 to 9 years	9
10 to 15 years	18
16 – 20 years	9
20 or more years	15
Information missing	10
Total %	100
Base (population)	31K
(Number interviewed)	(71)

(71 respondents: 524 had no in-home rehabilitation)

Although these figures suggest that the delay between onset and practical instruction is very protracted, they may in some cases be misleading. At YQ16 we asked about the time of onset of sight loss, but for many people it might be several years before sight loss was severe enough to request a home instruction visit.

19.6.4 Practical advice and instruction given

We asked: 'What sort of practical advice and instructions did they (home instructor) give you?' (CQ15). Many different items were mentioned; 'provision of a white cane', 26%; 'mention or provision of a talking book', 20%; 'use of various aids and devices' (for writing, cooker markers, telephone dials, etc), 18%; 'help getting about the house', 15%; 'help in the kitchen/with cooking', 13%; 'help arranging things around the house', 12%; 'suggested or taught braille', 9%; 'talk on registration', 7%; 'provided tape recorders', 4%.

19.6.5 Demand for practical advice and instruction in the home

As noted in section 19.6.1, the great majority of respondents (population estimate 724,000 registrably visually impaired people) had not received a practical in-home instruction visit from their SSD. These respondents were asked if they would have liked such help. (CQ16) As Table 19.7 shows, only 19% overall said 'yes'. Those least likely to want a visit were younger registered and older non-registered people. Twenty and 28 per cent of the registered aged 16 – 59 and 60 or over wanted a visit; the corresponding figures for the non-registered were 32 and 16 per cent.

Table 19.7 Demand for practical home instruction

'If it were possible, would you like to have someone from the social services to come and give you advice and instructions about day-to-day problems?' (CQ16)

	Age and registration status				Total
	Registered		Non-registered		
	16 – 59	60 +	16 – 59	60 +	
	%	%	%	%	%
Yes	20	28	32	16	19
No	76	66	60	73	71
Don't know	4	6	9	10	9
No information	0	1	0	2	2
Total %	100	100	100	100	100
Base (population)	24K	126K	45K	529K	724K
(Number interviewed)	(168)	(119)	(83)	(154)	(524)

(524 respondents: 71 had received home instruction)

19.6.6 Reasons for not wanting practical home instruction

Those who had not had practical instruction in the home and said that they did not want any were asked why (CQ17). The responses are shown in Table 19.8.

Table 19.8 Reasons for not wanting a home visit from social services to give practical advice about dealing with sight problems, by registration status and age

'Why do you say that?' (CQ17)

	Age and registration status				Total
	Registered		Non-registered		
	16 – 59	60 +	16 – 59	60 +	
	%	%	%	%	%
Don't need help yet	8	12	15	30	26
Not necessary, can cope	33	12	25	27	24
Family or other people help	9	29	4	18	19
Like independence	35	26	19	11	14
They couldn't do anything	3	4	4	6	5
Too old	0	8	0	3	4
Something else causes problem	0	8	6	2	3
They don't know enough	9	1	0	0	1
Other	26	16	22	22	21
Base (population)	18K	83K	27K	385K	512K
(Number interviewed)	(119)	(85)	(50)	(112)	(366)

(366 respondents: 71 had home instruction; 111 'yes', 47 'no' or 'don't know' at CQ16)

Some 26% responded that they 'don't need help yet'; 24% that instruction was unnecessary as they could cope as they were; 19% that they had 'family or other people to help'; 14% (rising to 31% among the registered) said that they liked to be independent.

Though no age difference was found for those simply reporting that such help was not needed as they could cope, more older respondents gave the answer 'don't need help yet' (26 to 12 per cent) implying that in the future some help might be needed. The appeal to the family or other people to help was also greater among older respondents, 20 to 6 per cent.

These answers indicate that, although the question concerned the need for practical instruction in the home, respondents regarded it as an enquiry about whether they were capable of carrying on as they were or needed additional help. The answers are therefore largely defensive, asserting the respondents' independence and suggesting that visits from the social services would be an unwelcome intrusion into the home.

19.7 Current visiting by social and welfare services field workers

All respondents were asked: 'Does anyone from the social or welfare services visit you at home *nowadays* to give you special help with your sight problem?' (CQ18) Overall, only 4% replied 'yes' (population projection 28,000), of whom 16,000 were non-registered people aged 60 or over. At 17%, visits were significantly more frequent among the registered blind aged 16 – 59, although the relatively small size of this sub-group means that this percentage translates into a population projection of only 3,000 (of the 4,000 of that age who were being visited).

The few who were being visited were asked: 'Do you feel they (SSD field workers) understand the sort of help needed by someone with a sight problem?' (CQ19) Almost everyone (90%) answered 'yes'.

19.8 Advice on devices and gadgets to aid daily living

All respondents were asked: 'We talked earlier about various devices and gadgets which are available for people with sight difficulties. I mean things like special clocks, watches and timers, markers for the cooker and things like that. Have you ever seen anyone who has given you advice about these kinds of devices and gadgets for people with sight problems?' (CQ20)

Overall, 8% (population projection 59,000) answered 'yes'. Across the various sub-groups, however, the percentage fell steeply: registered aged 16 – 59, 40% (population projection 12,000); registered aged 60 or over, 19% (27,000); non-registered aged 16 – 59, 11% (5,000); and non-registered aged 60 or over, 3% (15,000).

We asked (at CQ21) who gave advice on aids and gadgets. SSD personnel were mentioned most often: 'social worker for the blind/home teacher', 29%, 'social worker/welfare worker', 27%; 'mobility officer', 2%; 'rehabilitation officer', 2%; 'technical officer', 1%; 'other', 16% (largely unidentified people from the social services but including occupational therapist, low vision clinic, blind teacher at the Manpower Services Centre and pension adviser). 'Home helps' were mentioned by 2%. Voluntary sector sources of advice mentioned were: 'local blind association', 8%; 'other local association', 1%. RNIB was mentioned by 4% (population projection 2,000 overall), though among the registered aged 16 – 59 the total was 12% (population projection 1,000). A residual 'others' category amounting to 9% contained a heterogeneous range of advisers: staff at commercial college, hospital staff, school teachers, relative, job centre, regional association and training course staff.

In summary, while SSDs are the central source for dissemination of information about aids and devices, additional peripheral sources collectively account for about a quarter of the information flow. These include voluntary organisations but are not restricted to them. One of these additional sources is RNIB; its impact is most marked among the registered aged 16 – 59.

19.9 Counselling services

19.9.1 Numbers receiving counselling

Counselling as a professional activity, distinct from psychotherapy on the one hand and informal supportive listening and discussion on the other, has a relatively recent origin. What counts as counselling is a matter of definition. Before asking specifically about counselling we thought it necessary to describe to respondents our definition of the concept in the following terms: 'Now I'd like to ask you about something a little different. People can be anxious and worried when they lose their sight, or if their sight gets worse. In some areas social workers and other helpers spend time listening and talking over people's worries and feelings about their loss of sight. It's called counselling. Have you had any special counselling like this to help you cope with worries about losing your sight?' (CQ22)

Less than one per cent of our sample (population projection 4,000) gave a straightforward 'yes' to this question, all of whom were registered. A further 2% said that they had talked over their worries and feelings with visiting social workers informally, but not to the extent that they could be said to have received special counselling.

The very few (13 respondents) who had received counselling were asked (CQ23) who counselled them and how old they were when this first happened (CQ24). Percentaging and population projections are not valid on the small number of respondents involved, and any inferences drawn from the distribution of the replies must be regarded as very tentative. This said, 7 of the 13 respondents were registered aged 16 – 59, with the remainder spread over the other registered sub-groups. Those named as giving the counselling were social workers for the blind (6 interviews), mobility officers (2), home helps (2), someone from RNIB (2), other social worker (1). Nine respondents said that they received the counselling before the age of 60, three at 60 – 74, and one at 75 +.

19.9.2 Unsatisfied demand for counselling

We asked those who had not been counselled, almost the entire sample, the following question: 'Given the opportunity, would you have liked, or would you still like to have, special counselling to help you cope with worries about losing your sight?' (CQ25) Twenty-three per cent said 'yes', of whom nearly half (10%) said that they would still like to have counselling. Of the remainder, one third (51% of the total) mentioned specifically in their reply that they did not have worries about losing their sight.

The data clearly show that there are very substantial numbers of people who feel that counselling would help or would have helped them to cope with their worries about losing their sight. The population projection is 171,000, of whom 77,000 say that they would still like such a service. This 77,000 divides 5,000 and 21,000 registered aged 16 – 59 and 60 or over, 10,000 and 41,000 non-registered in these same age bands. The extent of the demand can be seen when compared with the 4,000 who have received counselling.

These findings provide clear evidence of a major unsatisfied need for a counselling service for visually impaired adults. Hardly any have access to a service of this kind, even though very large numbers feel that they would benefit from it. It is hard to imagine that loss of vision can be anything but a major psychological trauma. A counselling service providing emotional support would have practical as well as therapeutic benefits, helping people to cope with the wide range of adjustments necessary.

19.10 Feelings about SSD help

19.10.1 Satisfaction ratings

We asked all respondents: 'How satisfied are you with the help you are getting *nowadays* to cope with your sight problem?' (CQ26) A quarter of respondents (population projection 181,000) were unwilling or felt unable to give a satisfaction rating in answer to the question. Of the remaining respondents (467 respondents, population estimate 576,000), four levels of satisfaction were prompted with results as follows: 'very satisfied', 16%; 'quite satisfied', 54%; 'a bit dissatisfied', 16%; 'very dissatisfied', 14%. There was little difference between sub-groups, except that marginally more registered people aged 16 – 59 said that they were 'very satisfied' (25%).

As noted in section 19.4.3, satisfaction ratings in surveys (note 5) usually have a positive skew, and it is uncommon to obtain so many ratings outside the 'satisfied' category. These ratings must therefore be taken to indicate considerable dissatisfaction with the services being received. The quarter who failed to give a satisfaction rating suggests yet further dissatisfaction, so much so that they were unwilling directly to express this dissatisfaction. These 'don't know' responses came largely from the non-registered aged 60 or over.

19.10.2   How much was done to help?

Although our initial question (CQ26) did not mention SSDs specifically, since they are the main helping agency the responses may be taken to reflect attitudes towards them. The next question (CQ27) directly concerned SSDs, asking respondents to consider the amount of help they had received; the results are shown in Table 19.9.

Overall, 67% said that 'nothing at all' had been done, and a further 12% said that they 'did not know'. If we equate the latter percentage, which was fairly consistent between sub-groups, with the 'nothing at all' response, we can say that on a conservative estimate between two-thirds and four-fifths of the registrably visually impaired population feel that SSDs have done nothing at all to help them to adjust to their sight problems. The remainder divided equally between those who said that 'everything possible' had been done to help them (11%) and those who thought that 'something but not enough' had been done (10%).

Table 19.9   Assistance given by SSDs

'So altogether, how much would you say that your local social or welfare services have done to help you adjust to your sight problems? Would you say they have done nothing at all, or have done something but not enough, or have done everything possible to help you to adjust to your loss of sight?' (CQ27)

	All registered by age and residual vision						Total
	16 – 59		60 +		All	All	
	B	PS	B	PS	R	NR*	
	%	%	%	%	%	%	%
Nothing at all	33	54	32	38	35	77	67
Something but not enough	23	20	29	18	25	6	10
Everything possible	33	17	25	31	27	6	11
Don't know	11	9	14	13	13	11	12
Total %	100	100	100	100	100	100	100
Base (population)	18K	12K	91K	49K	170K	587K	757K
(Number interviewed)	(123)	(92)	(74)	(63)	(352)	(243)	(595)

*The non-registered can be considered together as there were no significant differences between age or residual vision sub-groups

The main divide was between the registered and the non-registered. Among the non-registered the totals saying 'nothing at all', 'something but not enough', 'everything possible' and 'don't know' were 77, 6, 6 and 11 per cent. The corresponding totals for the registered were 35, 25, 27 and 13 per cent.

One sub-group, registered partially sighted people aged 16 – 59, stands out as significantly different from the other registered sub-groups, with corresponding totals of 54, 20, 17 and 9 per cent. In numerical terms they are relatively small (population projection 12,000), but evidently they felt less satisfied with the help they were getting than others who are registered, including elderly partially sighted people. (See section 19.14.2 for further discussion.)

19.10.3   What more should have been done?

All those who said (at CQ27) 'nothing' or 'something but not enough' were asked 'What more should have been done?' (CQ28) Overall, 28% (15% of the registered, 31% of the non-registered) said 'don't know', 22% (7% of the registered, 25% of the non-registered) said that they 'don't need help'; a further 3% said that they 'can cope/manage'. Table 19.10 shows the breakdown of the responses.

Table 19.10   Additional help would have liked from social services at about the time of onset by registration status

'What more should have been done?' (CQ28)

| | Registration status | | Total |
| | R | NR | |
	%	%	%
Don't need help	7	25	22
Should have been offered help	10	10	10
Other practical help	14	6	7
More information generally	16	4	6
They can't help	5	4	5
Financial help	3	4	4
Visits/more visits from social workers	17	1	4
Information about...			
– aids and gadgets	5	3	4
– optical aids and glasses	#	3	3
– Talking Books	2	1	2
– registration	#	#	#
Can cope/manage	4	3	3
Nothing offered when needed it	4	1	2
Someone from social services to talk to/more often	8	1	2
Home helps	1	1	1
Respite for carer	1	1	1
Other	16	7	9
Don't know	15	31	28
Base (population) = 100%	101K	475K	576K
(Number interviewed)	(222)	(203)	(425)

(425 respondents: 170 said 'everything possible' or 'don't know' at CQ27)

The main specific items that registered people mentioned more often than the non-registered are as follows. The overall percentage mentioned is given first, followed by the percentages of registered and non-registered in brackets. Some would have liked to have had 'more information generally', 6% (16%, 4%); 'visits/more visits from social workers', 4% (17%, 1%); 'someone from social services to talk to/more often', 2% (8%, 1%); 'other practical help', 7% (14%, 6%). 'Other practical help' included occupational advice, reader for mail, more time with home help, while the general 'other' category, 9% (16%, 7%), included medical/health problems other than sight, free bus pass, leisure suggestions, help at the right time/at the start, more rural transport, better medical diagnosis, help buying spectacles.

There were several categories of reply that did not reveal any marked difference between the registered and non-registered: 'financial help' was mentioned by 4%, 'home helps' by 1%. Ten per cent simply stated that they 'should have been offered help'. None of the remaining categories had more than 4% of the replies. However, all these concerned information of different kinds. Information on 'aids and gadgets', 'optical aids and glasses', 'talking books' and 'registration' collectively accounted for 9%. Together with the 6% who mentioned 'more information generally', this reveals a not-insignificant segment of respondents who felt ill-informed by their local SSD.

19.11 Home helps

Only 1% of the respondents said (at CQ29) that they had not heard of home helps. Provision of a home help (CQ30) showed a straightforward relationship with age, and was unrelated to registration status or residual vision. In the age groups 16 – 59, 60 – 74 and 75 + the totals with home help were 11, 18 and 40 per cent respectively. Those who did not have a home help were asked (at CQ31) if they would like one. Ten per cent said that they would, a total that did not vary with either age or registration status.

19.12 Meals on wheels

Virtually all (99%) respondents said (at CQ32) that they had heard of meals on wheels, but only 12% said that they were receiving them. This service was solely related to age. In the age groups 16 – 59, 60 – 74 and 75 + the totals receiving meals on wheels were 1, 4 and 16 per cent respectively. Further demand for meals on wheels was minimal. Less than 3% of those not receiving meals on wheels said (at CQ34) that they would like to do so. There were no significant differences between sub-groups.

19.13 Overall visiting by SSDs

We asked all respondents: 'Thinking about all the reasons that the social or welfare services might visit, including meals on wheels and home helps, about how often would you say that someone from the social or welfare services visits you?' (CQ35)

The most striking feature of the answers, shown in Tables 19.10.a. and 19.10.b., is that a majority (53%) of visually impaired people say that someone from the social or welfare services never visits them. This total breaks down to 68, 59 and 50 per cent of those aged 16 – 59, 60 – 74 and 75 +. Fifty-nine per cent of the non-registered compared with 32% of the registered say this. With respect to both age and registration status, the totals who say that they are not visited are 59 and 26 per cent of the registered aged 16 – 59 and 60 or over and 71 and 58 per cent of the non-registered. Thus in only one sub-group, the registered aged 60 or over, is a majority (74%) visited by someone from the social or welfare services. There were no significant differences between registered blind and partially sighted people.

Table 19.10.a. Frequency of visits from the social services by age group

'Thinking about all the reasons that the social or welfare services might visit, including meals on wheels and home helps, about how often would you say that someone from the social or welfare services visits you?' (CQ35)

	Age			Total
	16 – 59	60 – 74	75 +	
	%	%	%	%
Never visited	68	59	50	53
Visited:				
Once or more a week	6	17	33	27
At least once a year	13	10	9	9
Less than once a year	13	14	8	11
All visited	32	41	50	47
Total %	100	100	100	100
Base (population)	77K	179K	501K	757K
(Number interviewed)	(299)	(124)	(172)	(595)

Table 19.10.b. Frequency of visits from the social services, by registration status and age (CQ35)

	Age and registration status				Total
	Registered		Non-registered		
	16 – 59	60 +	16 – 59	60 +	
	%	%	%	%	%
Never visited	59	26	71	58	53
Visited:					
Once or more a week	6	33	6	29	27
At least once a year	17	20	10	3	9
Less than once a year	18	21	13	10	11
All visited	41	74	29	42	47
Total %	100	100	100	100	100
Base (population)	30K	140K	49K	540K	757K
(Number interviewed)	(215)	(137)	(84)	(159)	(595)

These figures can also be examined in terms of the case-load profile for SSDs, that is in terms of the type and number of visually impaired people visited. Thus a total of 356,000 visually impaired people have been visited, of whom 330,000 are aged 60 or over; these latter divide 103,000 and 227,000 between the registered and non-registered. Among those aged 16 – 59, 26,000 have been visited, dividing 12,000 and 14,000 between the registered and non-registered. Doubling the number of visits to younger visually impaired people would not significantly increase the number of people visited. As noted (Table 19.10.b.), a large proportion (74%) of the registered aged 60 or over are already visited, while any attempt to increase visits to the non-registered aged 60 or over would be a vast task because of their large numbers (population projection 540,000).

The overall figures for frequency of visits were 27, 9 and 11 per cent for visits once or more a week, at least once a year, and less than once a year. These figures varied little with registration status. Age was the predominant factor governing visits at least weekly, the figures for the three age bands being 6, 17 and 33 per cent. Thus, our respondents were either visited relatively intensively, once or more a week, or else rarely. For example, among the 9% visited at least once a year, visits occurred once to three times a year rather than once a month. While more frequent visiting related, as already noted, only to age and not to registration status, less frequent visiting shows a greater relation to registration as well. Thus of the total of 20% visited less than once a week (for the most part much less often), the figures among the registered aged 16 – 59 and 60 or over were 35 and 41 per cent compared with 23 and 13 per cent of the non-registered in the same age groups.

The wording of our question was designed to encompass all kinds of visits from the social and welfare services to visually impaired people, not merely visits specifically connected with sight problems. Although, as noted, weekly or more frequent visits are in the main unrelated to registration, a very small proportion (4%) of visually impaired people are frequently visited to be given special help with their sight problem. We asked about such specialised visits at CQ18: 'Does anyone from the social or welfare services visit you at home *nowadays* to give you special help with your sight problem?' This 4% (reaching 11% of the registered under-60s) was strongly related to registration status. Generalising, although some 27% of visually impaired people receive weekly or more frequent visits from their SSD, most of these visits (23%) are related to the status of the client as an old person rather than because they are visually impaired.

19.14 Overview of SSD provision

This section brings together the data on service provision from sections 19.5 to 19.9 and 19.11 to 19.13 in order to examine the main patterns running through service provision across all the sub-groups. The material can be analysed from two distinct viewpoints: first, the total volume of provision of any service and its distribution across sub-groups; second, the extent to which the needs of particular sub-groups are met. Accordingly, the same data are presented showing, first, population projections for the number in each sub-group receiving the service and, second, this number as a percentage of the sub-group.

19.14.1   Registered and non-registered

Table 19.11.a. shows the total of the registered and the non-registered aged 16 – 59 and 60 or over receiving each service. Table 19.11.b. shows the same data as a percentage of the total in the sub-group.

In relative terms, as Table 19.11.b. reveals, the registered are about twice as aware as the non-registered (64 and 33 per cent) that SSDs can provide specialised help for visually impaired people. This corresponds with our finding that in relative terms the registered are much more likely to be recipients of specialised services. The registered aged 16 – 59 uniformly receive relatively more of each service. (The reason for the apparent exception, the initial onset visit (CQ5), is that because these data are percentaged on the total sample not just on those eligible, i.e. those who lost their sight as adults, there is no age group difference among the registered – see section 19.4.) Registration status is only irrelevant for non-specialised services to older people, such as meals on wheels and home helps.

Table 19.11.a.   Numbers in receipt of social and welfare services by registration status and age

		Age and registration status				Total
		Registered		Non-registered		
		16 – 59	60 +	16 – 59	60 +	
		(000)	(000)	(000)	(000)	(000)
CQ2	Aware SSD can help	21	88	18	172	299
CQ5	Received onset visit	7	60	1	42	109
CQ9	Offered rehabilitation	11	15	1	3	30
CQ12	Had home instruction	6	13	1	10	31
CQ18	Currently visited	3	9	1	16	28
CQ20	Advised on aids	12	27	5	15	59
CQ22	Counselling	1	3	0	0	4
CQ30	Has home help	2	44	5	183	236
CQ33	Has meals on wheels	1	18	0	69	88
CQ35	Visited by SSD	12	103	14	227	356
Base (population)		30K	140K	47K	540K	757K
(Number interviewed)		(215)	(137)	(84)	(159)	(595)

Table 19.11.b. Proportions in receipt of social and welfare services by registration status and age

		Age and registration status				Total
		Registered		Non-registered		
		16 – 59	60 +	16 – 59	60 +	
		%	%	%	%	%
CQ2	Aware SSD can help	69	63	38	33	39
CQ5	Received onset visit	23	43	2	8	14
CQ9	Offered rehabilitation	35	11	2	1	4
CQ12	Had home instruction	20	9	2	2	4
CQ18	Currently visited	10	6	2	3	4
CQ20	Advised on aids	40	19	11	3	8
CQ22	Counselling	3	2	0	0	#
CQ30	Has home help	7	31	11	34	31
CQ33	Has meals on wheels	3	13	0	13	12
CQ35	Visited by SSD	41	74	29	42	47
Base (population) = 100%		30K	140K	47K	540K	757K
(Number interviewed)		(215)	(137)	(84)	(159)	(595)

However, the concentration of specialised services among the registered is relative. From the point of view of SSDs, the non-registered aged 60 or over always form a substantial portion of the total numbers of clients receiving services. This is a result of the very large size of this group, even though the percentage of the group whose needs are met by the specialised services remains small. (The only exceptions are formal rehabilitation courses, which are very rarely offered to the non-registered, and the almost non-existing counselling services.) This applies both to those currently receiving specialised services and to those who have received them in the past. Once we move away from specialised services, the workload of SSDs among registrably visually impaired people is overwhelmingly concerned with visits to elderly people. Among elderly people, about three times as many non-registered as registered visually impaired people are visited once or more a week. Overall, SSD services are primarily directed at elderly people rather than at visually impaired people as such (section 19.13).

19.14.2 Registered blind and registered partially sighted recipients

Tables 19.12.a. and 19.12.b. repeat the information in Tables 19.11.a. and 19.11.b. but only show the data for registered blind or partially sighted respondents in the two age groups. One substantial difference is the higher proportion of registered blind people aged 16 – 59 who receive specialised services compared with registered partially sighted people of the same age. The differences among those aged 60 or over are marginal in each case i.e. they are not large enough to reach statistical significance.

Table 19.12.a. Numbers in receipt of social and welfare services by age and registration status

		Registered B or PS people in two age groups				Total
		16 – 59		60 +		
		B	PS	B	PS	
		(000)	(000)	(000)	(000)	(000)
CQ2	Aware SSD can help	14	7	59	29	109
CQ5	Received onset visit	5	2	43	18	68
CQ9	Offered rehabilitation	10	3	11	5	28
CQ12	Had home instruction	4	1	9	4	19
CQ18	Currently visited	3	1	5	2	11
CQ20	Advised on aids	9	2	20	8	39
CQ22	Counselling	1	0	1	1	3
CQ30	Has home help	2	1	25	20	48
CQ33	Has meals on wheels	1	0	12	5	18
CQ35	Visited by SSD	7	4	64	34	110
Base (population)		18K	12K	91K	49K	170K
(Number interviewed)		(123)	(92)	(74)	(63)	(352)

(352 respondents: 243 non-registered)

Table 19.12.b. Proportions in receipt of social and welfare services by age and registration status

		Registered B or PS people in two age groups				Total
		16 – 59		60 +		
		B	PS	B	PS	
		%	%	%	%	%
CQ2	Aware SSD can help	78	58	65	59	64
CQ5	Received onset visit	28	17	47	35	39
CQ9	Offered rehabilitation	56	17	12	10	16
CQ12	Had home instruction	24	8	10	8	11
CQ18	Currently visited	17	8	6	4	7
CQ20	Advised on aids	50	17	22	16	23
CQ22	Counselling	6	0	1	2	2
CQ30	Has home help	9	6	28	41	28
CQ33	Has meals on wheels	4	2	13	12	11
CQ35	Visited by SSD	33	41	71	69	65
Base (population) = 100%		18K	12K	91K	49K	170K
(Number interviewed)		(123)	(92)	(74)	(63)	(352)

(352 respondents: 243 non-registered)

Notes to Chapter 19

Note 1

Section 29 of the National Assistance Act, 1948, as amended by the Local Government Act, 1972, empowers a local authority to make arrangements for the welfare of substantially permanently handicapped people, including blind and partially sighted people. Some services are mandatory, such as the keeping of registers of persons to whom section 29 applies, the provision of a social work service, and advice and support facilities for social rehabilitation and adjustment to disability including assistance in overcoming limitations of mobility or communication. A much wider range of services is permissive: the local authority has a duty to provide them, but only if it is satisfied that there is a real need for such help.

The Social Services Inspectorate (SSI) (DHSS, 1988) study found huge variations in both the organisational arrangements and the standards of provision between the eight authorities inspected and between areas within authorities. 'In none of the authorities was there an observable relationship between the number of people needing help (as evidenced by the registers) and the deployment and training of staff.' Shore (1985) noted similarly that in 20 local authorities in England and Wales client:specialist ratios (the ratio of the numbers of specialist workers for visually impaired people to the numbers registered as blind or partially sighted) varied from 1:310 to 1:1,320. Both Shore's and the SSI study show that visually impaired people have so low a place on the priority of some local authorities that even mandatory duties are carried out to a minimal level and ineffectively.

Note 2

For an example of how prompts from a check list of items can inflate the apparent knowledge level of respondents see section 20.5.

Note 3

A DHSS inspection of eight authorities (DHSS, 1988) found that the main focus of work and the management of services specifically required by visually impaired people centred on the procedures incurred in registration following receipt of the certification of blindness or partial sight on form BD8. Ideally, having been examined by a consultant ophthalmologist and found eligible for registration, a visually impaired person should receive a visit from a field worker, who explains the significance of registration. He or she also provides details of benefits and services available, and, where needed, makes provision for social and emotional rehabilitation and adjustment to disability including assistance in overcoming limitations of mobility or communication.

The 1985 RNIB study conducted into local authority rehabilitation services for those on the blind register established just how far practice falls short of this ideal (Shore, 1985). Many authorities consider visually impaired people as clients only during the initial rehabilitation work and then cease to make contact. Furthermore, delays of months and even years can occur between registration examination and contact with the visually impaired person. In some places the SSD simply sent a letter confirming registration and giving a telephone number to use if any further information should be required. Shore found that for the majority of registered blind people the services provided amounted to little more than the supply of aids, such as a white cane, large-print telephone dial, tactile cooker markers and talking books.

Note 4

By 'overarching questions' is meant questions such as CQ2, 3, 9, 12, 16, 18, 20.

Note 5

Studies of how people use satisfaction ratings show that there is usually a marked bias towards positive satisfaction, with dissatisfaction rarely expressed, regardless of the precise question format and over a wide range of topic areas. For example, a major study of the *Quality of American life* obtained satisfaction ratings on seven-point scales ranging from 'completely satisfied' (7 points) to 'completely dissatisfied' (1 point) for fifteen life domains (housing, job, health, etc). For most domains 75% of respondents gave ratings of 6 or 7 and fewer than 10% ratings in the 1 – 3 range (Campbell and Converse, 1976, page 63). Another extensive American study used a seven-point delighted-terrible scale (points 7, 6, and 5 were labelled 'delighted', 'pleased' and 'mostly satisfied'; points 3, 2, 1 'mostly dissatisfied', 'unhappy', 'terrible') for an even larger number of life domains, including satisfaction with local government services. In almost all domains ratings fell predominantly into the top three categories, and only rarely were as many as 10% in the categories 1, 2, 3 or 4; one example was taxes paid (Andrews and Withey, 1976, Chapter 8). Among British studies, Abrams (1978) obtained ratings of satisfaction on an 11-point scale, 0 representing complete dissatisfaction and 10 complete satisfaction, for twelve life domains. The welfare services included received lower levels of rating than any other domain except 'financial situation', but even so 32% of responses were in the 8 – 10 range, only 4% in 0 – 1, and 16% in 0 – 3 ranges.

It has generally been found that older people express high satisfaction, and even people in disadvantaged circumstances do not necessarily express dissatisfaction. (One theory is that this results from lowered expectations, satisfaction being the gap between what one has and what one expects or feels entitled to.) Using a four-point scale very like ours, Abrams found that 67% of people aged 75 or more rated themselves as 'completely satisfied' with local organised social facilities, 10% 'fairly satisfied', and only 4 and 2 per cent respectively 'fairly and very dissatisfied, (17% could not say). Another British study of the *Quality of life of the elderly in residential care* found that over 80% of respondents rated themselves as 'very satisfied' or 'quite satisfied' with general facilities in their residential home; less than 5% said that they were 'very dissatisfied' (Peace, Hall and Hamblin, 1979, page 136).

20 Voluntary Organisations Involved with Visually Impaired People

20.1 Unprompted awareness

We asked all respondents the following unprompted question: 'Can you tell me which organisations you know of which help blind people and people with a sight problem?' (CQ45) As Table 20.1 shows, the Royal National Institute for the Blind (RNIB) was the most frequently mentioned, by 22% of respondents overall. Next most often mentioned were St Dunstan's, 9%; Guide Dogs for the Blind Association, 7%; local society for the blind, 6%; National Federation of the Blind, 2%; and the Partially Sighted Society, 2%. Thereafter a string of organisations was mentioned, but none by more than 0.5%: Torch Club, Sunshine Homes, Haigh fund/war blind, diabetic associations and the Citizens Advice Bureau.

The fact that RNIB was mentioned at the beginning of the interview may have inflated its unprompted awareness level of 22%. Even on a

Table 20.1 Spontaneous awareness of national organisations for visually impaired people, by registration status and age

'Can you tell me which organisations you know of which help blind people and people with a sight problem?' (CQ45)

	Age and registration status				Total
	Registered		Non-registered		
	16 – 59	60 +	16 – 59	60 +	
	%	%	%	%	%
RNIB	58	37	38	15	22
St Dunstan's	5	7	8	10	9
Guide Dogs Association	12	7	6	7	7
Local society for the blind	21	10	2	5	6
National Federation of the Blind	7	3	3	1	2
Partially Sighted Society	9	#	#	2	2
Social worker for the blind	8	1	2	0	1
None mentioned	14	38	35	55	49
Base (population) = 100%	29K	140K	48K	540K	757K
(Number interviewed)	(215)	(137)	(84)	(159)	(595)

conservative interpretation, however, its total is so far ahead of those of the other organisations mentioned as to indicate a considerable edge in awareness level (note 1).

Nearly half the respondents (49%) were unable to name any organisation spontaneously. In general the registered and the younger age groups tended to be more knowledgeable. Thus, of the registered, 14% of the under-60s but 38% of those aged 60 or over failed to mention any organisation; among the non-registered the corresponding figures were 35 and 55 per cent. The same awareness trends were found for most of the individual organisations mentioned (St Dunstan's being the exception). Mentions of RNIB reached 58% among the registered aged 16 – 59 and 37% among those aged 60 or over; the equivalent figures among the non-registered were 38 and 15 per cent. Taking these four sub-groups in the same order, the figures for local societies for the blind were 21, 10, 2 and 5 per cent; for National Federation of the Blind, 7, 3, 3 and 1 per cent; for the Partially Sighted Society 9, #, # and 2 per cent (# = less than 0.5%); Guide Dogs Association, 12, 7, 6 and 7 per cent; and St Dunstan's, 5, 7, 8 and 10 per cent. Partially sighted respondents did not show a greater awareness of the Partially Sighted Society than blind respondents.

20.2   The Royal National Institute for the Blind

20.2.1   Understanding of the initials RNIB

Those who said, either spontaneously at CQ45 or after prompting at CQ46 (population projection 404,000 people), that they had heard of RNIB were asked: 'Can you tell me what the letters "RNIB" stand for?' (CQ48) Just over half named all the words correctly; this is the equivalent of 192,000 people, 25% of the visually impaired population. This figure is consistent with the unprompted awareness result, 22%. Among those aged under 60, both registered and non-registered, the total stating all the words correctly was just over 80%. Among those aged 60 or over, the corresponding figures for the registered and non-registered were 65 and 42 per cent respectively.

The total naming all the words correctly declined with age: 82, 66 and 40 per cent among the three age bands 16 – 59, 60 – 74 and 75 and over.

Only about 15% of those asked did not name at least one word correctly. However, this is a poor test of prior knowledge, since the words 'blind' and 'institute' can easily be guessed.

20.2.2   People RNIB is thought to serve

All those who said, either spontaneously at CQ45 or after prompting at either CQ46 or CQ47 (554,000 people), that they had heard of RNIB were asked: 'I'd like to ask who you think RNIB aims to help. Do you think they aim to help...?' (CQ49)

The following items were then read out from a check list; the total replying 'yes' appears in brackets. 'People who are blind' (93%); 'people who are partially sighted' (77%); 'anyone who can't see well enough to read' (62%); 'anyone who is worried about their eyesight' (60%). These items showed little difference by registration status or residual vision.

Although these results are an accurate reflection of the people RNIB helps, they are nevertheless surprising. It has generally been assumed that, because the word 'blind' appears in RNIB's name, the majority of partially sighted people and people with better vision levels would believe that the organisation was unlikely to be able to help them. Our data suggest that partially sighted as well as blind people do believe that RNIB provides services to help them.

20.2.3   Services RNIB is thought to provide

20.2.3.1   Unprompted replies

Respondents (population projection 554,000 – all those who had heard of RNIB) were then asked (at CQ50 unprompted) about the services they thought RNIB provided. As shown in Table 20.2, over half the respondents (52%) failed to mention any. The highest failure (60%) was among the non-registered aged 60 or over, the lowest among the registered under-60s (21%). Even among the registered aged 60 or over, 41% failed to mention any services.

Most RNIB services were mentioned by the non-registered, but by only a small proportion. Guide dogs, a service that RNIB does not provide, were most often mentioned by the non-registered (12%, 6% by the registered). Other items that got some mention (between 4 and 8 per cent) among the non-registered were: Talking Books, braille, holidays and hotels, aids and gadgets, and white sticks.

To some extent, spontaneous mentions of services RNIB was believed to provide reflected usage of those services (section 15.6).

Registered respondents were more knowledgeable, particularly those aged under 60. The item they mentioned most frequently was aids and gadgets (39%), followed by Talking Books and braille (24% each),

Table 20.2 Spontaneous listing of RNIB services by registration status and age

'What sort of things do you know that RNIB does?' (CQ50)

	Age and registration status				Total
	Registered		Non-registered		
	16 – 59	60 +	16 – 59	60 +	
	%	%	%	%	%
Talking Books	24	19	7	8	11
Holidays and hotels for visually impaired people	20	15	8	8	10
Aids and gadgets	39	16	11	3	8
White sticks	8	5	4	7	6
Braille	24	7	8	5	6
Schools	22	6	3	3	4
Training courses	6	2	6	2	2
Talking newspapers/ magazines*	2	2	0	1	1
Rehabilitation centre	12	1	3	0	1
Employment information and training	11	1	6	#	1
Books in Moon	5	0	0	0	#
Guide dogs for the blind*	7	5	15	12	11
None above mentioned	21	41	39	60	52
Base (population) = 100%	27K	112K	36K	379K	554K
(Number interviewed)	(189)	(109)	(64)	(109)	(471)

(471 respondents: 124 not aware of RNIB)
*Not an RNIB service

schools (22%) and holidays and hotels (20%). At 12% each, rehabilitation and employment information and training also scored relatively well.

Among the registered aged 60 and over, the most frequently mentioned items were Talking Books (19%), aids and gadgets (16%) and holidays and hotels (15%).

About 6% in every sub-group mentioned the provision of white sticks.

The most striking finding is that being registered dramatically increases the chances of a visually impaired person knowing about an RNIB service. This is an important factor for RNIB as it seeks to improve the promotion of its products and services. However, of all the people who had heard of RNIB, half were unable to name a single service that the organisation provides. Even among the registered (i.e. those most likely to be knowledgeable) this was the case among a fifth of those aged 16 – 59 (21%) and two-fifths aged 60 or over (41%).

It is possible to identify individual services that might need more promotion among particular age groups. For example, it is encouraging to know that the under-60s were the most aware of services such as rehabilitation centres and employment information, the groups these services are chiefly aimed at, but overall levels of awareness are low. Items such as aids and gadgets could be most beneficial to older people, among whom knowledge was lamentably low. These findings indicate that RNIB faces a major communications challenge, requiring increased and focused promotion to bring beneficial results.

20.2.3.2 Prompted replies

The same respondents were then asked: 'I am going to read out various services provided for people with eyesight difficulties – some are provided by RNIB, some are not. Can you tell me for each one whether you think RNIB provides it. So, firstly, does it provide...?' (CQ51)

As Table 20.3 shows, the check-list contained eleven items, each of which was read out. Overall, the most acknowledged items were guide dogs (69%), articles and aids (67%), braille books (63%), training

Table 20.3 Prompted awareness of RNIB services by registration status and age

'I am going to read out various services provided for people with eyesight difficulties – some are provided by RNIB and some are not. Can you tell me for each one whether you think RNIB provides it...?' (CQ51)

	Age and registration status				Total
	Registered		Non-registered		
	16 – 59	60 +	16 – 59	60 +	
	%	%	%	%	%
Articles and aids	88	71	78	63	67
Braille books	91	65	85	62	63
Training courses	76	53	71	60	60
Talking Books	86	62	63	54	58
Schools	75	42	73	59	57
Rehabilitation centres	79	51	63	50	53
Holidays	59	43	34	55	52
Information and help with jobs	58	28	49	58	51
Talking newspapers*	37	42	49	41	41
Books in Moon	50	24	28	25	26
Guide dogs*	57	51	84	73	69
None above mentioned	#	11	8	15	13
Base (population) = 100%	27K	112K	36K	379K	554K
(Number interviewed)	(189)	(109)	(64)	(109)	(471)

(471 respondents: 124 not aware of RNIB)
*Not an RNIB service

courses (60%), schools (57%), holidays (52%), and information and help with jobs (51%). Even though the items were prompted one at a time, 13% of respondents were not prepared even to guess whether any of the eleven was a service provided by RNIB.

Because of 'false positives' (section 19.2.2), these prompted awareness levels almost certainly over-estimate true knowledge of RNIB services. Nevertheless, the figures do show encouraging levels of awareness of many RNIB services, while still leaving a huge gap for improvement. For instance, 42% of blind and partially sighted people do not realise that RNIB provides Talking Books.

20.3 Users of RNIB services

For each item a respondent said (at CQ51) that they thought was an RNIB service, they were asked (at CQ52) whether they had actually used that service, as shown in Table 20.4. Overall, only 18% of those who knew about RNIB said that they had made any use of its services. As a population projection, this is equivalent to just under 100,000 people, that is 13% of the estimated 757,000 visually impaired people living in private households. While serving 100,000 people represents a considerable achievement, the fact that only 13% of the target group is reached demonstrates a huge level of unawareness of the services RNIB provides for blind and partially sighted people.

At 13%, Talking Books were the most frequently mentioned overall (note 2), followed by articles and aids (6%), braille books (3%), talking newspapers (2%), rehabilitation centres (2%), and holidays, schools, training courses and information and help with jobs (1% each). However, to understand the distribution of RNIB services it is necessary to examine the specific sections of the visually impaired population that it currently serves or fails to serve.

20.3.1 Age and registration status

The registered, notably those aged 16 – 59, are the most extensive users of RNIB services. As Table 20.4 shows, 72% of the younger registered had used them, compared with 47% of those aged 60 or over and with only 14 and 5 per cent respectively of the non-registered.

The registered under-60s made fairly widespread use of the RNIB services listed. Articles and aids (46%) and Talking Books (42%) were the most widely used, followed by braille books (24%), rehabilitation centres (22%), information and help with jobs (16%), training courses (15%), schools (11%) and holidays (10%). Among the registered aged 60 or over, Talking Books (38%), articles and aids (15%) and braille books (8%) were the only items gaining significant mentions.

Table 20.4 Use of RNIB services, by registration status and age

'Can I just check have you actually used ... provided by RNIB?' (CQ52)

	Age and registration status				Total
	Registered		Non-registered		
	16 – 59	60 +	16 – 59	60 +	
	%	%	%	%	%
Talking Books	42	38	8	5	13
Articles and aids	46	15	6	0	6
Braille books	24	8	6	0	3
Rehabilitation centres	22	2	3	0	2
Talking newspapers*	4	6	1	1	2
Books in Moon	4	0	4	0	1
Holidays	10	4	0	0	1
Schools	11	1	3	0	1
Training courses	15	1	3	0	1
Information and help with jobs	16	1	2	0	1
Guide dogs*	4	0	0	0	#
Used one or more service	72	47	14	5	18
Not used any RNIB service	28	53	86	95	82
Base (population) = 100%	27K	112K	36K	379K	554K
(Number interviewed)	(189)	(109)	(64)	(109)	(471)

(471 respondents: 124 not aware of RNIB)
*Not an RNIB service

When prompting respondents about their awareness of RNIB services (Table 20.3 – CQ51), we deliberately included talking newspapers and guide dogs (not in fact provided by RNIB) as a check on true understanding.

Only 6% of the non-registered reported using any RNIB services. Among those aged 60 or over, use was limited to Talking Books (5%). Although the under-60s used a wider range of services, none was used very extensively, the highest being Talking Books. Articles and aids and braille books were mentioned by 6%, the remaining items receiving fewer mentions.

20.3.2   Residual vision

Table 20.5 analyses the use of RNIB services according to the residual vision level of users. Although the services are more widely used by people at blind registrable level, age produces a greater differentiation than residual vision level. Thus, 63% of blind people under 60 but only 22% of those aged 60 or over use RNIB services, compared with 24 and 10 per cent respectively of partially sighted people.

Table 20.5   Usage of RNIB services, by age and residual vision

'Can I just check have you actually used ... provided by the RNIB?' (CQ52)

	Age and residual vision				Total
	16 – 59		60 +		
	B	PS	B	PS	
	%	%	%	%	%
Talking Books	41	11	18	8	13
Articles and aids	42	11	6	3	6
Braille books	24	6	4	0	3
Rehabilitation centres	19	6	1	#	2
Talking newspapers*	3	2	3	1	2
Books in Moon	4	4	0	0	1
Holidays	11	0	2	#	1
Schools	10	4	1	0	1
Training courses	13	5	#	#	1
Information and help with jobs	15	4	1	0	1
Guide dogs*	4	0	0	0	#
Used one or more service	63	24	22	10	18
Not used any RNIB service	37	76	78	90	82
Base (population) = 100%	25K	38K	206K	285K	554K
(Number interviewed)	(125)	(128)	(103)	(115)	(471)

(471 respondents: 124 not aware of RNIB)

*Not an RNIB service

Take-up of RNIB services is higher among registrably blind than among registrably partially sighted people. This seems to contradict the general appreciation among visually impaired people of RNIB's role as reported above. However, a majority of registrably blind people aged 16 – 59 are registered as such, whereas the vast majority of people in the four other sub-groups are non-registered (section 3.1). The concentration in the use of RNIB services among younger people at blind registrable levels therefore reflects their registration status. Registration rather than sight level is the predominant factor determining the use of RNIB services.

20.3.3   User profiles and resource allocation

The data in Chapter 19 on the provision of specialised services by SSDs showed a similar concentration of take-up among the registered. The point made there (section 19.14) and indeed at many points in this survey is that this concentration is relative. In terms of the absolute numbers of users, the age skew in the visually impaired population is a powerful determining factor. For example, as Table 20.4 shows, 46% of the registered aged 16 – 59 use articles and aids compared with 15% of those aged 60 or over. However, the population projection for the under-60s is 12,000, while for those aged 60 or over it is almost 17,000.

As noted in section 19.14, even quite small percentages of elderly non-registered respondents represent very large numbers of users of SSD services. This results from the very large size of the non-registered (but registrable) elderly group. When examining RNIB services, we encountered the same phenomenon with respect to the age distribution of Talking Book users (section 8.3.1.1). However, the non-registered aged 60 or over have little impact on the age distribution of other RNIB services since, on the evidence in Table 20.4, this segment of the visually impaired population, massive though it is, makes very little use of RNIB services.

20.3.4   Sources of information about RNIB services

Those who mentioned (at CQ52) that they had used any RNIB service were asked: 'How did you come to hear about the services that RNIB provides?' (CQ53) As Table 20.6 shows, a wide variety of sources was named. A social or welfare worker (18%) was most often mentioned, with social worker for the blind scoring a further 6%. Another visually impaired person (10%) was the second most frequently mentioned source, while 8% each mentioned a sighted person and an RNIB

Table 20.6   Sources of information about RNIB services

'How did you come to hear about the services that RNIB provides?' (CQ53)

	Users of RNIB services
	%
Social/welfare worker	18
Another visually impaired person	10
Sighted person	8
RNIB Talking Book	8
Always known them	6
Social worker for the blind	6
Media, excluding *In Touch*	6
In Touch (radio programme)	5
Optician	4
Fundraiser	4
Doctor	2
Mobility officer	1
Rehabilitation officer	1
Other sources	30
Don't know	9
Base (population) = 100%	98K
(Number interviewed)	(209)

(209 respondents: only those using RNIB services were asked)

Talking Book. Other sources of information included the *In Touch* programme, opticians, fundraisers and doctors.

These findings help to explain why RNIB is more likely to be in contact with registered visually impaired people than with the non-registered. Approximately a quarter of visually impaired people (24%) heard about RNIB services from social services workers, and Chapter 19 showed that social workers are most likely to be in touch with the registered. Nevertheless, even though it is relatively high already, penetration of RNIB services among the registered still has growth potential. This emphasises the importance of social services workers as an essential link in the communication chain between RNIB and visually impaired people.

The media (11% including *In Touch*) provide an important opportunity for reaching the non-registered, as could perhaps opticians as well.

20.3.5 Initial expectations of RNIB contact

Following the enquiry (at CQ53) about how they came to hear about RNIB services, the same respondents (omitting those who experienced early onset of their sight problems) were asked: 'Did you expect RNIB to contact you to offer you help and advice?' (CQ54) Only 2% said that they had expected such contact. Almost all of these were registered, of whom 8% had this expectation.

20.4 Provision of names on the Social Services Register to RNIB

All respondents who said that they had heard of RNIB were asked: 'The registers for blind and partially sighted people are kept in confidence by the social services. Do you think the social services should give RNIB the names of people on the register?' (CQ55) Seventy-four per cent said 'yes', only 7% 'no', while the rest did not express any opinion. There was little difference among sub-groups.

We might expect the practice of referral to RNIB to increase in the future, given the permissions section of the BD8 form. However, although this represents an important step forward, it will not solve the major challenge for RNIB and other service-giving agencies to reach non-registered blind and partially sighted people.

Notes to Chapter 20

Note 1

In designing the survey, we debated whether to avoid mentioning RNIB beforehand in order to provide an unbiased measure of salience at this point in the interview. It was felt, however, that we could not be other than completely open from the start about the purpose of the survey. Therefore, in introducing it and themselves our interviewers were instructed to say that they were working on behalf of RNIB. However, this mention was made only at the beginning of the interview and was distanced by a mass of complicated and thought-provoking questions that would be fairly effective in burying most, even if not all, of the initial prompt. This interpretation is supported by independent surveys. Unprompted awareness of RNIB among the general population has oscillated in the three years 1987 to 1989 between 9 and 13 per cent, 10% being the most stable figure. However, these statistics relate to the general population, while our survey was of blind and partially sighted people. Thus an unprompted awareness level of 22% (CQ45) does not seem to be incredible, although it may be on the high side.

The results for prompted awareness (CQ46) are not reported as they were considered in retrospect not to be a fair measure of awareness of RNIB against other organisations. This was because in the prompts RNIB was mentioned only by its initials, whereas other organisations were mentioned by their full names.

Note 2

The 13% figure here corresponds to a population estimate of 74,000, which falls short of the estimated 90,000 in section 8.2.2 (Table 8.2). The reasons for this are uncertain. The discrepancy involves very few respondents, but they could carry different weights. One hypothesis, which could be checked on secondary analysis, is that a handful of respondents using Talking Books are unaware of the link with RNIB. The earlier enquiry into Talking Books (reported in Chapter 8) made no mention of RNIB, and only those who had knowledge of RNIB have been filtered into the questions reported in this section.

Part F

Method

21 Methodological Appendix

21.1 Borderline between registrable blind and partially sighted

The cut-off point used to categorise non-registered blind people covers the legal <3/60 (i.e. worse than 3/60) Snellen level and the next level <6/60 (or 3/60, i.e. no better than 3/60). People in the latter category can see the chart but cannot read the top line. They are not regarded as blind according to the statutory definition unless their field of vision is considerably contracted. However, the *de facto* spread of the registered blind across Snellen levels of 3/60 or even better is considerable. When this spread is considered, as below, it turns out that the higher cut-off point, – 3/60 but <6/60 – provides the best available estimate of the total number (192,000) of non-registered who could qualify for registration as blind. The crucial data are shown in Table 21.1. (Figure 2.1, Chapter 2, is based on these data percentaged within the columns.)

Table 21.1 Snellen categories and reported registration status

Registration status	Snellen category						Total
	<3/60	<6/60	6/60	6/36	6/24	6/24*	
Blind	77	15	5	3	1	1	102
Partially sighted	20	29	20	20	11	20	120
Base (population)	97	44	25	23	12	21	222

*But unable to read N12
Source: Data from OPCS master tape, as initially computed in 1986

Special factors may affect these data. The Snellen tests were taken in the home situation. Although we are dealing with reported rather than actual registration, there is a close correspondence between the two (section 2.4.2.1). The data have not been re-weighted to reflect population numbers. However, when the calculations noted below were re-worked using weighted data for Table 21.1 (working memo dated 17.3.89, see note 1), neither the blind/partially sighted cutting-point nor the population estimates for the blind and partially sighted groups (both non-registered and registered components) changed significantly.

The key point is that we assume registrability among the non-registered follows the distribution shown in Table 21.1. In this case, we can calculate from Table 21.1 the number and proportion of the non-registered who would be registrable as blind if treated similarly to the registered. For the joint category <3/60 and <6/60, although 65% [(77 + 15)/(97 + 44)] reported that they were registered blind, these constitute 90% [(77 + 15)/102] of all those so reporting. A cut at <3/60 would do less justice to the numbers of registered (and hence to the non-registered registrable) blind people. While the latter cut would result in a category consisting of 79% (77/97) of those reporting that they were registered blind, it would omit the 25% (25/102) of those reporting that they were registered blind who were at higher Snellen levels. Another reason why this cut is inadvisable, concerned with weighting, is given below.

Although the true figure for the non-registered registrable blind can be calculated using the inferences from data in Table 21.1, we cannot make the operational split in terms of it, since we only have Snellen data for the non-registered. Any cut made on the basis of Snellen data will put some partially sighted people into the blind category and leave some blind people in the partially sighted category. Thus, the <6/60 cut categorises as blind some 34% (49/141) who actually reported that they were registered as partially sighted. It should be noted that this dilution does not apply to all the 301,000 people in our blind category. The 109,000 people who were registered (LA sample) or reported that they were registered blind (OPCS sample) are categorised accordingly. The dilution applies to the remaining 192,000 non-registered about whom we are making inferences based on the data in Table 21.1. It turns out, however, that the true figure for the non-registered blind brings us back to the figure of 192,000. This is because the dilution element of 35% partially sighted at <6/60 happens to be balanced by the numbers of registered blind (and by inference the numbers of non-registered registrable blind) at Snellen levels of 3/60 or above. In detail, the working here was as follows:

We draw on population estimates for the non-registered in each Snellen category. (These are given in a working paper POPES2. The detailed working showing this is described in a working memo to Ian Bruce dated March 15 1989 (Appendix B, page 6, of Paper D), see note 1.) The proportions for the registered in Table 21.1 are applied to these overall estimates of the numbers of non-registered in the Snellen categories.

Thus according to Table 21.1 there are 141 in the first two Snellen categories (97 + 44). Of these the 77 <3/60 and the 15 <6/60 represent 55 and 11 per cent respectively registered blind. From POPES2 we obtained an estimate of 121,000 in these two categories. If these are divided as in Table 21.1, the result is 67,000 at <3/60 and 13,000 at 3/60 (i.e. <6/60), or 80,000 who are registrable blind among the non-registered from the first two categories <3/60 and <6/60. There will also be the dilution element in these two categories of 35% of 121,000 and 42,000 who will be registrable partially sighted.

However the remaining categories, although largely consisting of the partially sighted, each contain some blind. Thus there are, from Table 21.1, 20, 13 and 8 per cent of blind people in the categories 6/60, 6/36 and 6/24 (e.g. 20% is given by 5/25), which POPES2 shows to contain 43,000, 156,000 and 175,000 respectively. The result of multiplying through to obtain the total in these last three categories is 43,000. This roughly balances the 41,000 we need to subtract from the first two Snellen categories, $<3/60$ and $<6/60$. Thus the original estimate of 192,000 proves to be very near the mark.

There is a further reason for not wishing to separate the $<3/60$ from the 3/60 Snellen levels in our data. Our data set contained only 12 non-registered respondents at the $<3/60$ level, which is too small to carry substantial weights for projecting the population numbers. The combined category, with 70 respondents, provides a more reliable basis for weighting.

Finally, to complete the record, it should be noted that there were 16 (out of the 70) non-registered respondents placed in the blind category for whom no Snellen test data were available. They were classified on the basis of the questionnaire response scale, as described in section 21.7.

21.2 Snellen categories $<3/60$ and $<6/60$ in the OPCS home sight tests

Measurements below 6/60 Snellen were not attempted in the OPCS home sight tests. But those who had no light perception or said that they could not see the test card can be judged to have vision worse than 3/60 (World Health Organisation (WHO) categories 3, 4 and 5 of visual impairment, Cullinan, 1977), the level that normally counts for registration as blind, while those who could not read the top line of the card but could see the card can be considered as falling into the no better than 3/60 category, i.e. $<6/60$ category (WHO category 2).

21.2.1 Near vision criteria

'No better than N14', the criterion for membership of the RNIB Talking Book Service, means cannot read N12, ie. 'worse than N12'. Those we have termed N12s for short (section 2.4.2.2) correspond to the 'no better than N14' criterion.

21.3　Technical details on weighting

21.3.1　General aim and procedure

Weighting factors had to be applied first so as to restore older respondents, and those at higher residual vision levels, both under-represented in the RNIB interview sample, to their correct proportions. Results for each person interviewed were further multiplied by the appropriate weight to obtain population estimates for Great Britain.

Since part of the RNIB sample was representative of another probability sample (OPCS), and the remaining part was drawn from local authority registers, different weighting procedures were applied according to whether or not the respondents were registered. Published DOH figures were used to provide population estimates for re-weighting the registered blind and the registered partially sighted in both the LA and the OPCS sample. This allowed us to combine the registered sections of the two samples. For the non-registered, who all came from the OPCS sample, we applied the same weighting factors that were used to make population estimates in the OPCS disability survey.

21.3.2　Detailed procedure – the basic steps

a　Weight up those RNIB respondents obtained from the OPCS survey who reported that they were unregistered, to obtain the same numbers in each age/residual vision cell as were present in the original OPCS sample.

b　Apply to this sub-group the 30 weights (15 five-year age bands x 2 interview types) shown in Table 8.1, page 68 of the OPCS Disability Survey (Martin et al, 1988a).

Steps a and b gross up the non-registered segment of the sample to population numbers.

c　Weight up the respondents obtained from the local authority registers, together with respondents obtained from the OPCS sample who said that they were registered blind or partially sighted, to obtain the numbers in 15 age-bands, corresponding to those already published in the DHSS registers for the blind and partially sighted.

In applying the weights we assumed that OPCS respondents correctly reported their position with respect to registration. Such data we do have supports this (section 21.9).

Published DOH figures for registration include people in institutions. The necessary adjustment was made by a ratio worked out from the OPCS Disability Survey of those with a severe seeing disability in private households to those in communal establishments: this produced an approximation to the numbers in private households (section 21.3.3). Prevalence rates derived from DOH figures by Shankland Cox (1985) were used to obtain visually impaired population figures for the year 1985 in five-year age bands for England, Scotland and Wales combined.

In steps a and c there were 15 x 2 x 9 = 270 cells to which weights could in principle be applied (15 age bands, 2 types of OPCS interviewer sift, 9 Snellen test levels). Some of these cells were empty even in the original OPCS sample, and still more in the RNIB achieved sample. A procedure for collapsing neighbouring cells, by sift, by Snellen values on each side of the blind/partially sighted split or, in the last resort, by age bands, was developed.

OPCS excluded from the data it supplied to RNIB all individuals aged 16 – 24 as these were required for another follow-up study. For simplicity we have retained the description of the younger age band as 16 – 59 in the tables. This is strictly true only for the registered, where our LA sample did include four individuals between the ages of 16 and 20. For the non-registered there may be some very slight under-estimation because of the absence of the 16 – 24s.

However, the effect on our age breakdowns is insignificant. There are 77 respondents aged under 60 among the non-registered (all from the OPCS sample). We do not know how many 16 – 24s might have been obtained from the OPCS data had they not been excluded, but the number would have been far too few to draw any conclusions and would have made little difference to the overall percentages or population estimates in the 16 – 59 age band.

Further technical details on the weighting procedure can be obtained from an SPSS 'Document' saved with the program system file used to generate the weights, and also in a working appendix and box file of hard documents available for inspection at the RNIB Reference Library (see note 1).

21.3.3 Allowance for communal establishments

We had to take into account that DOH figures include people in institutions while our survey was of private households. No separate estimate of the numbers of institutionalised people in the DOH figures is possible. The best, possibly the only, information on this can be found in the published OPCS report which provides estimates of the numbers of people living in private households and communal establishments, with breakdowns by age, type of disability and severity levels (Martin et al, 1988a). We used the severity categories 3 – 10 for seeing difficulty (as the best approximation available to registrability) to arrive at our estimate of 21% of registrable visually impaired people living in communal establishments. A detailed working memo showing our steps in calculation is available (see note 1). Tables 21.2.a. and 21.2.b. show the results broken by age group; Table 21.2.a. gives data for disability in general and Table 21.2.b. specifically for visually impaired people.

Table 21.2.a. Proportion of all severely disabled people living in communal establishments

	Age			All
	16 – 59	60 – 74	75 +	
	%	%	%	%
Severity category				
3 – 10 More severe	5	5	17	9
1 – 2 Moderate	1	1	3	2
1 – 10 All	4	3	13	7

Table 21.2.b. Proportion of visually impaired people living in communal establishments

	Age			All
	16 – 59	60 – 74	75 +	
	%	%	%	%
Severity category				
3 – 10 More severe	22	12	25	21
1 – 2 Moderate	2	2	3	7
1 – 10 All	16	9	21	17

Source: OPCS Disability Survey, Report 1 (Martin, et al, 1988a)

As is to be expected, among those experiencing severe disability in general it is predominantly those aged 75 or over who live in institutions. It is of interest to note that for vision the relation between institutionalisation and age is curvilinear. As Table 21.2.b. shows, among visually impaired people the 16 – 59 age group is almost as likely to be living in communal establishments as the very old (22 and 25 per cent). Overall, registrable visually impaired people are more likely to be institutionalised than the disabled in general (21 and 9 per cent at severity levels 3 – 10); the gap is particularly noticeable for the 16 – 59 year-olds (22 and 5 per cent). These results were applied to DOH data and to our data in the following manner. Estimated population projections for those registered blind and partially sighted aged 16 or over in 1986 were 140,374 and 78,398 respectively. Of these, 79%, or 110,895 and 61,934 respectively, were living in private households. Our population estimates of 300,000 and 457,000 registrable blind and partially sighted people living in private households yield estimates of 380,000 and 579,000 people respectively, when adjusted upward by the same proportion to allow for those in institutions.

21.4 Significance tests

Sample survey estimates of population parameters always contain errors as a result of random variations, termed sampling error. When the sample has been drawn by strict probability methods it is possible to compute the likelihood of an error of any given size occurring. The essential aim is to avoid the danger of misinterpreting information from the survey by taking seriously small differences that are mostly the results of chance in the sampling. In policy surveys, whose readers are often searching for differences, this is a more likely source of error than the opposite one of ignoring differences which may be indicative of important contrasts.

This section is designed to help non-technical readers to understand when they should or should not consider the difference between two percentages to be significant. In addition, since population estimates are routinely made from the percentages in our survey, guidance is necessary in the allowance, the 'confidence interval', that should be set around the sample percentage value as an estimate of the true percentage in the population. Although related in probability theory, these two aspects will be considered separately.

21.4.1 Differences between percentages

Small differences between percentages can often be dismissed as 'statistically insignificant' at a given probability level. For example, non-significance at the 0.05 probability level means that such a difference can be expected to occur by chance more than five times in a hundred, or more than once in twenty times. A statistically significant result at the 0.05 probability level is one that can be expected to occur merely by chance not more than five times in a hundred. At this level, the probability that the finding has occurred by chance can be ignored with 95% confidence.

Statistical significance depends on the size of the sub-samples on which the percentages are based as well as on the difference between them. (Technically, a numerical measure of the variation because of sampling is provided by the quantity known as the standard error. The size of this varies as the square root of the sample or sub-sample sizes, and is also affected by other factors such as the use made of weighting and the type of survey estimate.)

Because the LA segment was selected by non-probability methods, statistical significance tests, and their associated probability levels, cannot strictly be applied to estimates from our total sample. Nevertheless we have used these tests as a guide to the emphasis to be placed on findings of small differences between percentage differences. Such uses of significance tests provide guidelines that avoid self-selection of issues, and provide a more rigorous selection process for the findings on which to focus attention. When in this report, therefore, we speak of differences that are 'statistically significant' or 'not statistically significant', we mean that tests depending on the assumption of random sampling have been made, so as to provide guidelines rather than to identify with precision confidence limits and probability levels.

As noted in Section 2.5, for example, we have collapsed adjacent categories in the standard six-category age/residual vision variable used in analyses when no significant differences could be observed between the percentages in these categories. A probability level of 0.05 was used as a criterion for this purpose.

The entries in the following tabulations may help to provide an intuitive grasp of the percentage differences that would or would not pass this screening for statistical significance.

Table 21.3 Examples of 95% confidence intervals when comparing two percentages (based on random samples)

Sample sizes		Region of percentages being compared		
n1	n2	50	40/60	10/90
250	250	9	7	5
250	100	12	9	7
100	100	14	11	8
100	50	16	12	8
50	50	18	13	9

Table 21.3 is read as follows. For percentages in the region of 50 based on samples of size 250, a difference of 9 could be accepted (with 95% confidence) as existing in the population from which the samples were drawn. Thus two percentages of 50 and 59 would be accepted as significantly different. Percentages of 50 and 57 would not be accepted as statistically significant. The confidence interval decreases somewhat as percentages depart from 50. For example, percentages in the region of 10 or 90, a difference of as little as 5% would be significant on samples of 250.

As the sample size decreases the allowance that must be made for chance differences increases. For example, with sample sizes of 50 the difference must be as large as 18 for statistical significance for percentages in the region of 50. For percentages in the region of 10 the difference has to be as large as 9 for sample sizes of 50.

In presenting tables in the text we have used these estimates as a rough guide and have not as a rule presented separate categories where any differences would fall well below statistical significance. When we have departed from this rule, for example when only small sample bases are available for important comparisons, we have pointed out the smallness of the bases and the need for caution in interpretation because of the possibility that the differences observed could be non-significant statistically, that is they could have arisen by chance.

Table 21.4 Confidence limits for a single percentage

Sample size	Percentage finding		
	50	70/30	90/10
	95% confidence limits $(+/-)$		
500	4	4	3
400	5	4	3
300	6	5	3
200	7	6	4
150	8	6	5
100	10	8	6
50	14	11	8

Table 21.4 is read as follows. An allowance of $+/-$ 4 should be made for a percentage finding of 50% on a sample size of 500. That is, the population value can be taken as lying between 54 and 46 per cent for this sample size with 95% confidence. (In other words, there is still a 5% or 1 in 20 chance that the population value could be outside these limits.) For a sample size of 100 the (95%) confidence limits would be $+/-$ 10 on a finding of 50% giving a confidence interval of between 40 and 60 per cent.

As percentages depart each side from 50, the confidence limits narrow somewhat for a given sample size. Thus for a 90% finding based on a sample of 100 the allowance would be $+/-$ 6, giving an expected population value between 84 and 96 per cent. The allowance for a 10% finding would be the same, $+/-$ 6%, but in this case the population values would be expected (with 95% confidence) to fall in the range 4 to 16 per cent.

Note that for the percentages based on weighted data in this report, the sample size relevant to the significance estimate is the unweighted numbers interviewed for the sub-group for which the percentages are computed. Note that below 100 one should be extremely careful in projecting population estimates for small percentages. On a sample of only 50 the confidence range for a finding of 10% could be as wide as 2 to 18 per cent.

BMRB fieldwork response rates

	Age group												Grand Total
	16 – 59				60 – 74				75 +				
	Total	B	PS	N/R	Total	B	PS	N/R	Total	B	PS	N/R	Total
Wave 1													
Set	160	34	36	90	114	22	29	63	250	40	46	164	524
Achieved	110	23	29	58	75	18	15	42	153	22	31	100	338
Response rate (%)	69	68	81	64	66	82	52	67	61	55	67	61	65
Wave 2													
Set	271	143	98	30	59	27	18	14	49	26	–	23	379
Achieved	188	106	59	23	40	20	11	9	29	15	–	14	257
Response rate (%)	69	74	60	77	68	74	61	64	59	58	–	61	68
Waves 1 and 2 combined													
Set	431	177	134	120	173	49	47	77	299	66	46	187	903
Achieved	298	129	88	81	115	38	26	51	182	37	31	114	595
Response rate (%)	69	73	66	68	66	78	55	66	61	56	67	61	66

21.5 Fieldwork response rates

The table titled 'BMRB fieldwork response' shows the response rates achieved in each of the two stages of the field work. These are shown for each of the blind, partially sighted and non-registered sub-groups within 3 age bands. The data from the table show that older respondents made up the bulk of interviews in the first wave with younger respondents predominating in the second wave.

Details were kept of any addresses where an interview could not be obtained. An analysis of the 308 non-effective interviews show the following reasons:

20%	Interview refused
20%	House empty/wrong address/moved
15%	No reply/no contact/out at all contacts
14%	Respondent dead
8%	Claimed not to have sight problem
7%	Respondent not well enough
6%	Respondent in hospital/residential home
5%	Away during fieldwork
5%	Miscellaneous/not known

21.6 Guide to questionnaire sections

The questionnaire was divided into 23 sections which were colour coded. The colours and question numbers in each section have been combined to form the question reference numbers used in the report. The questionnaire itself is not included in this report but copies may be obtained from RNIB's Reference Library.

Sections	Question numbers (used to identify questions in the text)
01 Introduction	IQ1-IQ4
Yellow	
02 Accommodation	YQ1-YQ12
03 Onset	YQ13-YQ19
04 Registration	YQ20-YQ28
05 Residual vision	YQ29-YQ47
Green	
06 Hearing	GQ1-GQ4
07 Health	GQ5-GQ11
08 Psychology	GQ12
09 Daily living skills	GQ13-GQ32

White
10	Large print	WQ1-WQ7
11	Braille	WQ8-WQ35
12	Tapes	WQ36-WQ71
13	Reading	WQ72-WQ84

Pink
14	Employment	PQ1-PQ40
15	Allowances	PQ41-PQ47
16	Psychological	PQ48

Blue
17	Mobility	BQ1-BQ34
18	Shopping and transport	BQ35-BQ42
19	Leisure	BQ44-BQ70
20	Psychology	BQ71

Buff
21	Social Services Department	CQ1-CQ44
22	RNIB	CQ45-CQ55

Grey
23	Demography	GR1-GR16

21.7   The questionnaire scale (QRVS7) for distance vision

21.7.1   Interview stage

The six questions forming the scale YQ29 to YQ34 are shown in Table 21.5. It would not have made sense to ask any of the later questions in the series of someone who said at YQ29 that they could not tell from the light where the windows were. So these people were 'filtered out', that is they were not asked the later questions. Similarly, because the questions form a graded series, it was not necessary, and could well have strained rapport, to ask a later question of someone who had said that they could not see at an earlier question. So these people were filtered out at the point at which they said they could not see.

21.7.2   Distribution of interviews over the QRVS7

The levels of residual vision marked by the six questions can thus be thought of as six points on a scale, or six rungs on a ladder. A respondent with no light perception (cannot see where the windows are, YQ29) does not climb on to the first rung of the ladder and is scored zero. A person who responds 'yes' to the fifth question, YQ32 (can see at arms length), will be on the fourth rung of the ladder, and must therefore have said 'yes' to the three earlier questions. If they now answer 'no' to YQ32 (i.e. they cannot see across a room), they stay on the fourth rung of the ladder and receive a score of 4.

Table 21.5 The questionnaire scale for residual vision (QRVS7)

	Residual vision level	(a) Scale	(b) Number at each scale point	
(YQ29)	Can't see windows (NLP) 'No' at YQ29	0	48	The respondents at each point are those who say
(YQ29)	Sees windows (LP only) (but not furniture) 'Yes' at YQ29	1	48	they can see to that point but not at the next level.
(YQ30)	Sees furniture (but not close up)	2	90	
(YQ31)	Sees close up (but not at arms length)	3	67	Respondents were not asked questions beyond the level at which
(YQ32)	Sees at arms length (but not across a room)	4	107	they said they could not see.
(YQ33)	Sees across room (But not across road)	5	139	
(YQ34)	Sees across road	6	96	
	Total		595	

Table 21.5 shows how the 595 respondents were distributed along the scale which, for brevity, is referred to as QRVS7.

Forty-eight respondents had no light perception (YQ29). A further 48 had light perception only; they said that they could tell from the light where the windows were (YQ29) but could not see the shapes of the furniture (YQ30) and received a score of 1. The total at each scale point marks the numbers of respondents who have reached that rung of the ladder but have gone no further. We can establish the number of respondents who said 'yes' to a given question by totalling those who reached a higher question and those who got as far as the scale point marked by the question. For example, 139 + 96 = 235 must have answered 'yes' to YQ33, since the 96 who reached the top of the scale must, logically, also have said 'yes' to the earlier question. (This in turn implies that 595 − 235 = 360 said 'no' or were filtered out before they got to YQ33.) Similarly, the number that 'sees close up' (to recognise a friend) at YQ31 are 67 + 107 + 139 + 96 = 409.

21.7.3   Relation of QRVS7 to Snellen values

The body of data we received from OPCS, from which we drew part of our sample, contains the results of Snellen tests (and also reading tests) carried out in the home. We did not repeat the Snellen tests in our survey, but were careful to replicate exactly the wording of any questions bearing on residual vision, including those used to construct QRVS7. The Snellen test data from the OPCS survey can therefore be used to show the relationship between QRVS7 and Snellen data, with the results shown in Tables 21.6.a. and 21.6.b.

Table 21.6.a.   Questionnaire residual vision scale (QRVS7) by Snellen test

	Results of Snellen tests						Total
	<3/60**	<6/60**	6/60	6/36	6/24	>6/24*	
			Number				
0 NLP***	33	–	–	–	–	–	33
1 Windows only	12	1	–	–	–	–	13
2 Furniture only	34	13	4	9	3	3	66
3 Close up only	18	15	10	7	3	8	61
4 Arms length only	31	34	16	27	27	5	140
5 Across room only	19	73	40	120	136	56	444
6 Sees across road	3	23	18	77	101	116	338
Total numbers	150	159	88	240	270	188	1095

Source: Data from OPCS master sample *See 2.4.2.2 **See 21.2 ***NLP-No light perception

Table 21.6.b.   Questionnaire residual vision scale by Snellen test

	Results of Snellen tests						Total
	<3/60	<6/60	6/60	6/36	6/24	>6/24	
			percentages (%)				
0 NLP	22	–	–	–	–	–	3
1 Windows only	8	1	–	–	–	–	1
2 Furniture only	23	8	5	4	1	2	6
3 Close up only	12	9	11	3	1	4	6
4 Arms length only	21	21	18	11	10	3	13
5 Across room only	13	46	45	50	50	30	41
6 Sees across road	2	14	20	32	37	62	31
Total %	100	100	100	100	100	100	100
Base numbers	150	159	88	240	270	188	1095

Data as in Table 21.6.a., with percentages taken within Snellen categories

21.7.4   Demarcation of blind and partially sighted on QRVS7

As with Snellen measures (section 2.4.2.3) there is no single cutting-point which exactly divides blind and partially sighted people. A cutting-point on QRVS7 between YQ31 and YQ32 (sees at close up but not at arms length – equivalent to dividing the scale 0 – 3, 4 – 6) yields 34% blind and 66% partially sighted for the population as a whole. This compares with the 40/60 per cent split obtained with demarcations based on the combined Snellen and registration criteria actually adopted for this report (section 2.4.2.3).

At one point in the design stage, we were short of respondents in the registrable blind category from the OPCS master frame (section 2.2.3.1) and had to consider how to classify those few OPCS respondents for whom no Snellen test data had been obtained. For this purpose we took the cutting-point on QRVS7 at a more generous level, one point higher at YQ32 (sees at arms length but not across a room, equivalent to dividing the scale 0 – 4, 5 – 6), even though this cutting-point yielded the proportions 54/46 per cent for the blind/partially sighted division.

The working paper 'Note on QRVS7' should be consulted for more detail of our initial thinking on QRVS7 (see note 1).

21.8   Numbers interviewed by registration status

The data shown in Table 3.1 are weighted (section 2.4.1). The numbers actually interviewed in each age/residual vision/registration group are shown in Table 21.7.

Table 21.7   Number of interviewed registrable and registered visually impaired adults by age

	Age			Total
	16 – 59	60 – 74	75 +	
Registered				
Registered B	123	41	33	197
Registered PS	92	29	34	155
Total registered	215	70	67	352
Non-registered				
Registrable B	14	14	42	70
Registrable PS	70	40	63	173
Total non-registered	84	54	105	243
Total registrable VI	299	124	172	595

21.9   Reliability of reported registration

21.9.1   Self-reports compared with actual registration

The local authority sub-sample is tabulated in this report by actual registration status. By comparing this with self-reported registration status we obtain a useful check on the validity of the latter, as shown in Table 21.8.

Table 21.8 Comparison of the registration status on the LA record and reported registration for the LA sub-sample

	Actual registration status from local authority records		
	Blind	Partially sighted	
Self-reported registration status			
Blind	120	10	
Partially sighted	10	58	
Don't know status	1	2	
Don't know if registered	8	0	
Total, LA sub-sample	139	70	209
OPCS sub-sample			386
Total interviews			595

Local authority respondents had previously been approached by their local SSDs to give them an opportunity to decline to be interviewed. But registration as such was not mentioned by the interviewer until the questions (YQ20 and YQ24) that provided the data for Table 21.8. The data show that very few (8) did not know that they were registered (or said that they were not), only one person was uncertain about their registration status and that, although more people are mistaken about their registration category, they too are very much in a minority (20 out of 209). Only 46 of the 209 local authority sample were aged 60 or over (because of the requirements of the top-up sample), but nevertheless the data support the view that errors of self-reported registration status are not serious.

21.9.2 Consistency of self-reports about registration status

The second line of evidence comes from the 386 respondents in the OPCS sub-sample. They reported their registration status on two separate occasions, at the original OPCS fieldwork stage, towards the end of 1985, and again in the re-interviews by RNIB (mostly towards the end of 1986). It is unlikely that respondents would be able to recall 15 to 18 months later their reply on the first occasion, so the consistency of their replies, as shown in Table 21.9, provides a test-retest measure of the reliability of the reported registration variable.

Table 21.9 Consistency of replies about registration status in 1985 and 1986/7

		1985 replies			
		Reg B	Reg PS	Non-Reg	
	Reg B	57	9	8	74
1986/7	Reg PS	7	58	14	79
replies	Non-Reg	1	11	221	233
	COLUMN	65	78	243	386

For weighting purposes we classified OPCS respondents as registered if they said that they were registered blind or partially sighted in 1985; there were 143 in all (65 + 78 in Table 21.9). This procedure was designed to minimise the chances of error. It is possible but not certain that the 17 people who said that they were 'Reg B' in 1986/7 but either 'Non-Reg' or 'Reg PS' in 1985 could have been responding factually. The same applies to the 14 'Non-Reg' in 1985 who reported as 'Reg PS' in 1986/7. But the 12 who said that they were not registered in 1986/7 but had been in 1985 would appear to be definitely mistaken. (The same is probably true of the 7 who said that they were 'Reg B' in 1985 but 'Reg PS' in 1986/7.) However, the majority of respondents (336 in all) appear in the diagonal cells of the table which indicate consistency of reply. It is possible that they could have been consistently wrong. But while proof of reliability is not sufficient to establish validity, it is nevertheless a necessary condition for it. This second demonstration of the reliability of reports of registration status, in a sub-sample in which all age groups are well represented, thus further strengthens the assumption that, in the absence of factual data on registration status, reported registration status provides an acceptably accurate proxy variable.

Note to Chapter 21

Note 1

There are several working memos and documents which detail many of the decisions that we have made in this research. To have included the details here would have made an already long report even longer; much of the detail will only be of interest to those who wish to use the data for secondary analysis or those considering some replication of the study. These papers will be kept for inspection in the RNIB Reference Library.

References

Place of publication is London unless otherwise stated

Abrams, M., 1978. *Beyond three score years and ten*, Age Concern

Andrews, F.M., and Withey, S.B, 1976. *Social indicators of well-being*, Plenum Press, New York and London

BBC, 1982 and 1991. *The In Touch Handbook*, Broadcasting Support Services

Bradshaw, J., 1972. 'The concept of social need', *New Society*, 19, pp. 640 – 3

Bruce, I., and McKennell, A.C., 1986. 'RNIB general needs survey', *New Beacon*, 830, pp. 165 – 8

Campbell, A.E., and Converse, R.E., 1976. *The quality of American life*, Russell Sage Foundation, New York

Carroll, T.J., 1961. *Blindness: what it is, what it does and how to live with it*, Little, Brown, Boston, Massachusetts

Central Statistical Office, 1990. *Annual Abstract of Statistics: 1990 Edition*, HMSO

Central Statistical Office, 1988. *Social Trends 18*, HMSO

Central Statistical Office, 1990. *Social Trends 20*, HMSO

Clayton, S., 1983. 'Social need revisited', *Journal of Social Policy*, 12, pp. 215 – 34

Clark-Carter, D.D., et al, 1981. *The visually handicapped in the City of Nottingham*, Blind Mobility Research Unit, University of Nottingham

Cullinan, T. R., 1977. *The epidemiology of visual disability: studies of visually disabled people in the community*, HSRU report 28, Health Services Research Unit, University of Kent, Canterbury

Department of Health and Social Security, 1988. *A wider vision: report of the inspection of the management and organisation of services for people who are blind and partially sighted*, carried out by the Social Services Inspectorate

Edge, S., 1987. *Visually handicapped people in Hampshire*, Hampshire Association for the Care of the Blind, Eastleigh, Hampshire

Epstein, J., 1980. *Information needs of the elderly*, a study commissioned by the Department of Health and Social Security and carried out by the Research Institute for Consumer Affairs (RICA)

Graham, P.A., et al, 1968. 'Evaluation of postal detection of registrable blindness', *British Journal of Preventative and Social Medicine*, 22, pp. 238 – 41

Gray, P., and Todd, J.E., 1968. *Mobility and reading habits of the blind*, (OPCS) HMSO

Hall, L., 1982. *Who are Britain's blind people?*, RNIB

Harris, A., 1971. *Handicapped and impaired in Great Britain*, (OPCS) HMSO

Hunt, A., 1978. *The elderly at home*, (OPCS) HMSO

Martin, J., Meltzer, H., and Elliot, D., 1988a. *The prevalence of disability among adults. OPCS surveys of disability in Great Britain. Report 1*, HMSO

Martin, J. and White, A., 1988b. *The financial circumstances of disabled adults living in private households. OPCS surveys of disability in Great Britain. Report 2*, HMSO

Martin, J., White, A., and Meltzer, H., 1989. *Disabled adults: services, transport and employment. OPCS surveys of disability in Great Britain. Report 4*, HMSO

OPCS 1985, General Household Survey 1985, HMSO

OPCS 1986, General Household Survey 1986, HMSO

OPCS 1988, General Household Survey 1988, HMSO

Peace, S. M., Hall J. F. and Hamblin, G.R., 1979. *The quality of life of the elderly in residential care*, North London Polytechnic

Shankland Cox, 1985. *Initial demographic study: a review of available data on the visually disabled population*, RNIB

Shore, P., 1985. *Local authority social rehabilitation services to visually handicapped people*, RNIB

Smith, G., 1980. *Social need, policy, practice and research*, Routledge and Kegan Paul

Tobin, M., and Hill, E., 1984. 'Blind in Birmingham: a pilot survey of needs and knowledge of available services', *New Beacon*, 68, pp. 61 – 6

Printed in the United Kingdom for HMSO
Dd294386 10/91 C20 G3390 10170